Influence of Deoxynivalenol and Zearalenone in Feed on Animal Health

Influence of Deoxynivalenol and Zearalenone in Feed on Animal Health

Editors

Maciej Gajęcki
Magdalena Gajęcka

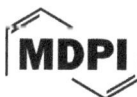

Basel • Beijing • Wuhan • Barcelona • Belgrade • Novi Sad • Cluj • Manchester

Editors

Maciej Gajęcki
Department of Veterinary
Prevention and Feed Hygiene
University of Warmia
and Mazury
Olsztyn
Poland

Magdalena Gajęcka
Department of Veterinary
Prevention and Feed Hygiene
University of Warmia
and Mazury
Olsztyn
Poland

Editorial Office
MDPI
St. Alban-Anlage 66
4052 Basel, Switzerland

This is a reprint of articles from the Special Issue published online in the open access journal *Toxins* (ISSN 2072-6651) (available at: www.mdpi.com/journal/toxins/special_issues/mycotoxins_feed).

For citation purposes, cite each article independently as indicated on the article page online and as indicated below:

Lastname, A.A.; Lastname, B.B. Article Title. *Journal Name* **Year**, *Volume Number*, Page Range.

ISBN 978-3-0365-8493-5 (Hbk)
ISBN 978-3-0365-8492-8 (PDF)
doi.org/10.3390/books978-3-0365-8492-8

© 2023 by the authors. Articles in this book are Open Access and distributed under the Creative Commons Attribution (CC BY) license. The book as a whole is distributed by MDPI under the terms and conditions of the Creative Commons Attribution-NonCommercial-NoDerivs (CC BY-NC-ND) license.

Contents

About the Editors vii

Preface ix

Maciej T. Gajęcki and Magdalena Gajęcka
The Multidirectional Influence of Feed-Borne Deoxynivalenol and Zearalenone on Animal Health
Reprinted from: *Toxins* 2023, *15*, 419, doi:10.3390/toxins15070419 1

Magdalena Gajęcka, Iwona Otrocka-Domagała, Paweł Brzuzan, Michał Dąbrowski, Sylwia Lisieska-Żołnierczyk and Łukasz Zielonka et al.
Immunohistochemical Expression (IE) of Oestrogen Receptors in the Intestines of Prepubertal Gilts Exposed to Zearalenone
Reprinted from: *Toxins* 2023, *15*, 122, doi:10.3390/toxins15020122 5

Magdalena Gajęcka, Łukasz Zielonka, Andrzej Babuchowski and Maciej Tadeusz Gajęcki
Exposure to Low Zearalenone Doses and Changes in the Homeostasis and Concentrations of Endogenous Hormones in Selected Steroid-Sensitive Tissues in Pre-Pubertal Gilts
Reprinted from: *Toxins* 2022, *14*, 790, doi:10.3390/toxins14110790 21

Marta Mendel, Wojciech Karlik, Urszula Latek, Magdalena Chłopecka, Ewelina Nowacka-Kozak and Katarzyna Pietruszka et al.
Does Deoxynivalenol Affect Amoxicillin and Doxycycline Absorption in the Gastrointestinal Tract? Ex Vivo Study on Swine Jejunum Mucosa Explants
Reprinted from: *Toxins* 2022, *14*, 743, doi:10.3390/toxins14110743 39

Magdalena Mróz, Magdalena Gajęcka, Paweł Brzuzan, Sylwia Lisieska-Żołnierczyk, Dawid Leski and Łukasz Zielonka et al.
Carry-Over of Zearalenone and Its Metabolites to Intestinal Tissues and the Expression of CYP1A1 and GSTπ1 in the Colon of Gilts before Puberty
Reprinted from: *Toxins* 2022, *14*, 354, doi:10.3390/toxins14050354 53

Oky Setyo Widodo, Makoto Etoh, Emiko Kokushi, Seiichi Uno, Osamu Yamato and Dhidhi Pambudi et al.
Practical Application of Urinary Zearalenone Monitoring System for Feed Hygiene Management of a Japanese Black Cattle Breeding Herd—The Relationship between Monthly Anti-Müllerian Hormone and Serum Amyloid A Concentrations
Reprinted from: *Toxins* 2022, *14*, 143, doi:10.3390/toxins14020143 75

Magdalena Mróz, Magdalena Gajęcka, Katarzyna E. Przybyłowicz, Tomasz Sawicki, Sylwia Lisieska-Żołnierczyk and Łukasz Zielonka et al.
The Effect of Low Doses of Zearalenone (ZEN) on the Bone Marrow Microenvironment and Haematological Parameters of Blood Plasma in Pre-Pubertal Gilts
Reprinted from: *Toxins* 2022, *14*, 105, doi:10.3390/toxins14020105 91

Krisztina Majer-Baranyi, Nóra Adányi and András Székács
Biosensors for Deoxynivalenol and Zearalenone Determination in Feed Quality Control
Reprinted from: *Toxins* 2021, *13*, 499, doi:10.3390/toxins13070499 111

Wojciech Barański, Magdalena Gajęcka, Łukasz Zielonka, Magdalena Mróz, Ewa Onyszek and Katarzyna E. Przybyłowicz et al.
Occurrence of Zearalenone and Its Metabolites in the Blood of High-Yielding Dairy Cows at Selected Collection Sites in Various Disease States
Reprinted from: *Toxins* 2021, *13*, 446, doi:10.3390/toxins13070446 129

Magdalena Gajęcka, Michał S. Majewski, Łukasz Zielonka, Waldemar Grzegorzewski, Ewa Onyszek and Sylwia Lisieska-Żołnierczyk et al.
Concentration of Zearalenone, Alpha-Zearalenol and Beta-Zearalenol in the Myocardium and the Results of Isometric Analyses of the Coronary Artery in Prepubertal Gilts
Reprinted from: *Toxins* **2021**, *13*, 396, doi:10.3390/toxins13060396 . . . . **141**

Magdalena Gajęcka, Magdalena Mróz, Paweł Brzuzan, Ewa Onyszek, Łukasz Zielonka and Karolina Lipczyńska-Ilczuk et al.
Correlations between Low Doses of Zearalenone, Its Carryover Factor and Estrogen Receptor Expression in Different Segments of the Intestines in Pre-Pubertal Gilts—A Study Protocol
Reprinted from: *Toxins* **2021**, *13*, 379, doi:10.3390/toxins13060379 . . . . **157**

About the Editors

Maciej Gajęcki

DVM—Professor of Veterinary Sciences at the Department of Veterinary Prevention and Feed Hygiene, Faculty of Veterinary Medicine, University of Warmia and Mazury in Olsztyn, Poland. He completed a full-time Master's degree program at the Faculty of Veterinary Medicine, University of Agriculture and Technology in Olsztyn, and received a Master of Science degree in Veterinary Medicine in 1973. From May 1973 to September 1975, he was employed at the state-owned Animal Health Care Center and Commercial Pig Farm. Since 1981, he has been employed at the University of Warmia and Mazury in Olsztyn. During his professional career, he has been awarded a doctoral degree in Veterinary Sciences, a postdoctoral degree in Veterinary Sciences and the academic title of Professor of Veterinary Sciences. Over the last 27 years, the research interests of Professor Gajecki and his co-workers have centered around the effects exerted by zearalenone on farm animals (gilts), companion animals (female dogs), and humans (female patients). Professor Gajecki has conducted studies investigating the influence of zearalenone on the health of the reproductive tract and zearalenone mycotoxicosis in female patients, with a particular emphasis on the mycotoxin's effects on the mammary gland. As part of his professional activities, Professor Gajecki provided advisory service to the Ministry of Agriculture and Rural Development. He was President of the Sanitary-Epizootic Council at the General Veterinary Inspectorate (prevention and control of bovine spongiform encephalopathy and Aujeszky's disease). He is also the Director of postgraduate specialization studies in veterinary prevention and feed hygiene at the Polish National Veterinary Chamber. He has been elected three times as the Chairman of Polish delegates participating in annual meetings of the Ad Hoc Intergovernmental Codex Task Force on Animal Feeding (established by the Codex Alimentarius Commission) in Copenhagen.

Magdalena Gajęcka

DVM—Professor of Veterinary Sciences at the Department of Veterinary Prevention and Feed Hygiene, Faculty of Veterinary Medicine, University of Warmia and Mazury in Olsztyn, Poland (including a 10th semester at the Faculty of Veterinary Medicine, Complutense University in Madrid, Spain) and received a Master of Science degree in Veterinary Medicine in 2001. In 2002, she completed postgraduate studies in analytics in environmental protection at the Faculty of Chemistry, Nicolaus Copernicus University in Toruń. In June 2005, she completed postgraduate specialization studies in veterinary prevention and feed hygiene at the Polish National Veterinary Chamber. In 2006, awarded a doctoral degree in Veterinary Sciences at the Faculty of Veterinary Medicine, University of Warmia and Mazury in Olsztyn, after successfully defending a doctoral dissertation entitled "The Effect of Experimental Zearalenone Mycotoxicosis on the Female Canine Reproductive Tract". In 2014, she was awarded a postdoctoral degree in Veterinary Sciences at the Faculty of Veterinary Medicine, University of Warmia and Mazury in Olsztyn, after publishing a monothematic series of publications regarded as an outstanding research achievement, entitled "The Effect of Short-Term Zearalenone Mycotoxicosis on Changes in Selected Tissues of Female Dogs". In 2019, she was awarded the academic title of Professor of Veterinary Sciences. Professor Gajecka's research interests focus on feed hygiene, with a particular emphasis on animal waste management, the applicability of natural feed additives and feed materials, distribution and disposal of medicated feeds, safety and quality of animal feedstuffs, mycotoxicosis —implications for animal and human health, zearalenone mycotoxicosis: plants–animals–humans, diagnostic significance of selected Fusarium mycotoxicoses, zearalenone as a destructor of endocrine homeostasis of steroid hormones in female patients.

Preface

Zearalenone, deoxynivalenol, and their metabolites are among the most frequently encountered mycotoxins in plant materials. Their presence compromises the health quality of foodstuffs and feedstuffs, and increases the risk of ischemia and reperfusion injury, stress-related intestinal disorders, as well as endocrine, metabolic, and immune disorders. These problems are resolved on an individual basis by selecting the appropriate combination of measures. The symptoms and health consequences of high mycotoxin doses are generally known. However, small doses can cause disease without clinical symptoms or they can interact with the host body at various stages of life. Due to this ambiguous dose–response relationship, the symptoms associated with high mycotoxin doses cannot be easily extrapolated to low doses. The interactions between mycotoxins and between mycotoxins and physiological processes in cells, tissues, and microorganisms are also problematic. Mycotoxins present in feed come into direct contact with the intestinal mucosa. A healthy gastrointestinal tract comprises active cells and tissues with high-protein metabolic turnover rates. Cells and tissues are often targeted by mycotoxins. Some mycotoxins inhibit protein synthesis. For instance, deoxynivalenol ingested in small doses inhibits the uptake of substrates responsible for protein transport across intestinal walls. On the other hand, zearalenone has estrogenic properties, and low doses of this mycotoxin stimulate proliferative processes. Mycotoxins also influence the activity of local and general immune systems, and their adverse effects become manifested in immunosuppressed hosts. Mycotoxins can also suppress the host's immune system, thus increasing the risk of disorders caused by microorganisms, intestinal enzymes, and other toxins in the digestive tract without the clinical symptoms that are characteristic of mycotoxicoses.

Therefore, this study, presented in the Special Issue of *Toxins*, attempted to evaluate selected body systems and functional biomarkers of animals for varying doses of mycotoxins causing mycotoxicosis. I hope that the knowledge gained will deepen our understanding of the impact of mycotoxins on animal health and will facilitate decision-making in risk management.

The editors are grateful to all authors who contributed to the Special Issue. We would like to thank all expert peer reviewers for rigorously evaluating the submitted manuscripts. We are also grateful to the MDPI management team and staff for their valuable contributions, organizational input, and editorial support.

Maciej Gajęcki and Magdalena Gajęcka
Editors

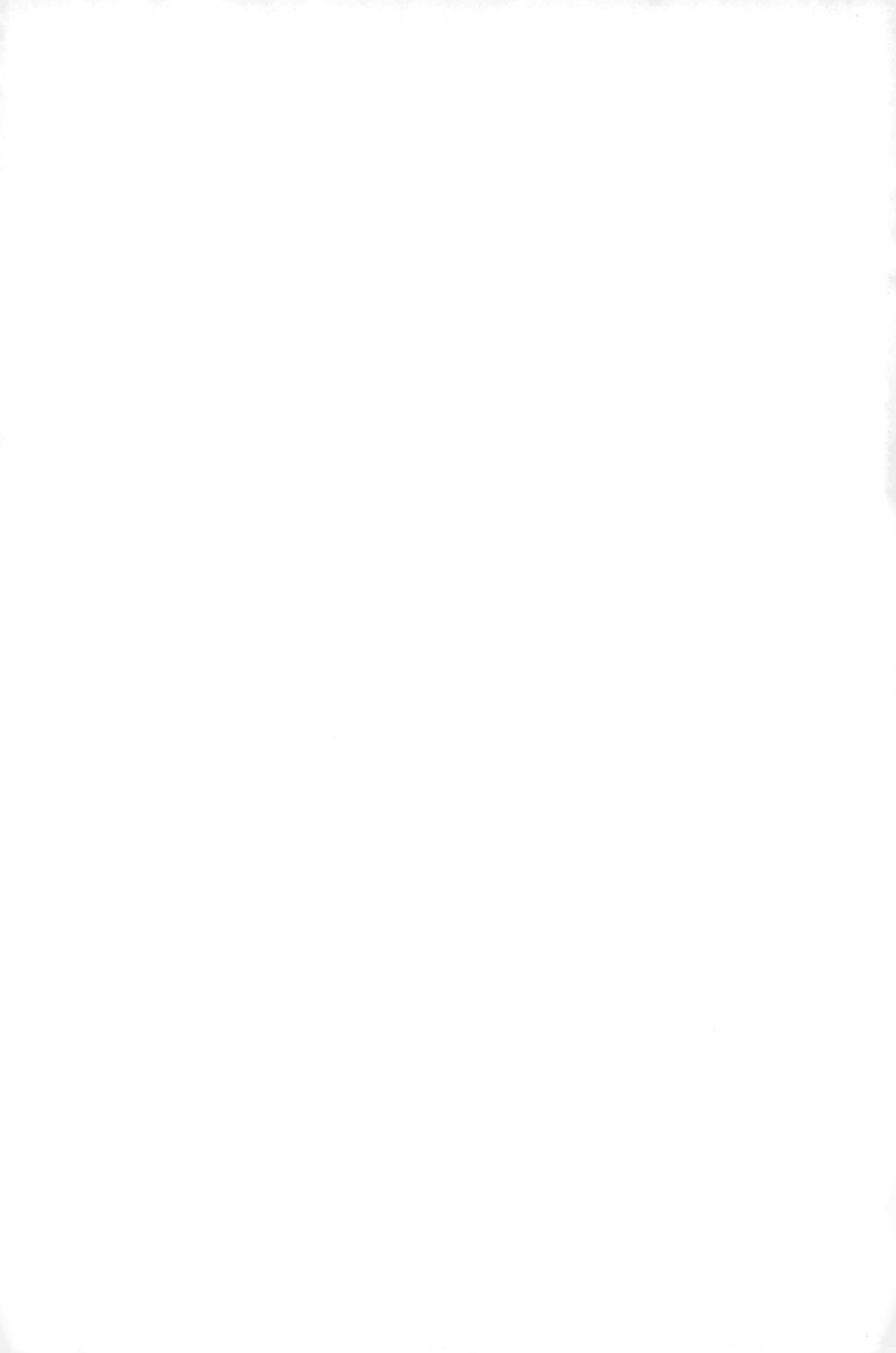

Editorial

The Multidirectional Influence of Feed-Borne Deoxynivalenol and Zearalenone on Animal Health

Maciej T. Gajęcki and Magdalena Gajęcka *

Department of Veterinary Prevention and Feed Hygiene, Faculty of Veterinary Medicine, University of Warmia and Mazury in Olsztyn, Oczapowskiego 13, 10-718 Olsztyn, Poland; gajecki@uwm.edu.pl
* Correspondence: mgaja@uwm.edu.pl; Tel.: +48-89-523-32-37; Fax: +48-89-523-36-18

Mycotoxins are secondary fungal metabolites which pose a significant threat for global food and feed security [1], due to their adverse effects on human and animal health [2], high chemical stability and ubiquitous presence [3]. The simultaneous exposure to several mycotoxins produced by the same or different fungal species exacerbates the risk of food and feed toxicity [4,5]. According to research, plant materials are often contaminated with both DON and ZEN, and the health risks associated with simultaneous exposure to both mycotoxins constitute an interesting topic of study [6,7].

Present in plant material, DON and ZEN belong to a large group of fusarium mycotoxins [8] which are produced by various fungal species, including *Fusarium*, *Myrothecium*, *Cephalosporium*, *Verticimonosporium* and *Stachybotrys* [3]. To date, the following mechanisms of toxicity of these mycotoxins have been identified in cells or proteins: (i) DON binds to the 60S ribosome subunit at the molecular level and induces ribotoxic stress, which activates protein kinase and, consequently, inhibits protein synthesis, and provokes endoplasmic reticulum stress [9], cell signalling, cell differentiation, cell proliferation and cell death [5,10]; (ii) ZEN [11] exerts toxic effects by binding to and activating both ERs, disrupting the cell cycle and inducing DNA fragmentation, which leads to the production of micronuclei and chromosomal aberrations [4,5,10].

Mycotoxicosis are ambiguous subclinical disorders that affect livestock herds [12,13]. These disorders can be caused by the chronic impairment of general bodily functions [14] or the increased susceptibility of specific tissues [15,16]. Acute poisoning and severe mycotoxicosis are less frequently reported. Complex toxicological interactions (additive effects, synergism, potentiation, and antagonism between mycotoxins) and the dose absorbed [17] undoubtedly affect health and reproductive processes [18]. Depending on the absorbed dose, the interactions between co-occurring mycotoxins or between mycotoxins and specific tissues in mammals [19–21] may require further investigation and risk assessments [22] based on an analysis of the biological activity of individual mycotoxins [12,16,17].

Low-dose exposure usually leads to subclinical states characterized by specific effects which are manifested by (i) the modulation of feminization processes in sexually immature gilts (which inhibits the somatic development of reproductive system tissues); (ii) disruptions in the neuroendocrine coordination of reproductive competence [14–16,19,23]; (iii) the balance between intestinal cells and the expression of selected genes encoding enzymes that participate in biotransformation processes in the large intestine [24]; and (iv) flexible, adaptive responses to low mycotoxin doses. Zearalenone (ZEN) and deoxynivalenol (DON) also induce non-specific effects that do not always decrease the feed conversion efficiency [20,21] and do not lead to a deterioration in the animals' overall health [25]. In addition, some mycotoxins, including DON, inhibit the activity of biologically active substances [18]. Therefore, their effects are determined by the dose and the duration of exposure.

According to the literature, systems for monitoring mycotoxins in animals should not be based solely on the results of blood tests [12,15]. A solution that delivers reliable results has been proposed in in one of the published studies [12]. The cited study demonstrated that blood samples from clinically healthy cows and/or cows with subclinical symptoms of ZEN mycotoxicosis should be collected from the caudal vein medium (prehepatic blood vessel) for toxicological tests. Samples collected from this site increase the probability that subclinical ZEN mycotoxicosis will be reliably diagnosed.

The monitoring system is a highly practical tool for identifying contaminated herds in the field and for evaluating the impact of chronic exposure on herd health and productivity. Other matrices, such as urine, can also be effectively used for this purpose [16].

However, preventive measures involving other matrices, such as feed materials (primary and partially processed products), are always preferable [13]. This type of monitoring relies on biosensor technologies that offer fast, highly selective, and highly sensitive detection methods, require minimal sample pre-treatment, and reduce reagent consumption. This article reviews recent advances in the development of biosensors for the quantification of DON and ZEN in cereals and feed, which substantially contribute to feed safety.

The articles published in the Special Issue entitled "Influence of Deoxynivalenol and Zearalenone in Feed on Animal Health" document the in vivo effects of low or very low doses of ZEN and its metabolites on mammals. These effects can vary, and remain insufficiently investigated. The above observations could also apply to other mycotoxins, including DON. Sexually immature gilts respond differently to mycotoxins. The ratio of α-ZEL (alpha-zearalenol) to β-ZEL (beta-zearalenol), where β-ZEL is the predominant compound, could be one of the first biomarkers of mycotoxin contamination. The value of this parameter is different in other age groups. This effect is ambiguous because β-ZEL contributes to a minor increase in body weight, while slowing down the sexual maturation of immature gilts. Initially, ZEN levels are very low, and metabolites are not detected in the blood serum (especially at the MABEL dose), which confirms that gilts have a high physiological demand for exogenous estrogen-like substances. These substances are fully utilized by immature gilts. Exposure to higher mycotoxin doses generates "free ZEN", which plays different, not always positive roles. The concentrations of estradiol and "free ZEN" increase proportionally to the ZEN dose, which decreases progesterone and testosterone levels [26]. At the same time, the metabolic profile points to a greater loss of energy and protein (stimulation), which suggests that feed is used more efficiently (weight gain) and that mycotoxins are highly involved in biotransformation and detoxification processes. Changes in the metabolic profile fluctuate over time. In the initial period of exposure, metabolic activity is relatively high, which could also be attributed to the compensatory effect. In successive periods, energy-intensive processes initiate adaptive mechanisms. These mechanisms could also be triggered by the increasing involvement of β-ZEL in the final biotransformation process.

The results of selected diagnostic tests could be used as biomarkers of prolonged low-dose ZEN mycotoxicosis in sexually immature gilts in precision veterinary medicine.

The question that arises is whether cereal grains contaminated with such low doses of ZEN and DON should be detoxified or eliminated from feed production. The results of the study suggest that such low mycotoxin doses should be tolerated due to their potentially stimulating effects on sexually immature gilts in commercial farms.

Author Contributions: Conceptualization, M.T.G.; writing—original draft preparation, M.G. All authors have read and agreed to the published version of the manuscript.

Acknowledgments: The editors are grateful to all authors who contributed to the Special Issue. We would like to thank all expert peer reviewers for rigorously evaluating the submitted manuscripts. We are also grateful to the MDPI management team and staff for their valuable contributions, organizational input, and editorial support.

Conflicts of Interest: The authors declare no conflict of interest.

References

1. Bryła, M.; Pierzgalski, A.; Zapaśnik, A.; Uwineza, P.A.; Ksieniewicz-Woźniak, E.; Modrzewska, M.; Waśkiewicz, A. Recent Research on Fusarium Mycotoxins in Maize—A Review. *Foods* **2022**, *11*, 3465. [CrossRef] [PubMed]
2. Viegas, S.; Assunção, R.; Martins, C.; Nunes, C.; Osteresch, B.; Twarużek, M.; Kosicki, R.; Grajewski, J.; Ribeiro, E.; Viegas, C. Occupational Exposure to Mycotoxins in Swine Production: Environmental and Biological Monitoring Approaches. *Toxins* **2019**, *11*, 78. [CrossRef] [PubMed]
3. Zhou, H.; George, S.; Hay, C.; Lee, J.; Qian, H.; Sun, X. Individual and combined effects of Aflatoxin B1, Deoxynivalenol and Zearalenone on HepG2 and RAW 264.7 cell lines. *Food Chem. Toxicol.* **2017**, *103*, 18–27. [CrossRef]
4. Knutsen, H.-K.; Alexander, J.; Barregård, L.; Bignami, M.; Brüschweiler, B.; Ceccatelli, S.; Cottrill, B.; Dinovi, M.; Edler, L.; Grasl-Kraupp, B.; et al. Risks for animal health related to the presence of zearalenone and its modified forms in feed. *EFSA J.* **2017**, *15*, 4851. [CrossRef]
5. Payros, D.; Alassane-Kpembi, I.; Pierron, A.; Loiseau, N.; Pinton, P.; Oswald, I.P. Toxicology of deoxynivalenol and its acetylated and modified forms. *Arch. Toxicol.* **2016**, *90*, 2931–2957. [CrossRef]
6. Medina, A.; Akbar, A.; Baazeem, A.; Rodriguez, A.; Magan, N. Climate change, food security and mycotoxins: Do we know enough? *Fungal Biol. Rev.* **2017**, *31*, 43–154. [CrossRef]
7. Zachariasova, M.; Dzuman, Z.; Veprikova, Z.; Hajkova, K.; Jiru, M.; Vaclavikova, M.; Zachariasova, A.; Pospichalova, M.; Florian, M.; Hajslova, J. Occurrence of multiple mycotoxins in European feedingstuffs, assessment of dietary intake by farm animals. *Anim. Feed Sci. Tech.* **2014**, *193*, 124–140. [CrossRef]
8. Statsyuk, N.V.; Popletaeva, S.B.; Shcherbakova, L.A. Post-Harvest Prevention of Fusariotoxin Contamination of Agricultural Products by Irreversible Microbial Biotransformation: Current Status and Prospects. *BioTech* **2023**, *12*, 32. [CrossRef]
9. You, L.; Zhao, Y.; Kuca, K.; Wang, X.; Oleksak, P.; Chrienova, Z.; Nepovimova, E.; Jaćević, V.; Wu, Q.; Wu, W. Hypoxia, oxidative stress, and immune evasion: A trinity of the trichothecenes T-2 toxin and deoxynivalenol (DON). *Arch. Toxicol.* **2021**, *95*, 1899–1915. [CrossRef]
10. Gajęcka, M.; Brzuzan, P.; Otrocka-Domagała, I.; Zielonka, Ł.; Lisieska-Żołnierczyk, S.; Gajęcki, M.T. The Effect of 42-Day Exposure to a Low Deoxynivalenol Dose on the Immunohistochemical Expression of Intestinal ERs and the Activation of CYP1A1 and GSTP1 Genes in the Large Intestine of Pre-pubertal Gilts. *Front. Vet. Sci.* **2021**, *8*, 64459. [CrossRef]
11. Ropejko, K.; Twarużek, M. Zearalenone and Its Metabolites-General Overview, Occurrence, and Toxicity. *Toxins* **2021**, *13*, 35. [CrossRef] [PubMed]
12. Barański, W.; Gajęcka, M.; Zielonka, Ł.; Mróz, M.; Onyszek, E.; Przybyłowicz, K.E.; Nowicki, A.; Babuchowski, A.; Gajęcki, M.T. Occurrence of Zearalenone and Its Metabolites in the Blood of High-Yielding Dairy Cows at Selected Collection Sites in Various Disease States. *Toxins* **2021**, *13*, 446. [CrossRef]
13. Majer-Baranyi, K.; Adányi, N.; Székács, A. Biosensors for Deoxynivalenol and Zearalenone Determination in Feed Quality Control. *Toxins* **2021**, *13*, 499. [CrossRef] [PubMed]
14. Mróz, M.; Gajęcka, M.; Przybyłowicz, K.E.; Sawicki, T.; Lisieska-Żołnierczyk, S.; Zielonk, Ł.; Gajęcki, M.T. The Effect of Low Doses of Zearalenone (ZEN) on the Bone Marrow Microenvironment and Haematological Parameters of Blood Plasma in Pre-Pubertal Gilts. *Toxins* **2022**, *14*, 105. [CrossRef] [PubMed]
15. Gajęcka, M.; Zielonka, Ł.; Babuchowski, A.; Gajęcki, M.T. Exposure to Low Zearalenone Doses and Changes in the Homeostasis and Concentrations of Endogenous Hormones in Selected Steroid-Sensitive Tissues in Pre-Pubertal Gilts. *Toxins* **2022**, *14*, 790. [CrossRef] [PubMed]
16. Widodo, O.S.; Etoh, M.; Kokushi, E.; Uno, S.; Yamato, O.; Pambudi, D.; Okawa, H.; Taniguchi, M.; Lamid, M.; Takagi, M. Practical Application of Urinary Zearalenone Monitoring System for Feed Hygiene Management of a Japanese Black Cattle Breeding Herd—The Relationship between Monthly Anti-Müllerian Hormone and Serum Amyloid A Concentrations. *Toxins* **2022**, *14*, 143. [CrossRef]
17. Gajęcka, M.; Mróz, M.; Brzuzan, P.; Onyszek, E.; Zielonka, Ł.; Lipczyńska-Ilczuk, K.; Przybyłowicz, K.E.; Babuchowski, A.; Gajęcki, M.T. Correlations between Low Doses of Zearalenone, Its Carryover Factor and Estrogen Receptor Expression in Different Segments of the Intestines in Pre-Pubertal Gilts—A Study Protocol. *Toxins* **2021**, *13*, 379. [CrossRef]
18. Mendel, M.; Karlik, W.; Latek, U.; Chłopecka, M.; Nowacka-Kozak, E.; Pietruszka, K.; Jedziniak, P. Does Deoxynivalenol Affect Amoxicillin and Doxycycline Absorption in the Gastrointestinal Tract? Ex Vivo Study on Swine Jejunum Mucosa Explants. *Toxins* **2022**, *14*, 743. [CrossRef]
19. Gajęcka, M.; Majewski, M.S.; Zielonka, Ł.; Grzegorzewski, W.; Onyszek, E.; Lisieska-Żołnierczyk, S.; Juśkiewicz, J.; Babuchowski, A.; Gajęcki, M.T. Concentration of Zearalenone, Alpha-Zearalenol and Beta-Zearalenol in the Myocardium and the Results of Isometric Analyses of the Coronary Artery in Prepubertal Gilts. *Toxins* **2021**, *13*, 396. [CrossRef]
20. Gajęcka, M.; Otrocka-Domagała, I.; Brzuzan, P.; Dąbrowski, M.; Lisieska-Żołnierczyk, S.; Zielonka, Ł.; Gajęcki, M.T. Immunohistochemical Expression (IE) of Oestrogen Receptors in the Intestines of Prepubertal Gilts Exposed to Zearalenone. *Toxins* **2023**, *15*, 122. [CrossRef]
21. Mróz, M.; Gajęcka, M.; Brzuzan, P.; Lisieska-Żołnierczyk, S.; Leski, D.; Zielonka, Ł.; Gajęcki, M.T. Carry-Over of Zearalenone and Its Metabolites to Intestinal Tissues and the Expression of CYP1A1 and GSTπ1 in the Colon of Gilts before Puberty. *Toxins* **2022**, *14*, 354. [CrossRef] [PubMed]

22. Pierzgalski, A.; Bryła, M.; Kanabus, J.; Modrzewska, M.; Podolska, G. Updated Review of the Toxicity of Selected Fusarium Toxins and Their Modified Forms. *Toxins* **2021**, *13*, 768. [CrossRef] [PubMed]
23. Balló, A.; Busznyákné Székvári, K.; Czétány, P.; Márk, L.; Török, A.; Szántó, Á.; Máté, G. Estrogenic and Non-Estrogenic Disruptor Effect of Zearalenone on Male Reproduction: A Review. *Int. J. Mol. Sci.* **2023**, *24*, 1578. [CrossRef] [PubMed]
24. Gonkowski, S.; Gajęcka, M.; Makowska, K. Mycotoxins and the Enteric Nervous System. *Toxins* **2020**, *12*, 461. [CrossRef] [PubMed]
25. Gajęcka, M.; Otrocka-Domagała, I.; Brzuzan, P.; Zielonka, Ł.; Dąbrowski, M.; Gajęcki, M.T. Influence of deoxynivalenol and zearalenone on the immunohistochemical expression of oestrogen receptors and liver enzyme genes in vivo in prepubertal gilts. *Arch. Toxicol.* **2023**, 1–14. *Online ahead of print*. [CrossRef]
26. Schmidhauser, M.; Hankele, A.-K.; Ulbrich, S.E. Reconsidering "low-dose"—Impacts of oral estrogen exposure during preimplantation embryo development. *Mol. Reprod. Dev.* **2023**, 1–14. [CrossRef]

Disclaimer/Publisher's Note: The statements, opinions and data contained in all publications are solely those of the individual author(s) and contributor(s) and not of MDPI and/or the editor(s). MDPI and/or the editor(s) disclaim responsibility for any injury to people or property resulting from any ideas, methods, instructions or products referred to in the content.

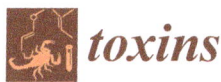

Article

Immunohistochemical Expression (IE) of Oestrogen Receptors in the Intestines of Prepubertal Gilts Exposed to Zearalenone

Magdalena Gajęcka [1,*], Iwona Otrocka-Domagała [2], Paweł Brzuzan [3], Michał Dąbrowski [1], Sylwia Lisieska-Żołnierczyk [4], Łukasz Zielonka [1] and Maciej Tadeusz Gajęcki [1]

[1] Department of Veterinary Prevention and Feed Hygiene, Faculty of Veterinary Medicine, University of Warmia and Mazury in Olsztyn, Oczapowskiego 13, 10-718 Olsztyn, Poland
[2] Department of Pathological Anatomy, Faculty of Veterinary Medicine, University of Warmia and Mazury in Olsztyn, Oczapowskiego 13, 10-718 Olsztyn, Poland
[3] Department of Environmental Biotechnology, Faculty of Environmental Sciences and Fisheries, University of Warmia and Mazury in Olsztyn, Oczapowskiego 13, 10-718 Olsztyn, Poland
[4] Independent Public Health Care Centre of the Ministry of the Interior and Administration, and the Warmia and Mazury Oncology Centre in Olsztyn, al. Wojska Polskiego 37, 10-228 Olsztyn, Poland
* Correspondence: mgaja@uwm.edu.pl

Abstract: This study was conducted to determine if a low monotonic dose of zearalenone (ZEN) affects the immunohistochemical expression (IE) of oestrogen receptor alpha (ERα) and oestrogen receptor beta (ERβ) in the intestines of sexually immature gilts. Group C (control group; n = 18) gilts were given a placebo. Group E (experimental group; n = 18) gilts were dosed orally with 40 μg ZEN /kg body weight (BW), each day before morning feeding. Samples of intestinal tissue were collected post-mortem six times. The samples were stained to analyse the IE of ERα and Erβ in the scanned slides. The strongest response was observed in ERα in the duodenum (90.387—average % of cells with ERα expression) and in ERβ in the descending colon (84.329—average % of cells with ERβ expression); the opposite response was recorded in the caecum (2.484—average % of cells with ERα expression) and the ascending colon (2.448—average % of cells with ERα expression); on the first two dates of exposure, the digestive tract had to adapt to ZEN in feed. The results of this study, supported by a mechanistic interpretation of previous research findings, suggest that ZEN performs numerous functions in the digestive tract.

Keywords: zearalenone; immunohistochemistry; oestrogen receptors; gilts before puberty

Key Contribution: Qualitative changes were manifested by a shift in oestrogen receptor expression levels from absorption level 0 to 3; particularly in ERβ expression in the descending colon.

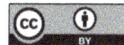

1. Introduction

Oestrogens and oestrogen-like substances found in the natural environment including the mycoestrogen ZEN, affect the developing reproductive and non-reproductive tissues [1,2]. Oestrogens are synthesised by the body, but they are also present in the environment, in the form of xenobiotics and naturally occurring compounds (undesirable substances) [3]. Most of these substances (not necessarily pollutants) are known as endocrine disruptors (EDs) [4], and they are usually found in soil, air, water, food and feed (i.e., the environment) [5,6]. Phytoestrogens (genistein, coumestrol) and the mycoestrogen ZEN (fungal metabolite) are naturally occurring EDs [7–9].

Zearalenone and α-zearalenol (α-ZEL) have an oestrogen-like structure. However, they are not steroids and do not originate from sterane structures [10]. EDs such as zearalenone are involved in several processes [11,12] that influence the endocrine system [13] and induce side effects [14]: (i) in prepubertal gilts, EDs compete with endogenous oestrogens for the binding sites of oestrogen receptors (ERs), which can alter mRNA expression levels and protein synthesis and reduce the efficacy of endogenous steroids [10,15–17]; (ii) EDs can bind to the inactive receptor (i.e., blocking it), thereby preventing the binding of natural hormones to that receptor (antagonistic effect) [11,17]; (iii) EDs reduce the levels of circulating natural hormones because they bind to blood transporting proteins, [2]; and (iv) EDs can also affect the body's metabolism by influencing the rates of synthesis, decomposition, and release of natural hormones [10,18–20].

When ingested, ZEN can prevent or delay the clinical and subclinical spread of oestrogen-dependent tumours [2,21,22]. Sex hormones and exogenous oestrogen-like chemicals are frequently implicated in the aetiology of tumours in various tissues [8]. Many oestrogen-sensitive tumours are termed oestrogen receptor-positive tumours because ERs are mediators of oestrogens or oestrogen-like substances that cause cancer [14,21]. Zearalenone may be a selective oestrogen receptor modulator, but its binding affinity for ERs is 10,000 times lower than that of 17-oestradiol (E_2) [2]. Zearalenone has agonistic or antagonistic effects on target tissues, depending on the type of ER [1,2]. The chemopreventive effect of ZEN can be attributed to its antagonistic influence on ERs [18]. There is evidence that ZEN can inhibit circulating oestrogen precursors and slow the development and progression of oestrogen-dependent tumours by binding to ERs, and ERs can probably also inhibit the activity of steroid hormones that convert circulating hormones to E_2 [18,23].

Elements of the oestrogen response have been investigated in studies involving endogenous oestrogens and oestrogen-containing drugs [12,13,18]. When endogenous oestrogens exert genomic effects via ERs, oestrogen response elements bind with ERs or other response elements in the neighbouring genes that respond directly to oestrogens [3]. The resulting bonds influence the transcription of oestrogen-responsive genes. Mycoestrogens trigger similar responses by binding to ERs and initiating molecular cascades that alter gene expression [8]. Zearalenone is involved in molecular mechanisms, but its oestrogenic activity remains insufficiently investigated. Previous research has demonstrated that the presence of ZEN in feed or food affects the mRNA expression of ERs [8,24] and the activity of other genes encoding metabolic processes in enterocytes [25,26]. Subclinical symptoms of ZEN mycotoxicosis can cause changes in hormonal signalling when enterocytes in different intestinal segments are exposed to this mycotoxin [19]. The role of zearalenone in the digestive system should be evaluated to determine possible risks for gilts before puberty [2,27–30]. Therefore, this experiment aimed to find out whether a low monotonic dose of ZEN affects the immunohistochemical expression (IE) of ERα and ERβ in the gut of prepubertal gilts. The findings may contribute to a mechanistic understanding of changes in ERα and ERβ expression.

2. Results

2.1. Clinical Observations

Clinical manifestations of ZEN mycotoxicosis were not noted during the experiment. However, histopathological analyses, ultrastructural analyses, and analyses of the metabolic profile of samples taken from same gilts frequently revealed changes in certain tissues or cells. These findings have been posted in various articles [2,19,20,31–35].

2.2. Optical Density

The brown background staining of the slides (Figures 1 and 2) was not specific to all intestinal segments, and it may have occurred in staining assays examining the ERα and ERβ expression in DAB-stained gastrointestinal tissues (most samples exhibited lightbrown, non-specific staining).

The effect of six-week exposure to ZEN on the expression levels of the selected ERs was determined in selected segments of the gastrointestinal tract (GI) of gilts in the control and experimental groups using a four point scale (negative—0; weak and homogeneous—1; mild or moderate and homogeneous—2; intense or strong and homogeneous—3) (Figures 3 and 4). Expression levels were compared between the dates of sample collection in specific sections of the intestines. Meaningful differences in the IE of ERα were not observed in the descending colon in the control group and in the ascending colon and descending colon in the experimental group. Meaningful differences in the IE of ERβ were not noted in the caecum and ascending colon in group C, and in the duodenal cap, the third section of the duodenum and the caecum in group E. The intestinal sections where no significant differences were found are not presented graphically.

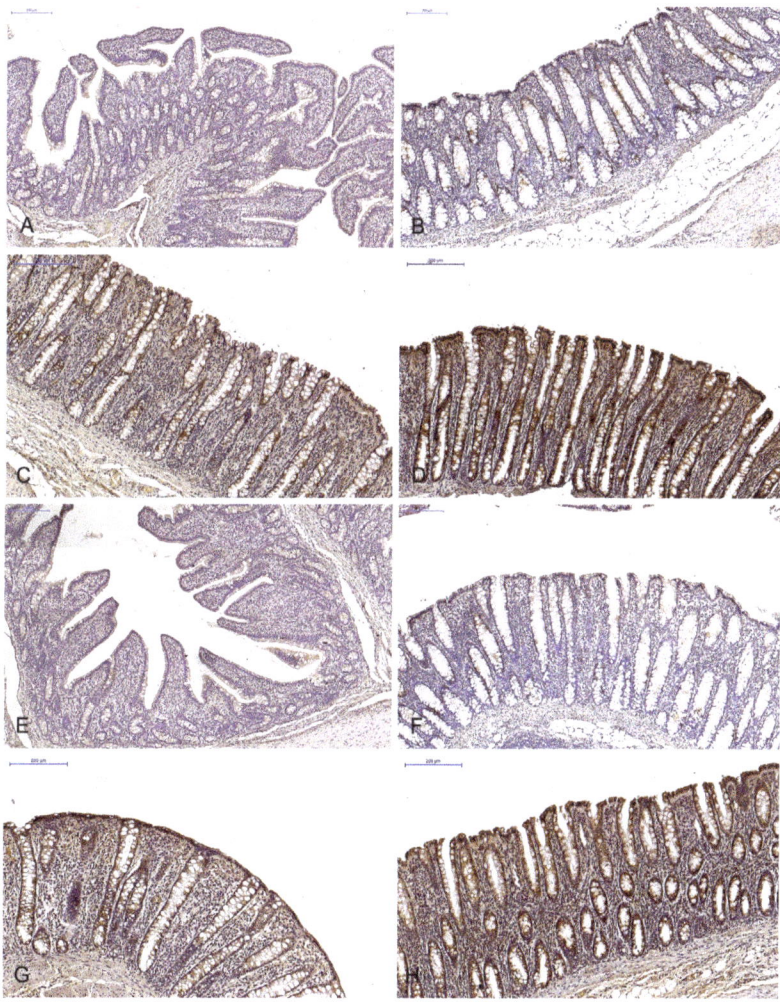

Figure 1. Scanned slides showing the IE of ERα in the descending colon in group C ((**A**)—0; (**B**)—+; (**C**)—++; (**D**)—+++) and group E ((**E**)—0; (**F**)—+; (**G**)—++;. (**H**)—+++). HE.

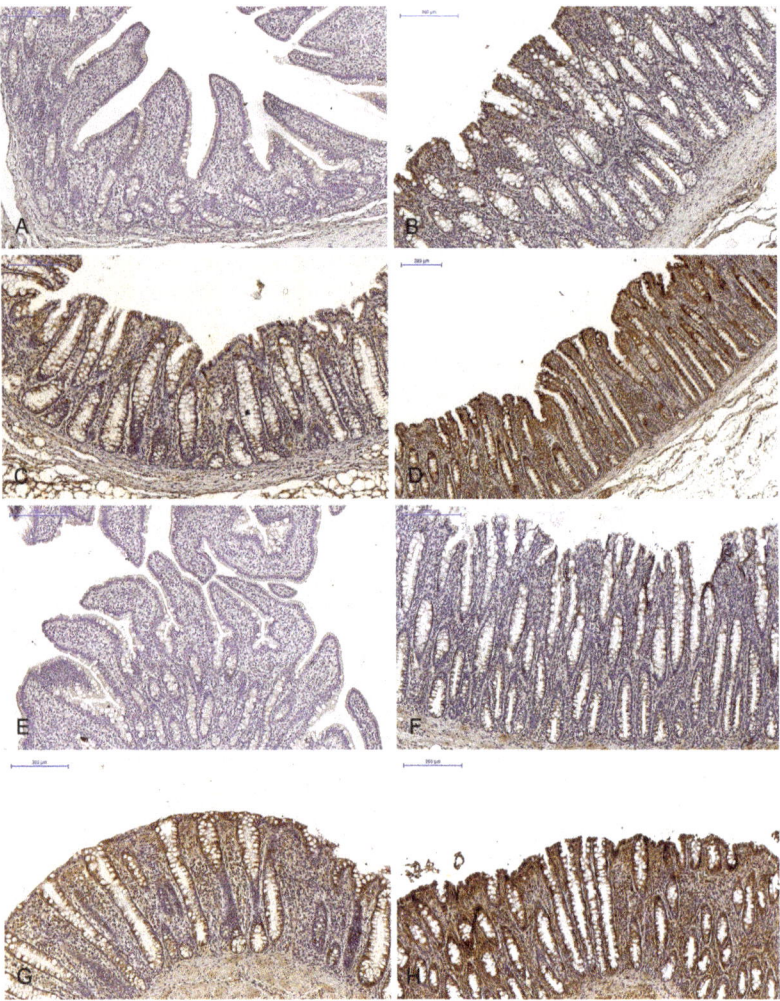

Figure 2. Scanned slides showing the IE of ERβ in the descending colon in group C ((**A**)—0; (**B**)—+; (**C**)—++; (**D**)—+++) and group E ((**E**)—0; (**F**)—+; (**G**)—++; (**H**)—+++). HE.

On each date of analysis, ERα was more highly expressed in the control group than in the experimental group, especially at absorbance level 0 (Figure 3A–D). Significant differences in ERα expression were found in the control group at different absorption levels, but absorption was significantly more pronounced on dates I, II, and VI. Significant differences in ERα expression were also observed at other absorption levels, but the noted values were much lower than at absorption level 0, and they were only found in the small intestine (Figure 3A–D). In the control group, the average ERα expression was highest at absorbance level 0, and it increased when the digesta entered the caudal segment of the small intestine.

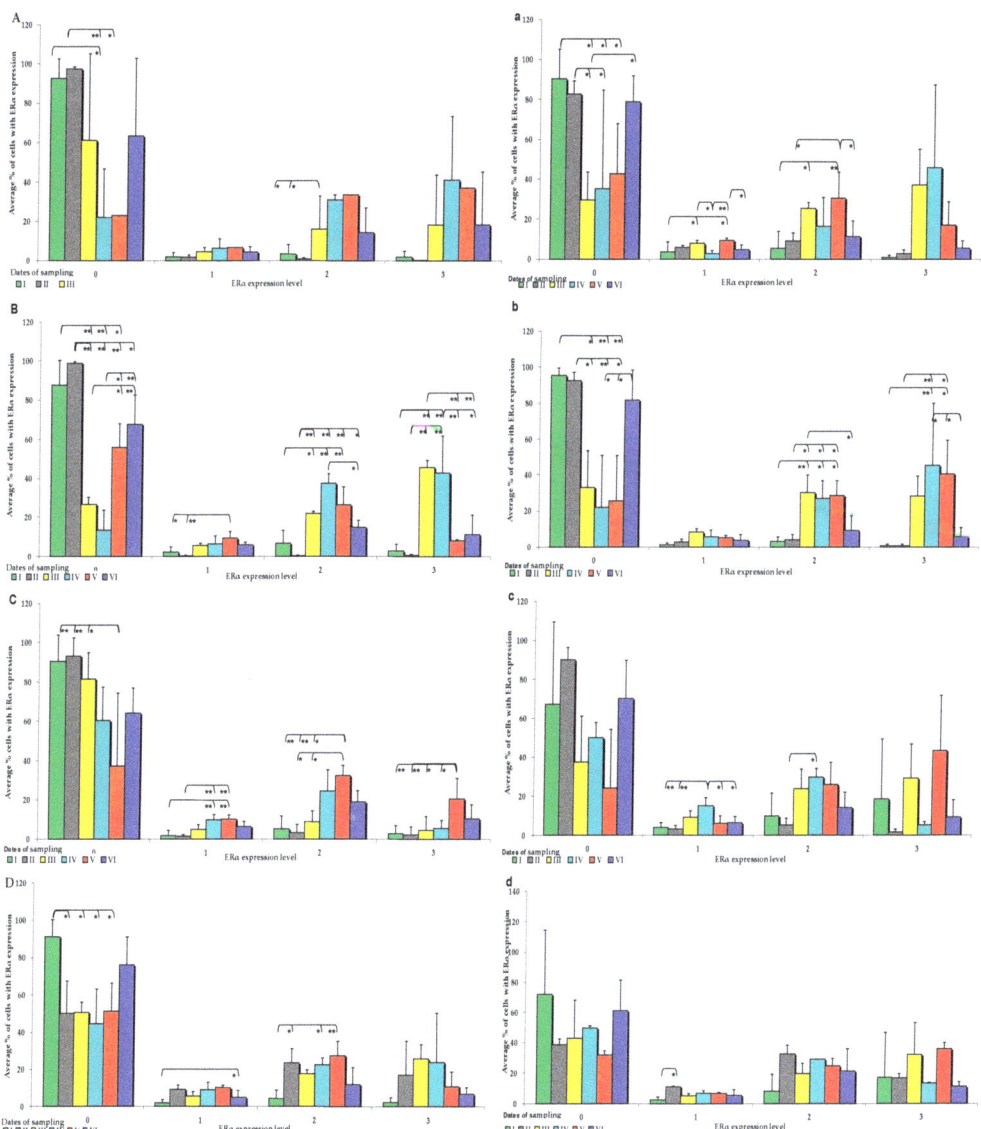

Figure 3. IE of ERα (based on a 4-point grading scale: negative—0; weak and homogeneous—1; mild or moderate and homogeneous—2; intense or strong and homogeneous—3) in the intestines of sexually immature gilts from the control group: (**A**) in the duodenal cap on selected dates of exposure; (**B**)—in the third section of the duodenum on selected dates of exposure; (**C**) in the jejunum on selected dates of exposure; (**D**) in the caecum on selected dates of exposure. In the intestines of sexually immature gilts from the experimental group: (**a**) in the duodenal cap on selected dates of exposure; (**b**) in the third section of the duodenum on selected dates of exposure; (**c**) in the jejunum on selected dates of exposure only in the weak(1) and mild (2) grades; (**d**) in the caecum on selected dates of exposure only in the weak grade (1). Expression was presented as ± (confidence interval) and SE (standard error) for some samples. * $p \leq 0.05$ and ** $p \leq 0.01$ compared with the residual groups.

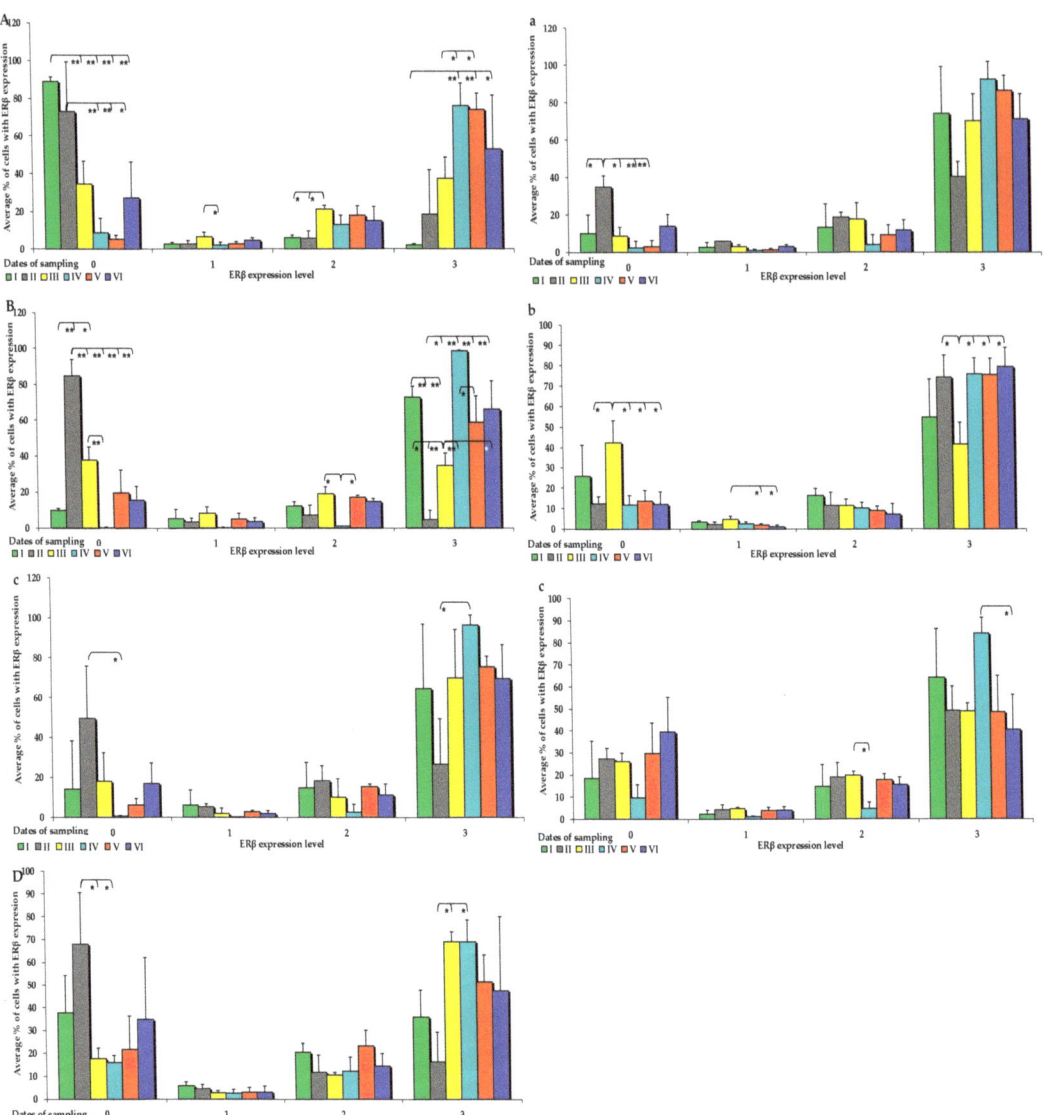

Figure 4. IE of ERβ (based on a 4-point grading scale: negative—0; weak and homogeneous—1; mild or moderate and homogeneous—2; intense or strong and homogeneous—3) in the intestines of sexually immature gilts from the control group: (**A**) in the duodenal cap on selected dates of exposure; (**B**) in the third section of the duodenum on selected dates of exposure; (**C**) in the jejunum on selected dates of exposure only in the negative (0) and intense (3) grades; (**D**) in the descending colon on selected dates of exposure only in the negative (0) and intense (3) grades; in the intestines of sexually immature gilts from the experimental group: (**a**) in the jejunum on selected dates of exposure only in the negative grade (0); (**b**) in the ascending colon on selected dates of exposure; (**c**) in the descending colon on selected dates of exposure only in the mild (2) and intense (3) grades. Expression was presented as ± (confidence interval) and SE (standard error) for some samples. * $p \leq 0.05$ and ** $p \leq 0.01$ compared with the residual groups.

An analysis of the IE of ERα revealed that it was suppressed in most intestinal segments on all dates in group E (0 points on a 4-point scale), but significant differences were detected only on dates I, II, and VI (Figure 3a). ERα was more highly expressed in the ascending and descending colon at absorption level 3 in the experimental group than in the control group. However, in group E, ERα expression was suppressed at all absorption levels (Figure 3a–d). Differences in the ERα expression were noted in the control group, but only in selected segments of the small intestine, particularly in both parts of the duodenum examined in the study (Figure 3a,b). Similarly to group C, ERα expression was induced in the experimental group at absorbance level 0, whereas at absorbance level 3, the levels of ERα expression in the analysed intestinal segments were higher in the experimental group than in the control group.

In group C, the IE of ERβ was suppressed in both segments of the duodenum, jejunum, and descending colon (Figure 4A–D). The average values of ERβ expression in the control group and in the experimental group followed a certain trend. In group E, ERβ expression was observed at absorbance level 3, and ERβ was more strongly expressed in all analysed tissues, but its expression was more suppressed at absorbance level 0. However, these differences were not significant. An immunohistochemical analysis of ERβ expression in the examined intestinal segments, compared with ERα expression, revealed completely different results. In group E, ERβ was more strongly expressed, especially at absorption level 3 and, interestingly, in the jejunum and colon (Figure 4a–c). However, significant differences between the groups were found only on dates I, II, and III, especially in the examined segments of the duodenum, which can be explained by the fact that ERβ saturation was lower in the duodenum than in the other intestinal segments.

2.3. The Prognostic Value of the ERs Expression Profile

A total of 432 samples were analysed to determine the ER expression indicator (P-ERs). In many of the analysed samples, there were no significant differences in ER expression. The mean values of P-ERs were 42 ± 27 for ERα and 38 ± 26 for ERβ. P-ERs values were not normally distributed (Table 1).

Table 1. ERα and ERβ expression at various absorption levels in the analysed sections of the GI tract in pre-pubertal gilts.

Group	Absorption	Duodenal Cap	Third Part of Duodenum	Jejunum	Caecum	Ascending Colon	Descending Colon
			ERα				
Group C	0	C	C	C	C	C	D
	1	A	A	A	A	A	A
	2	B	B	B	B	B	A
	3	B	B	A	A	A	A
Group E	0	C	C	C	C	C	D
	1	A	A	A	A	A	A
	2	B	B	B	B	B	B
	3	B	B	B	B	B	B
			ERβ				
Group C	0	C	B	B	B	B	B
	1	A	A	A	A	A	A
	2	B	B	B	B	B	B
	3	C	C	D	C	C	C

Table 1. Cont.

Group	Absorption	Duodenal Cap	Third Part of Duodenum	Jejunum	Caecum	Ascending Colon	Descending Colon
			ERα				
Group E	0	B	B	B	B	B	B
	1	A	A	A	A	A	A
	2	B	B	B	A	A	B
	3	C	C	D	D	D	C

Abbreviation: In group E, the value of P-ERα was 35, reaching 8 in the lower quartile and 62 in the upper quartile. The analysed expression values were divided into four subgroups based on the values of the median, and the upper and lower quartiles: A—very low P-ERα (P-Erα ≤ 8), B—low P-ERα (8 ≤ P-ERα < 35), C—high P-ERα (35 ≤ P-Erα < 62), and D—very high P-ERα (P-Erα ≥ 62) (Table 1). In group E, very low (A), low (B), high (C), and very high (D) values of P-ERα were noted in six (25%), 12 (50%), five (21%), and one (4%) cases, accordingly. The statistical analysis was carried out for different mean, median, upper and lower quartile cut-off points, but no meaningful differences were noted.

2.3.1. P-ER Values for ERα

In group C, the P-ERα value was 42, reaching 15 in the lower quartile and 69 in the upper quartile. An analysis of the median and the upper and lower quartiles revealed that the expression values could be divided into four subgroups: A—very low P-ERα (P-ERα <15), B—low P-ERα (15 ≤ P -ERα < 42), C—high P-ERα (42 ≤ P-ERα < 69) and D—very high P-ERα (P-Erα ≥69) (Table 1). In group C, very low (A), low (B), high (C), and very high (D) P-ERα values were found in 11 (46%), seven (29%), five (21%), and one (4%) cases, respectively. The statistical analysis was conducted for different means, medians, upper and lower quartiles of the separation points, but no meaningful differences were observed.

The results of the analyses involving the uptake of only Erα or ERβ are difficult to interpret. The values of P-ERs (Table 1) provide new information on the presence of a low ZEN dose in the diet. These were very similar in both groups, but at absorption level 3, an increase in P-ERs was observed in group E, resulting in a shift from quartile A to quartile B from the jejunum directly to the descending colon. The results described above and previous research findings suggest that ZEN may compensate for E_2 deficiency by triggering ERα [27].

2.3.2. P-ER Values for ERβ

In group C, the P-ERβ worth was 35, reaching 9 in the lower quartile and 61 in the upper quartile. Based on the average value of the median, and the upper and lower quartiles, expression values were divided into four subgroups: A—very low P-ERβ (P—ERβ ≤ 9), B—low P-ERβ (9 ≤ P-ERβ < 35), C—high P-ERβ (35 ≤ P-ERβ < 61), and D—very high P-ERβ (P-Erβ ≥ 61) (Table 1). In group C, very low (A), low (B), high (C), and very high (D) levels of P-ERβ were found in six (25%), 11 (46%), 6 (25%), and one (4%) cases, respectively. The statistical analysis was carried out for different means, medians, upper and lower quartiles, but no meaningful differences were found.

In group E, the P-ERβ value was 38, reaching 12 in the lower quartile and 64 in the upper quartile. Based on the values of the median, the upper and lower quartiles and expression values were divided into four subgroups: A—very low P-ERβ (P-Rβ < 12), B—low P-ERβ (12 ≤ P-ERβ < 38), C—high P-ERβ (38 ≤ P-ERβ < 64) and D—very high P-ERβ (P-Erβ ≥ 64) (Table 1). In the experimental group, very low (A), low (B), high (C), and very high (D) P-ERβ values were known in eight (33%), 10 (42%), three (12%), and three (12%) cases, respectively. The statistical analysis was carried out for different means, medians, upper and lower quartiles, but no meaningful differences were found.

The values of P-ERβ (Table 1) shifted to the right from quartile C to quartile D at absorption level 3 in the caecum and the ascending colon. An analysis of the expression of both receptors demonstrated that the P-ERα levels shifted significantly to the lower quartiles (to the left) in animals exposed to low ZEN doses.

3. Discussion

This study confirmed our recent observations that low ZEN doses improve somatic [36] and reproductive health (our previous mechanistic studies) [2,19,37]. On the first day of exposure, ZEN exerted a stimulatory effect on the body, with the exception of the reproductive system [18,38]. This effect was minimised after the second or third day of exposure, probably due to: (i) the negative effects of extragonadal compensation for oestrogen synthesis [39,40] by androgen conversion or the acquisition of exogenous oestrogens or oestrogen-like substances [2,9,41]; (ii) adaptive mechanisms [37]; (iii) higher energy and protein utilisation, indicating more efficient feed conversion (productivity in group E) [41–43]; or (iv) detoxification processes (biotransformation) [3]. The last argument is difficult to confirm since an analysis of the carry-over factor in the GI tract of the same animals did not reveal the inherence of α- ZEL or β- ZEL (ZEN metabolites) in the intestinal walls or that the registered levels were below the detection limit [20,25]. According to López-Calderero et al. [44], a higher ERα/ERβ ratio indicates that proliferative processes are stimulated or silenced, and it is unrelated to apoptosis [38]. Similar observations were made by Cleveland et al. [45] and Williams et al. [46]. These results suggest that low levels of ZEN in the diet stimulate proliferative processes in the gastrointestinal tract of prepubertal gilts, especially in the colon. In sexually mature animals, this is a good predictor of weight gain or the time needed to reach slaughter weight [41], and it suggests that the gastrointestinal tract regulates somatic health [9,38]. Thus, the digestive system acts as a "second brain" [47] as it performs numerous functions including a modulatory role between the intestinal contents and tissues vis. the central nervous system [48]. These findings also suggest that ZEN and endogenous oestrogens control growth, differentiation and other important functions in tissues including in the gastrointestinal tract [2] of prepubertal gilts with suprahypsiological oestrogen levels [18]. The above also suggests that oestrogen signalling (e.g., ZEN and its metabolites), regardless of its origin, is the major regulator of genomic mechanisms. Oestrogen receptors play a special role: (i) they are activated by ligand-dependent and ligand-independent pathways; (ii) they act as transcription factors that activate and trigger the expression of all sensitive genes; and (iii) the feedback loop regulated by oestrogens contributes to the maintenance or modification of all genomic processes.

3.1. Oestrogen Receptors

The biological effects of oestrogens are determined by the type of ERs including the classical nuclear ERα and ERβ as well as the G-protein-coupled ERs (GPER; its expression has not been analysed). Therefore, the levels of different ERs determine the effects of endogenous and exogenous oestrogens on cells (tissues).

3.1.1. Oestrogen Receptor Alpha

The expression of ERα in the control group could be attributed to the physiological deficiency of E_2 in the gilts before puberty [4,24,49], which could point to suprahypsiological hormone levels rather than hypoestrogenism [18,50]. Zearalenone mycotoxicosis contributes to an increase in steroid levels (endogenous steroids such as E_2, progesterone, and testosterone as well as exogenous steroids such as ZEN), which may restore or enhance ER signalling in cells [18,51], but only in relation to hormone-dependent ERs [27]. As a result, ERα expression is not stimulated but deregulated [51]. Most importantly, circulating steroid hormones are bioavailable (not bound to carrier proteins) and their cellular effects are observed at very low concentrations of approximately 0.1–9 pg/mL E_2 [49]. The concentrations of active hormones are determined by the age and health status of animals [2,8,18,24,52].

Various conclusions can be drawn from the observations of the role of ERα in mammals and the results of the experimentally induced ZEN mycotoxicosis. According to Suba [38], both high and low levels of E_2 stimulate the expression and transcriptional activity of ERs to restore or enhance ER signalling in cells, which was not observed in the current study.

However, the IE of ERα was suppressed to a greater extent. Low ZEN doses in the diet decrease the IE of ERα, which directly affects the somatic (higher weight gain) [41] and reproductive health (delayed sexual maturity [53]) of animals. It should also be noted that low serum E_2 levels may induce compensatory effects to increase the expression and transcriptional activity of ERs, while increased synthesis of endogenous E_2 may compensate for low ER signalling [54]. However, it remains uncertain as to whether low ZEN doses are sufficient to meet the requirements of sexually immature gilts. The present findings suggest that this may be the case, with positive implications for pig farmers.

3.1.2. Oestrogen Receptor Beta

According to the literature, intense ERβ expression or a high level of absorption (3 points on a 4-point grading scale) contributes significantly to gut health, especially colon health, and intensifies metabolic processes [55,56]. In turn, ERβ silencing increases the risk of duodenal inflammation and enhances oncogenesis not only in the gastrointestinal tract, but also in the reproductive system [22,40,45,46,57]. Deletion processes suggest that ERβ has anti-inflammatory and anti-carcinogenic properties, and exerts chemopreventive effects in the colon [58], which was confirmed in a study of low-dose ZEN mycotoxicosis [59].

Apart from the previously published research on the effects of E_2 deficiency in prepubertal animals, another issue should be addressed. Williams et al. [46] and Gajęcka et al. [59] reported that selected phytoestrogens (silymarin and silibinin) and mycoestrogens (ZEN) have a selective affinity for ERβ [60,61]. This is the result of the increased expression of the ERβ gene, suggesting that natural exogenous dietary oestrogens may have anti-inflammatory properties [35]. These oestrogens also exert chemopreventive effects [22], and they can reverse minor carcinogenic changes in the colon [62]. Calabrese et al. [63] found that a mixture of phytoestrogens and lignans reduced the size and number of duodenal polyps and exerted therapeutic effects in this segment of the gastrointestinal tract [64].

As stated in the research objective, this study was conducted to determine if low ZEN doses naturally occurring in feeds could produce similar effects, and the present results suggest that it is possible. This conclusion is also consistent with the results of previous studies conducted as part of the same research project [2,19,29,31–36,52].

3.1.3. ER Expression Indicator

In animals exposed to ZEN, the P-ER levels differed between quartiles. In group E, the P-ERα values shifted from quartile A to quartile B, while the P-ERβ values shifted from quartiles B and C to quartiles A and D. The expression levels of ERα confirm that low ZEN doses can exert oestrogenic effects on the studied ERs.

The endogenous ligand that triggers ERβ [27] and the cells that are activated by specific receptors could not be identified based on the existing knowledge. For this reason, the influence of ZEN on ERβ is difficult to interpret. It seems that E_2 does not bind to ERα and ERβ with equal affinity, but it binds to oestrogen response elements. However, ERβ is a much weaker transcriptional activator than ERα. In turn, the oestrogen response element activator protein-1 is responsible for the proliferation processes induced by E_2. Nevertheless, E_2 has no effect on ERβ, which may indicate that ERβ can modulate ERα activity in cells where both receptors are co-expressed. However, in many cells, ERβ is expressed in the absence of ERα, and in these cells, ERβ remains active independently of ERα [56]. This is the case in epithelial cells of the colon [65], where ERβ-driven enhanced metabolic processes occur [55].

Preclinical models have shown that ERα activity can be modulated by ERβ, which inhibits oestrogen-dependent proliferation and promotes apoptosis [66]. There is evidence that uncontrolled proliferation, progression, and/or failure to respond to treatment may disrupt oestrogen signalling. ERα may be associated with proliferative disorders, and it can be used to determine the efficacy of hormone therapy. In contrast, ERβ is present in healthy colonic mucosa and its expression is significantly delayed in colonic proliferative disorders [44,56].

3.1.4. Summary

The observed silencing of ERs indicates that: (i) low monotonic doses of ZEN elicited the strongest responses on analytical dates III, IV, and VI, whereas on the last date, the prepubertal gilts developed tolerance to the analysed undesirable substance; (ii) ERα expression was increased in the duodenum and ERβ expression was increased in the descending colon; (iii) the opposite was observed in the caecum and the ascending colon; and (iv) the gastrointestinal tract of sexually immature gilts was adapted to the presence of ZEN in the feed after the first two exposure dates. Due to the very low concentrations of E_2, ZEN was bound to ERs and triggered qualitative changes in ERs during the successive weeks of the experiment (activation?). Qualitative changes were manifested by a shift in the ER expression levels from absorption level 0 to 3, especially ERβ expression in the descending colon. The observed shift in ERβ expression suggests that zearalenone and its metabolites are involved in the control of proliferation and apoptosis in enterocytes.

4. Materials and Methods

4.1. Experimental Animals

The experiment was carried out at the Department of Veterinary Prevention and Feed Hygiene of the Faculty of Veterinary Medicine of the University of Warmia and Mazury in Olsztyn, Poland, on 36 clinically healthy gilts with an initial body weight (BW) of 25 ± 2 kg. Pre-puberty gilts were kept in groups and had ad lib access to water.

4.2. Experimental Feed

The feed administered to animals (Table 2) was analysed for the presence of ZEN and DON. Mycotoxin content was determined by standard separation techniques using immunoaffinity columns (Zearala-TestTM Zearalenone Testing System, G1012, VICAM, Watertown, MA, USA; DON-TestTM DON Testing System, VICAM, Watertown, MA, USA) and high-performance liquid chromatography (HPLC) (Hewlett Packard, type 1050 and 1100) [67] with fluorescence and/or ultraviolet detection techniques. The detection limit was 3.0 ng/g for ZEN [19] and 1.0 ng/g for DON [36].

Table 2. Mixture of diets for pre-pubertal gilts (first stage of rearing).

Percentage Content of Feed Ingredients		Nutritional Value of Diets	
Barley (*Hordeum* L.)	27.65	Metabolizable energy MJ/kg	12.575
Wheat (*Triticum monococcum* L.)	17.5	Total protein (%)	16.8
Triticale (*Triticosecale* Wittm. ex A.Camus)	15.0	Digestible protein (%)	13.95
Maize (*Zea mays* L.)	17.5	Lysine (g/kg)	9.975
Soybean meal, 46%	16.0	Methionine + Cysteine (g/kg)	6.25
Rapeseed meal	3.5	Calcium (g/kg)	8.05
Limestone	0.35	Total phosphorus (g/kg)	5.75
Premix [1]	2.5	Available phosphorus (g/kg)	3.1
		Sodium (g/kg)	1.5

Abbreviation: Composition of the vitamin-mineral premix per kg: vitamin A—500.000 IU; iron—5000 mg; vitamin D3—100.000 IU; zinc—5000 mg; vitamin E (alpha-tocopherol)—2000 mg; manganese—3000 mg; vitamin K—150 mg; copper ($CuSO_4 \cdot 5H_2O$)—500 mg; vitamin B1—100 mg; cobalt—20 mg; vitamin B2—300 mg; iodine—40 mg; vitamin B6—150 mg; selenium—15 mg; vitamin B12—1500 µg; niacin—1200 mg; pantothenic acid—600 mg; L-threonine—2.3 g; folic acid—50 mg; tryptophan—1.1 g; biotin—7500 µg; phytase + choline—10 g; ToyoCerin probiotic + calcium—250 g; magnesium—5 g.

4.3. Experimental Design

The animals were allocated to an experimental group (E = ZEN; n = 18) and a control group (C, n = 18) [68,69]. The animals in group E were orally administered ZEN at a dose of 40 µg/kg BW (Table 3). The pigs in group C were given a placebo. At the time when this test was designed, the above value complied with the recommendations of the European Food Safety Authority (CR 2006/576/EC—2006 [70]) and No-Observed-Adverse-Effect Level (NOAEL) dose. The mycotoxin was administered every morning before feeding, in gel capsules that dissolved in the stomach. In group C, pigs received identical gel capsules, but without the mycotoxin.

Table 3. Diurnal feed intake in a restricted feeding regime (kg/day) and the average zearalenone concentration per kg feed (µg ZEN/kg feed).

Week of Exposure	Feed Intake	Total ZEN Dose	
	kg/Day	µg ZEN/kg BW	µg ZEN/kg Feed
I	1.1	280	1014
II	1.0	560	972
III	1.3	840	1014
IV	1.6	1120	987
V	1.9	1400	995
VI	1.7	1680	957

Zearalenone was biosynthesised at the Faculty of Chemistry at the University of Life Sciences in Poznań. The trial lasted 42 days. Zearalenone doses were adapted to the BW of gilts. Zearalenone was served in capsules to avoid potential problems resulting from unequal feed intake. Zearalenone samples were dissolved in 500 µL 96% C_2H_5OH (96% ethyl SWW 2442-90, Polskie Odczynniki Chemiczne SA, Poland) to obtain the required dose (converted to BW). The solutions were kept at 20 °C for twelve hours. The gilts were weighed at weekly intervals to adjust the ZEN dose of each animal. Three gilts from each group (six animals in total) were euthanised on days 7 (date I), 14 (date II), 21 (date III), 28 (date IV), 35 (date V), and 42 (date VI) by intravenous administration of sodium pentobarbital (Fatro, Ozzano Emilia BO, Italy). Directly after cardiac arrest, part of the intestinal tissue were taken and prepared for analysis.

4.4. Reagents

ZEN was obtained from the Faculty of Chemistry, University of Life Sciences in Poznań based on an earlier developed methodology [71,72] presented in other studies [73].

4.5. Chemicals and Equipment

The chromatographic analysis of ZEN was conducted at the Faculty of Chemistry, University of Biosciences in Poznań based on an earlier developed methodology [73].

4.6. Tissue Samples

On each experimental day, intestinal tissue samples (approx. 1 × 1.5 cm) were collected from the succeeding segments of the GI tract of gilts: the duodenum—the first part and the third section; the jejunum and ileum—the middle part; the large intestine—the middle parts of the ascending colon, transverse colon and descending colon; and the caecum—1 cm from the ileocecal valve. The samples were rinsed with phosphate buffer.

4.7. Immunohistochemistry

4.7.1. Localisation of ERα and ERβ

Tissue samples were fixed in four percent paraformaldehyde and embedded in paraffin. Two samples from each test section were stained to determine the ERα and ERβ expression. In the negative control, the primary antibody was omitted. To unmask the antigens, the sections were placed in citrate buffer (Sigma-Aldrich, Saint Louis, MO, USA) and cooked for 20 min in a microwave oven at 800 W. The sections were coated with ready-to-use DAKO REALTM Peroxidase Blocking Solution (DAKO, Glostrup, Denmark) and reacted for 15 min. Non-specific antigen binding areas were blocked with 2.5% normal goat serum solution. The sections were reacted overnight at a temperature of 6 °C with the following primary antibodies: Mouse Anti-Human Oestrogen Receptor α (Clone: 1D5, DAKO Santa Clara, CA, USA) and Mouse Anti-Oestrogen Receptor β (Clone: 14C8, Abcam, Cambridge, UK), diluted to 1:60 and 1:20, respectively. After the reaction, the specimens were rinsed three times with PBS (Sigma-Aldrich, Saint Louis, MO, USA) at five-minute intervals. Secondary antibodies conjugated with horseradish peroxidase-labelled micropolymer (ImmPRESS™ HRP Universal Antibody, Vector Laboratories, Burlingame, CA, USA) were applied to the specimens. The sections were coloured by incubation with DAB (DAKO, Glostrup, Denmark) for 3 min, and H_2O_2 was added to visualise the activity of the bound enzyme (brown colour). The sections were washed with water and contrast stained with Mayer's haematoxylin solution (Sigma-Aldrich, Saint Louis, MO, USA). The primary antibody was ignored in the negative control. Negative controls (solvent-coated slides only, no primary antibody) and positive controls were converted together with the slides [74]. The pig's ovary was used as a positive control for ERβ [75].

4.7.2. Scanning of the Coloured Slides

The expressions of ERα and ERβ were analysed on the scanned slides (Pannoramic MIDI scanner, 3DHISTECH, Budapest, H) using the NuclearQuant programme (3DHISTECH, H). The slides were converted into digital images (Figures 1 and 2). The profile of nuclear detection and staining intensity were as previously described [59].

4.8. Statistical Analysis

The activity of ERα and ERβ in the GI tract of pigs was presented on the basis of ± and SD for each sample. The results were compiled using the Statistica programme (StatSoft Inc., USA). Based on the applied ZEN dose and the duration of its application, the arithmetic means for systems with repeatable measurements were compared using one-way analysis of variance. The homogeneity of variance in the compared groups was checked with the Brown–Forsythe test. Differences between groups were analysed using Tukey's honestly significant difference test ($p < 0.05$ or $p < 0.01$).

Author Contributions: The experiments were designed and planned by M.G. and M.T.G. The experiments were conducted by I.O.-D., P.B., S.L.-Ż. and M.G. The data were analysed and interpreted by M.D. and M.G. The manuscript was written by M.G. and critically revised by Ł.Z. and M.T.G. All authors have read and agreed to the published version of the manuscript.

Funding: The study was supported by the Polish Ministry of Science and Higher Education as part of Project No. 12-0080-10/2010. The project was financially supported by the Minister of Education and Science under the program entitled "Regional Initiative of Excellence" for the years 2019–2023, Project No. 010/RID/2018/19, amount of funding PLN 12,000,000.

Institutional Review Board Statement: All experimental procedures involving animals were carried out in compliance with Polish regulations setting forth the terms and conditions of animal experimentation for 2010–2013 (opinion no. 88/2009 of the local Ethics Committee for Animal Experimentation at the University of Warmia and Mazury in Olsztyn, Poland of 16 Dec 2009). All of the investigators are authorised to perform experiments on animals.

Informed Consent Statement: Not applicable.

Data Availability Statement: Not applicable.

Conflicts of Interest: The authors declare no conflict of interest.

References

1. Han, X.; Huangfu, B.; Xu, T.; Xu, W.; Asakiya, C.; Huang, K.; He, X. Research Progress of Safety of Zearalenone: A Review. *Toxins* **2022**, *14*, 386. [CrossRef] [PubMed]
2. Gajęcka, M.; Zielonka, Ł.; Gajęcki, M. Activity of zearalenone in the porcine intestinal tract. *Molecules* **2017**, *22*, 18. [CrossRef]
3. Mahato, D.K.; Devi, S.; Pandhi, S.; Sharma, B.; Maurya, K.K.; Mishra, S.; Dhawan, K.; Selvakumar, R.; Kamle, M.; Mishra, A.K.; et al. Occurrence, Impact on Agriculture, Human Health, and Management Strategies of Zearalenone in Food and Feed: A Review. *Toxins* **2021**, *13*, 92. [CrossRef]

4. Hampl, R.; Kubatova, J.; Starka, L. Steroids and endocrine disruptors -History, recent state of art and open questions. *J. Steroid Biochem. Mol. Biol.* **2016**, *155*, 217–223. [CrossRef]
5. Crain, D.A.; Janssen, S.J.; Edwards, T.M.; Heindel, J.; Ho, S.; Hunt, P.; Iguchi, T.; Juul, A.; McLachlan, J.A.; Schwartz, J.; et al. Female reproductive disorders: The roles of endocrinedisrupting compounds and developmental timing. *Fertil. Steril.* **2008**, *90*, 911–940. [CrossRef]
6. Yurino, H.; Ishikawa, S.; Sato, T.; Akadegawa, K.; Ito, T.; Ueha, S.; Inadera, H. Endocrine disrupters (environmental estrogens) enhance autoantibody production by B1 cells. *Toxicol. Sci.* **2004**, *81*, 139–147. [CrossRef] [PubMed]
7. Grgic, D.; Varga, E.; Novak, B.; Müller, A.; Marko, D. Isoflavones in Animals: Metabolism and Effects in Livestock and Occurrence in Feed. *Toxins* **2021**, *13*, 836. [CrossRef]
8. Kowalska, K.; Habrowska-Górczyńska, D.E.; Piastowska-Ciesielska, A.W. Zearalenone as an endocrine disruptor in humans. *Environ. Toxicol. Phar.* **2016**, *48*, 141–149. [CrossRef]
9. Sun, L.; Dai, J.; Xu, J.; Yang, J.; Zhang, D. Comparative Cytotoxic Effects and Possible Mechanisms of Deoxynivalenol, Zearalenone and T-2 Toxin Exposure to Porcine Leydig Cells In Vitro. *Toxins* **2022**, *14*, 113. [CrossRef] [PubMed]
10. Lathe, R.; Kotelevtsev, Y.; Mason, J.I. Steroid promiscuity: Diversity of enzyme action. *J. Steroid Biochem.* **2015**, *151*, 1–2. [CrossRef]
11. Barton, M. Not lost in translation: Emerging clinical importance of the G protein-coupled estrogen receptor GPER, Review Article. *Steroids* **2016**, *111*, 37–45. [CrossRef]
12. Frizzell, C.; Ndossi, D.; Verhaegen, S.; Dahl, E.; Eriksen, G.; Sŕrlie, M.; Ropstad, E.; Muller, M.; Elliott, C.T.; Connolly, L. Endocrine disrupting effects of zearalenone, alpha- and beta-zearalenol at the level of nuclear receptor binding and steroidogenesis. *Toxicol. Lett.* **2011**, *206*, 210–217. [CrossRef] [PubMed]
13. Yang, R.; Wang, Y.M.; Zhang, L.; Zhao, Z.M.; Zhao, J.; Peng, S.Q. Prepubertal exposure to an oestrogenic mycotoxin zearalenone induces central precocious puberty in immature female rats through the mechanism of premature activation of hypothalamic kisspeptin-GPR54 signalling. *Mol. Cell. Endocrinol.* **2016**, *437*, 62–74. [CrossRef] [PubMed]
14. Taheri, M.; Shoorei, H.; Dinger, M.E.; Ghafouri-Fard, S. Perspectives on the Role of Non-Coding RNAs in the Regulation of Expression and Function of the Estrogen Receptor. *Cancers* **2020**, *12*, 2162. [CrossRef] [PubMed]
15. Adibnia, E.; Razi, M.; Malekinejad, H. Zearalenone and 17 β-estradiol induced damages in male rats reproduction potential; evidence for ERα and ERβ receptors expression and steroidogenesis. *Toxicon* **2016**, *120*, 133–146. [CrossRef] [PubMed]
16. Pizzo, F.; Caloni, F.; Schreiber, N.B.; Cortinovis, C.; Spicer, L.J. In vitro effects of deoxynivalenol and zearalenone major metabolites alone and combined, on cell proliferation, steroid production and gene expression in bovine small-follicle granulose cells. *Toxicon* **2016**, *109*, 70–83. [CrossRef] [PubMed]
17. Longobardi, C.; Damiano, S.; Ferrara, G.; Montagnaro, S.; Meucci, V.; Intorre, L.; Bacci, S.; Esposito, L.; Piscopo, N.; Rubino, A.; et al. Zearalenone (ZEN) and Its Metabolite Levels in Tissues of Wild Boar (Sus scrofa) from Southern Italy: A Pilot Study. *Toxins* **2023**, *15*, 56. [CrossRef]
18. Rykaczewska, A.; Gajęcka, M.; Onyszek, E.; Cieplińska, K.; Dąbrowski, M.; Lisieska-Żołnierczyk, S.; Bulińska, M.; Obuchowski, A.; Gajęcki, M.T.; Zielonka, Ł. Imbalance in the Blood Concentrations of Selected Steroids in Prepubertal Gilts Depending on the Time of Exposure to Low Doses of Zearalenone. *Toxins* **2019**, *11*, 561. [CrossRef]
19. Zielonka, Ł.; Gajęcka, M.; Żmudzki, J.; Gajęcki, M. The effect of selected environmental Fusarium mycotoxins on the ovaries in the female wild boar (Sus scrofa). *Pol. J. Vet. Sci.* **2015**, *18*, 391–399. [CrossRef]
20. Zhang, Q.; Huang, L.; Leng, B.; Li, Y.; Jiao, N.; Jiang, S.; Yang, W.; Yuan, X. Zearalenone Affect the Intestinal Villi Associated with the Distribution and the Expression of Ghrelin and Proliferating Cell Nuclear Antigen in Weaned Gilts. *Toxins* **2021**, *13*, 736. [CrossRef]
21. Obremski, K.; Gonkowski, S.; Wojtacha, P. Zearalenone—Induced changes in lymphoid tissue and mucosal nerve fibers in the porcine ileum. *Pol. J. Vet. Sci.* **2015**, *18*, 357–365. [CrossRef] [PubMed]
22. Lee, G.A.; Hwang, K.A.; Choi, K.C. Roles of Dietary Phytoestrogens on the Regulation of Epithelial-Mesenchymal Transition in Diverse Cancer Metastasis. *Toxins* **2016**, *8*, 162. [CrossRef] [PubMed]
23. Barton, M. Position paper: The membrane estrogen receptor GPER—Clues and questions. *Steroids* **2012**, *77*, 935–942. [CrossRef]
24. Fruhauf, S.; Novak, B.; Nagl, V.; Hackl, M.; Hartinger, D.; Rainer, V.; Labudová, S.; Adam, G.; Aleschko, M.; Moll, W.D.; et al. Biotransformation of the Mycotoxin Zearalenone to its Metabolites Hydrolyzed Zearalenone (HZEN) and Decarboxylated Hydrolyzed Zearalenone (DHZEN) Diminishes its Estrogenicity In Vitro and In Vivo. *Toxins* **2019**, *11*, 481. [CrossRef] [PubMed]
25. Guerre, P. Mycotoxins an Gut Microbiota Interactions. *Toxins* **2020**, *12*, 769. [CrossRef]
26. Freire, L.; Sant'Ana, A.S. Modified mycotoxins: An updated review on their formation, detection, occurrence, and toxic effects. *Food Chem. Toxicol.* **2018**, *111*, 189–205. [CrossRef]
27. Warner, M.; Gustafsson, J.A. DHEA—A precursor of ERß ligands. *J. Steroid Biochem.* **2015**, *145*, 245–247. [CrossRef]
28. Soler, L.; Oswald, I.P. The importance of accounting for sex in the search of proteomic signatures of mycotoxin exposure. *J. Proteomics* **2018**, *178*, 114–122. [CrossRef]
29. Song, T.; Zhou, X.; Ma, X.; Jiang, Y.; Yang, W.; Liu, F.; Liu, M.; Huang, L.; Jiang, S. Zearalenone Promotes Uterine Development of Weaned Gilts by Interfering with Serum Hormones and Up-Regulating Expression of Estrogen and Progesterone Receptors. *Toxins* **2022**, *14*, 732. [CrossRef]
30. Wan, B.; Yuan, X.; Yang, W.; Jiao, N.; Li, Y.; Liu, F.; Liu, M.; Yang, Z.; Huang, L.; Jiang, S. The Effects of Zearalenone on the Localization and Expression of Reproductive Hormones in the Ovaries of Weaned Gilts. *Toxins* **2021**, *13*, 626. [CrossRef]

31. Lewczuk, B.; Przybylska-Gornowicz, B.; Gajęcka, M.; Targońska, K.; Ziółkowska, N.; Prusik, M.; Gajęcki, M.T. Histological structure of duodenum in gilts receiving low doses of zearalenone and deoxynivalenol in feed. *Exp. Toxicol. Pathol.* **2016**, *68*, 157–166. [CrossRef] [PubMed]
32. Nowak, A.; Śliżewska, K.; Gajęcka, M.; Piotrowska, M.; Żakowska, Z.; Zielonka, Ł.; Gajęcki, M. The genotoxicity of caecal water from gilts following experimentally induced Fusarium mycotoxicosis. *Vet. Med.* **2015**, *60*, 133–140. [CrossRef]
33. Piotrowska, M.; Śliżewska, K.; Nowak, A.; Zielonka, Ł.; Żakowska, Z.; Gajęcka, M.; Gajęcki, M. The effect of experimental Fusarium mycotoxicosis on microbiota diversity in porcine ascending colon contents. *Toxins* **2014**, *6*, 2064–2081. [CrossRef] [PubMed]
34. Przybylska-Gornowicz, B.; Tarasiuk, M.; Lewczuk, B.; Prusik, M.; Ziółkowska, N.; Zielonka, Ł.; Gajęcki, M.; Gajęcka, M. The Effects of Low Doses of Two Fusarium Toxins, Zearalenone and Deoxynivalenol, on the Pig Jejunum. A Light and Electron Microscopic Study. *Toxins* **2015**, *7*, 4684–4705. [CrossRef] [PubMed]
35. Przybylska-Gornowicz, B.; Lewczuk, B.; Prusik, M.; Hanuszewska, M.; Petrusewicz-Kosińska, M.; Gajęcka, M.; Zielonka, Ł.; Gajęcki, M. The Effects of Deoxynivalenol and Zearalenone on the Pig Large Intestine. A Light and Electron Microscopic study. *Toxins* **2018**, *10*, 148. [CrossRef]
36. Mendel, M.; Karlik, W.; Latek, U.; Chłopecka, M.; Nowacka-Kozak, E.; Pietruszka, K.; Jedziniak, P. Does Deoxynivalenol Affect Amoxicillin and Doxycycline Absorption in the Gastrointestinal Tract? Ex Vivo Study on Swine Jejunum Mucosa Explants. *Toxins* **2022**, *14*, 743. [CrossRef]
37. Gajęcka, M.; Tarasiuk, M.; Zielonka, Ł.; Dąbrowski, M.; Nicpoń, J.; Baranowski, M.; Gajęcki, M.T. Changes in the metabolic profile and body weight of pre-pubertal gilts during prolonged monotonic exposure to low doses of zearalenone and deoxynivalenol. *Toxicon* **2017**, *125*, 32–43. [CrossRef]
38. Suba, Z. Key to estrogen's anticancer capacity. *Acad. Lett.* **2021**. submitted.
39. Grenier, B.; Applegate, T.J. Modulation of intestinal functions following mycotoxin ingestion: Meta analysis of published experiments in animals. *Toxins* **2013**, *5*, 396–430. [CrossRef]
40. Suba, Z. Estrogen Withdrawal by Oophorectomy as Presumed Anticancer Means is a Major Medical Mistake. *J. Family Med. Community Health* **2016**, *3*, 1081.
41. Thapa, A.; Horgan, K.A.; White, B.; Walls, D. Deoxynivalenol and Zearalenone—Synergistic or Antagonistic Agri-Food Chain Co-Contaminants? *Toxins* **2021**, *13*, 561. [CrossRef]
42. Bryden, W.L. Mycotoxin contamination of the feed supply chain: Implications for animal productivity and feed security. *Anim. Feed Sci. Technol.* **2012**, *173*, 134–158. [CrossRef]
43. Hickey, G.L.; Craig, P.S.; Luttik, R.; de Zwart, D. On the quantification of intertest variability in ecotoxicity data with application to species sensitivity distributions. *Environ. Toxicol. Chem.* **2012**, *31*, 1903–1910. [CrossRef]
44. López-Calderero, I.; Carnero, A.; Astudillo, A.; Palacios, J.; Chaves, M.; Benavent, M. Prognostic relevance of estrogen receptor-α Ser167 phosphorylation in stage II-III colon cancer patients. *Hum. Pathol.* **2014**, *45*, 2437–2446. [CrossRef] [PubMed]
45. Cleveland, A.G.; Oikarinen, S.I.; Bynoté, K.K.; Marttinen, M.; Rafter, J.J.; Gustafsson, J.Å.; Roy, S.K.; Pitot, H.C.; Korach, K.S.; Lubahn, D.B.; et al. Disruption of estrogen receptor signaling enhances intestinal neoplasia in Apc(Min/+) mice. *Carcinogenesis* **2009**, *30*, 1581–1590. [CrossRef]
46. Williams, C.; DiLeo, A.; Niv, Y.; Gustafsson, J.Å. Estrogen receptor beta as target for colorectal cancer prevention. *Cancer Lett.* **2016**, *372*, 48–56. [CrossRef]
47. Uvnäs-Moberg, K. The gastrointestinal tract in growth and reproduction. *Sci. Am.* **1989**, *261*, 78–83. [CrossRef] [PubMed]
48. Kozieł, M.J.; Ziaja, M.; Piastowska-Ciesielska, A.W. Intestinal Barrier, Claudins and Mycotoxins. *Toxins* **2021**, *13*, 758. [CrossRef]
49. Vandenberg, L.N.; Colborn, T.; Hayes, T.B.; Heindel, J.J.; Jacobs, D.R.; Lee, D.-H.; Shioda, T.; Soto, A.M.; vom Saal, F.S.; Welshons, W.V.; et al. Hormones and endocrine-disrupting chemicals: Low-dose effects and nonmonotonic dose responses. *Endoc. Rev.* **2012**, *33*, 378–455. [CrossRef]
50. Lawrenz, B.; Melado, L.; Fatemi, H. Premature progesterone rise in ART-cycles. *Reprod. Biol.* **2018**, *18*, 1–4. [CrossRef]
51. Suba, Z. Amplified crosstalk between estrogen binding and GFR signaling mediated pathways of ER activation drives responses in tumors treated with endocrine disruptors. *Recent Pat. Anticancer Drug Discov.* **2018**, *13*, 428–444. [CrossRef]
52. Lee, H.J.; Park, J.H.; Oh, S.Y.; Cho, D.H.; Kim, S.; Jo, I. Zearalenone-Induced Interaction between PXR and Sp1 Increases Binding of Sp1 to a Promoter Site of the eNOS, Decreasing Its Transcription and NO Production in BAECs. *Toxins* **2020**, *12*, 421. [CrossRef]
53. Bayala, B.; Zoure, A.A.; Baron, S.; de Joussineau, C.; Simpore, J.; Lobaccaro, J.M.A. Pharmacological Modulation of Steroid Activity in Hormone-Dependent Breast and Prostate Cancers: Effect of Some Plant Extract Derivatives. *Int. J. Mol. Sci.* **2020**, *21*, 3690. [CrossRef]
54. Suba, Z. Diverse pathomechanisms leading to the breakdown of cellular estrogen surveillance and breast cancer development: New therapeutic strategies. *Drug Design Devel. Ther.* **2014**, *8*, 1381–1390. [CrossRef]
55. Savva, C.; Korach-André, M. Estrogen Receptor beta (ERβ) Regulation of Lipid Homeostasis—Does Sex Matter? *Metabolites* **2020**, *10*, 116. [CrossRef]
56. Wen, X.; Zhu, M.; Li, Z.; Li, T.; Xu, X. Dual effects of bisphenol A on wound healing, involvement of estrogen receptor β. *Ecotoxic. Environ. Saf.* **2022**, *231*, 113207. [CrossRef] [PubMed]
57. Giroux, V.; Lemay, F.; Bernatchez, G.; Robitaille, Y.; Carrier, J.C. Estrogen receptor β deficiency enhances small intestinal tumorigenesis in ApcMin/+ mice. *Int. J. Cancer* **2008**, *123*, 303–311. [CrossRef] [PubMed]

58. Saleiro, D.; Murillo, G.; Benya, R.V.; Bissonnette, M.; Hart, J.; Mehta, R.G. Estrogen receptor-β protects against colitis-associated neoplasia in mice. *Int. J. Cancer* **2012**, *131*, 2553–2561. [CrossRef]
59. Jakimiuk, E.; Radwińska, J.; Woźny, M.; Pomianowski, A.; Brzuzan, P.; Wojtacha, P.; Obremski, K.; Zielonka, Ł. The Influence of Zearalenone on Selected Hemostatic Parameters in Sexually Immature Gilts. *Toxins* **2021**, *13*, 625. [CrossRef]
60. Jia, M.; Dahlman-Wright, K.; Gustafsson, J.Å. Estrogen receptor alpha and beta in health and disease. *Best Pract. Res. Clin. Endocrinol. Metab.* **2015**, *29*, 557–568. [CrossRef] [PubMed]
61. El-Shitany, N.A.; Hegazy, S.; El-Desoky, K. Evidences for antiosteoporotic and selective estrogen receptor modulator activity of silymarin compared with ethinylestradiol in ovariectomized rats. *Phytomedicine* **2010**, *17*, 116–125. [CrossRef]
62. Barone, M.; Tanzi, S.; Lofano, K.; Scavo, M.P.; Pricci, M.; Demarinis, L.; Papagni, S.; Guido, R.; Maiorano, E.; Ingravallo, G.; et al. Dietary-induced ERbeta upregulation counteracts intestinal neoplasia development in intact male ApcMin/+ mice. *Carcinogenesis* **2010**, *31*, 269–274. [CrossRef] [PubMed]
63. Calabrese, C.; Pratico, C.; Calafiore, A.; Coscia, M.; Gentilini, L.; Poggioli, G.; Gionchetti, P.; Campieri, M.; Rizzello, F. Eviendep (R) reduces number and size of duodenal polyps in familial adenomatous polyposis patients with ileal pouch-anal anastomosis. *World J. Gastroenterol.* **2013**, *19*, 5671–5677. [CrossRef]
64. Pasternak, J.A.; Aiyer, V.I.A.; Hamonic, G.; Beaulieu, A.D.; Columbus, D.A.; Wilson, H.L. Molecular and Physiological Effects on the Small Intestine of Weaner Pigs Following Feeding with Deoxynivalenol-Contaminated Feed. *Toxins* **2018**, *10*, 40. [CrossRef] [PubMed]
65. Wada-Hiraike, O.; Imamov, O.; Hiraike, H.; Hultenby, K.; Schwend, T.; Omoto, Y.; Warner, M.; Gustafsson, J.Å. Role of estrogen receptor beta in colonic epithelium. *Proc. Natl. Acad. Sci. USA* **2006**, *103*, 2959–2964. [CrossRef] [PubMed]
66. Oturkar, C.C.; Gandhi, N.; Rao, P.; Eng, K.H.; Miller, A.; Singh, P.K.; Zsiros, E.; Odunsi, K.O.; Das, G.M. Estrogen Receptor-Beta2 (ERβ2)–Mutant p53–FOXM1 Axis: A Novel Driver of Proliferation, Chemoresistance, and Disease Progression in High Grade Serous Ovarian Cancer (HGSOC). *Cancers* **2022**, *14*, 1120. [CrossRef] [PubMed]
67. Zwierzchowski, W.; Gajęcki, M.; Obremski, K.; Zielonka, Ł.; Baranowski, M. The occurrence of zearalenone and its derivatives in standard and therapeutic feeds for companion animals. *Pol. J. Vet. Sci.* **2004**, *7*, 289–293.
68. Heberer, T.; Lahrssen-Wiederholt, M.; Schafft, H.; Abraham, K.; Pzyrembel, H.; Henning, K.J.; Schauzu, M.; Braeunig, J.; Goetz, M.; Niemann, L.O.; et al. Zero tolerances in food and animal feed-Are there any scientific alternatives? A European point of view on an international controversy. *Toxicol. Lett.* **2007**, *175*, 118–135. [CrossRef]
69. Smith, D.; Combes, R.; Depelchin, O.; Jacobsen, S.D.; Hack, R.; Luft, J. Optimising the design of preliminary toxicity studies for pharmaceutical safety testing in the dog. *Regul. Toxicol. Pharm.* **2005**, *41*, 95–101. [CrossRef]
70. The Commission of the European Communities. Commission Recommendation 2006/576/EC, of 17 August 2006 on the Presence of Deoxynivalenol, Zearalenone, Ochratoxin A, T-2 and HT-2 and Fumonisins in Products Intended for Animal Feeding. *Off. J. Eur. Union Series L* **2006**, *229*, 7–9.
71. Kostecki, M.; Goliński, P.; Chełkowski, J. Biosynthesis, isolation, separation and purification of zearalenone, deoxynivalenol and 15-acetyldeoxynivalenol. *Mycotoxin Res.* **1991**, *7*, 156–159. [CrossRef]
72. Kostecki, M.; Goliński, P.; Chełkowski, J. Biosynthesis, isolation, separation and purification of nivalenol, fusarenone-X and zearalenone. *Mycotoxin Res.* **1991**, *7*, 160–164. [CrossRef] [PubMed]
73. Gajęcka, M.; Waśkiewicz, A.; Zielonka, Ł.; Golinski, P.; Rykaczewska, A.; Lisieska-Żołnierczyk, S.; Gajęcki, M.T. Mycotoxin levels in the digestive tissues of immature gilts exposed to zearalenone and deoxynivalenol. *Toxicon* **2018**, *153*, 1–11. [CrossRef] [PubMed]
74. Norrby, M.; Madej, A.; Ekstedt, E.; Holm, L. Effects of genistein on oestrogen and progesterone receptor, proliferative marker Ki-67 and carbonic anhydrase localisation in the uterus and cervix of gilts after insemination. *Anim. Reprod. Sci.* **2013**, *138*, 90–101. [CrossRef]
75. Słomczyńska, M.; Woźniak, J. Differential distribution of estrogen receptor-beta and estrogen receptor-alpha in the porcine ovary. *Exp. Clin. Endocrinol. Diabetes* **2001**, *109*, 238–244. [CrossRef] [PubMed]

Disclaimer/Publisher's Note: The statements, opinions and data contained in all publications are solely those of the individual author(s) and contributor(s) and not of MDPI and/or the editor(s). MDPI and/or the editor(s) disclaim responsibility for any injury to people or property resulting from any ideas, methods, instructions or products referred to in the content.

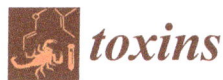

Article

Exposure to Low Zearalenone Doses and Changes in the Homeostasis and Concentrations of Endogenous Hormones in Selected Steroid-Sensitive Tissues in Pre-Pubertal Gilts

Magdalena Gajęcka [1,*], Łukasz Zielonka [1], Andrzej Babuchowski [2] and Maciej Tadeusz Gajęcki [1]

[1] Department of Veterinary Prevention and Feed Hygiene, Faculty of Veterinary Medicine, University of Warmia and Mazury in Olsztyn, Oczapowskiego 13, 10-718 Olsztyn, Poland
[2] Dairy Industry Innovation Institute Ltd., Kormoranów 1, 11-700 Mrągowo, Poland
* Correspondence: mgaja@uwm.edu.pl

Abstract: This study was undertaken to analyze whether prolonged exposure to low-dose zearalenone (ZEN) mycotoxicosis affects the concentrations of ZEN, α-zearalenol (α-ZEL), and β-zearalenol (β-ZEL) in selected reproductive system tissues (ovaries, uterine horn—ovarian and uterine sections, and the middle part of the cervix), the hypothalamus, and pituitary gland, or the concentrations of selected steroid hormones in pre-pubertal gilts. For 42 days, gilts were administered per os different ZEN doses (MABEL dose [5 µg/kg BW], the highest NOAEL dose [10 µg/kg BW], and the lowest LOAEL dose [15 µg/kg BW]). Tissue samples were collected on days seven, twenty-one, and forty-two of exposure to ZEN (exposure days D1, D2, and D3, respectively). Blood for the analyses of estradiol and progesterone concentrations was collected in vivo on six dates at seven-day intervals (on analytical dates D1–D6). The analyses revealed that both ZEN and its metabolites were accumulated in the examined tissues. On successive analytical dates, the rate of mycotoxin accumulation in the studied tissues decreased gradually by 50% and proportionally to the administered ZEN dose. A hierarchical visualization revealed that values of the carry-over factor (CF) were highest on exposure day D2. In most groups and on most exposure days, the highest CF values were found in the middle part of the cervix, followed by the ovaries, both sections of the uterine horn, and the hypothalamus. These results suggest that ZEN, α-ZEL, and β-ZEL were deposited in all analyzed tissues despite exposure to very low ZEN doses. The presence of these undesirable compounds in the examined tissues can inhibit the somatic development of the reproductive system and compromise neuroendocrine coordination of reproductive competence in pre-pubertal gilts.

Keywords: zearalenone; low doses; gonads; hypothalamus; pituitary gland; steroid hormones; pre-pubertal gilts

Key Contribution: Even the MABEL dose of ZEN can cross the blood-brain barrier. Low-dose ZEN mycotoxicosis accelerates somatic development and delays sexual maturation in gilts.

1. Introduction

Raw materials and feed components of plant origin are often contaminated with undesirable substances such as mycotoxins [1], which pose a health risk to humans [2] and various livestock species, pigs in particular [3]. The symptoms and health (toxicological) risks associated with exposure to high doses of these compounds have been investigated with regard to a limited number of mycotoxins, including ZEN and its metabolites: α-ZEL and β-ZEL [4–7]. In light of the hormesis paradigm, which posits that low doses of undesirable substances exert beneficial effects on the body [8,9], the consequences of prolonged exposure to low concentrations of mycotoxins (which are frequently found in animal feed) should be studied. Numerous studies involving mammals have been undertaken to identify potential physiological dysfunctions resulting from exposure to

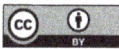

the pure parent compound [10–15] without metabolites, or to modified mycotoxins [9], particularly in the reproductive [16] and hormonal systems [10].

The existing research indicates that exposure to low ZEN concentration may cause side effects that are hard to predict [17]. The observed changes are influenced by the administered dose and duration of exposure [18]. Low mycotoxin doses can elicit surprising effects: for example, the body's failure to detect undesirable substances such as mycotoxins [19]. Long-term exposure to orally administered ZEN leads to increased mycotoxin accumulation in target cells [13,14] and induces the compensatory effect [20] by altering the analyzed indicators, for example, in the reproductive system [21], changing the activity of the hypothalamic-pituitary-gonadal (HPG) axis [22,23] and disrupting hormonal homeostasis in pre-pubertal animals. Homeostasis is restored [24] in subsequent stages of exposure [10]. These factors, as well as the promiscuity [25] of ZEN and its known metabolites [17], and the type and intensity of physiological reaction in gilts exposed to this mycotoxin, point to the need for further study into the effects of low dietary zearalenone doses.

Based on the results of our prior studies [10,14,15], a low ZEN dose was defined by examining whether clinical symptoms of ongoing mycotoxicosis were present. Three ZEN doses were proposed based on our previous work and a review of the literature: (i) the lowest dose which elicits clinical symptoms [3] (>10 μg ZEN/kg of body weight, BW), defined as the lowest observed adverse effect level (LOAEL) [19]; (ii) the highest dose which does not elicit clinical symptoms (subclinical states) (= 10 μg ZEN/kg BW), defined as the no observed adverse effect level (NOAEL) [26]; and (iii) the lowest measurable dose which enters into positive interactions with the host organism in different stages of life (<10 μg ZEN/kg BW), defined as the minimal anticipated biological effect level (MABEL) [6,27,28].

Since zearalenone is a mycoestrogen, the dose-reaction paradigm has been subverted and replaced with the low dose hypothesis [17]. This applies, in particular, to hormonally active chemical compounds [29]. The ambiguous dose-response relationship prevents a direct, monotonic extrapolation or meta-analysis of the risks (including clinical symptoms and the results of laboratory analyses) associated with the transition from a high to a low dose [3,24]. On the other hand, ZEN's toxicity can be attributed to its chemical structure and ability to interact with steroid hormone receptors in many internal organs [30]. Zearalenone can also cross the barrier between the cerebral capillary blood and the interstitial fluid of the brain and affects neurons in the central nervous system [31,32]. Recent research has shown that exposure to ZEN disturbs the synthesis of neuronal factors and enzymes in brain neurons. In pigs (including pre-pubertal gilts), reproductive functions are controlled by complex regulatory networks which integrate peripheral and internal signals, thus affecting brain regions that control, e.g., the HPG axis [33]. By binding to specific receptors on gonadotropic cells in the pituitary gland, ZEN and/or its metabolites block these signals, which inhibits the biosynthesis and release of two gonadotropins—the luteinizing hormone (LH) and the follicle-stimulating hormone (FSH) [23]—and decreases the amplitude of LH pulsation [34]. LH and FSH are essential for gonadal development and fertility, and they bind to gonadal receptors to regulate gametogenesis and steroidogenesis [35,36].

Based on the above observations and a review of the literature, we hypothesized that ZEN present in feed materials at very low concentrations is accumulated in the reproductive systems, hypothalamus, and pituitary glands of pre-pubertal gilts. Thus, the aim of this study was to determine whether exposure to low doses of zearalenone (MABEL dose [5 μg/kg BW], the highest NOAEL dose [10 μg/kg BW], and the lowest LOAEL dose [15 μg/kg BW]) administered per os to sexually immature gilts over a period of 42 days affects the levels of zearalenone, alfa-ZEL, and beta-ZEL in selected reproductive system tissues (ovaries, uterine horn—ovarian and uterine sections, and the middle part of the cervix), the hypothalamus and pituitary gland, along with whether it affects the peripheral blood levels of two steroid hormones: estradiol and progesterone.

2. Results

The presented results were obtained as part of a large-scale experiment which did not reveal clinical signs of ZEN mycotoxicosis. However, differences were frequently observed in the values of the carry-over factor (CF) of zearalenone and its metabolites in intestinal tissues, in CYP1A1 and GSTπ1 expression in the large intestine, in selected serum biochemical profiles, in the myocardium and the coronary artery, in cecal water genotoxicity, in selected steroid concentrations, in intestinal microbiota parameters, and in the weight gain of animals. Samples gathered from the same animals were analyzed. Previous findings were published in several publications [10–15,17,37].

2.1. Experimental Feed

Experimental diets did not contain any mycotoxins, or their amounts were below the limit of detection (LOD). The concentrations of masked and/or modified mycotoxins were not determined.

2.2. Results of Laboratory Analyses

2.2.1. Concentrations of ZEN and Its Metabolites in Selected Tissues

The CF values of ZEN and its metabolites differed considerably (see Tables 1–3, Figures 1–3, Figures S1–S3) not only on different exposure dates, but also between groups and the analyzed tissues. These differences are evident in the resulting tree maps, where hierarchical data are presented by a series of nested rectangles (see Figures S1–S3).

In all groups, mean ZEN concentrations decreased in all analyzed tissues on successive exposure dates (see Table 1). In group ZEN5 (MABEL dose), significant differences were found in the uterine horn (ovarian and uterine sections) and the middle part of the cervix on D2 and D3 relative to D1. In group ZEN10 (NOAEL dose), significant differences were observed in the uterine section of the uterine horn on D2 and D3, and in the ovarian section of the uterine horn only on D2, in comparison to D1. In group ZEN15 (LOAEL dose), significant differences were noted in the ovarian section of the uterine horn on D2 and D3 vs. D1, and in the middle part of the cervix on D3 vs. D1.

The statistical analysis of ZEN concentrations (see Table 1) in the analyzed tissues, on different exposure dates and in different groups, revealed that ZEN levels increased with a rise in the administered ZEN dose. On D1, significant differences in the ovarian and uterine sections of the uterine horn, in the middle part of the cervix, and in the hypothalamus were observed in group ZEN15 vs. groups ZEN5 and ZEN10. Groups ZEN5 and ZEN10 also differed in ZEN concentrations in the middle part of the cervix. On D2, significant differences were also found between group ZEN15 and groups ZEN5 and ZEN10, excluding both sections of the uterine horn in group ZEN5. On D3, significant differences were observed only in the ovaries, the ovarian section of the uterine horn, and the middle part of the cervix.

The hierarchical analysis revealed that ZEN levels were highest on exposure date D1 in all analyzed tissues and in all groups. In all groups and on all exposure dates, the evaluated parameter was highest (see Figures S1–S3) in the ovaries (proportional to the administered dose; Figure 1), followed by the middle part of the cervix, and, interestingly, the pituitary gland.

Insignificant differences were noted between groups on D1, and between exposure dates in group ZEN5 (MABEL dose) (see Table 2). A comparison of α-ZEL levels in groups and on different exposure dates indicates that mean α-ZEL concentrations increased in proportion to the ZEN doses administered in groups, and to exposure dates, which probably could be attributed to the biotransformation of ZEN. The concentrations of the parent compound (see Table 1) in groups and on different exposure dates followed the opposite trend.

Table 1. The CF and the mean (±) concentrations of ZEN (ng/g) in the reproductive system tissues, hypothalamus and pituitary glands of sexually immature gilts.

Exposure Dates	Feed Intake [kg/day]	Total ZEN Doses in Groups [µg/kg BW]	Tissue	Group ZEN5 [ng/g]	Group ZEN10 [ng/g]	Group ZEN15 [ng/g]
D1	0.8	80.5/161.9/242.7	Ovaries	83.15 ± 99.60	54.29 ± 51.37	451.67 ± 433.14
			Uterine horn, ovarian section	10.71 ± 5.13 [xx]	7.46 ± 3.24 [xx]	55.00 ± 17.00
			Uterine horn, uterine section	7.47 ± 1.52 [x]	11.44 ± 5.24	62.08 ± 51.33
			Middle part of the cervix	18.06 ± 5.07 [xx]	3.93 ± 0.93 [xx yy]	75.19 ± 5.77
			Hypothalamus	4.88 ± 2.13 [x]	4.43 ± 2.54 [x]	16.76 ± 9.44
			Pituitary gland	13.77	12.66	14.26
D2	1.1	101.01/196.9/298.2	Ovary	33.40 ± 26.09	79.67 ± 19.94	194.56 ± 138.81
			Uterine horn, ovarian section	3.20 ± 3.32 [a]	2.03 ± 0.88 [a x]	13.40 ± 10.66 [aa]
			Uterine horn, uterine section	3.67 ± 1.95 [a]	2.20 ± 0.53 [aa, x]	7.41 ± 4.60
			Middle part of the cervix	4.17 ± 3.11 [aa xx]	4.46 ± 2.35 [b]	45.35 ± 26.09
			Hypothalamus	4.39 ± 2.81 [x]	2.38 ± 0.81 [x]	17.07 ± 11.52
			Pituitary gland	6.81	8.63	9.02
D3	1.6	128.3/481.4/716.7	Ovary	16.80 ± 15.69 [xx]	29.06 ± 17.79 [xx]	110.38 ± 26.91
			Uterine horn, ovarian section	2.80 ± 1.71 [a xx]	3.60 ± 1.84 [x]	10.17 ± 2.37 [aa]
			Uterine horn, uterine section	3.17 ± 1.80 [aa]	2.73 ± 1.19 [a]	2.47 ± 1.51
			Middle part of the cervix	1.51 ± 0.67 [aa xx]	4.86 ± 2.89 [xx]	23.17 ± 5.91 [a]
			Hypothalamus	3.45 ± 1.20	6.93 ± 5.65	10.02 ± 2.72
			Pituitary gland	7.28	6.10	9.25

Abbreviations: D1—exposure day 7; D2—exposure day 21; D3—exposure day 42. Experimental groups: Group ZEN5—5 µg ZEN/kg BW; Group ZEN10—10 µg ZEN/kg BW; Group ZEN15—15 µg ZEN/kg BW. In the pituitary gland, ZEN concentrations were assayed in aggregate samples. The differences were regarded as statistically significant at [a], [b], [x] $p \leq 0.05$ and [aa], [xx], [yy] $p \leq 0.01$; [a], [aa] significant difference between exposure date D1 and exposure dates D2 and D3; [x], [xx] significant difference between group ZEN15 and groups ZEN5 and ZEN10; [yy] significant difference between group ZEN5 and group ZEN10.

In group ZEN10 (NOAEL dose) (see Table 2), significant differences in α-ZEL concentrations were observed in the ovaries and the uterine section of the uterine horn on D2 and D3, and in the middle part of the cervix on D3 relative to D1. Significant differences in the examined parameters were also noted in the uterine section of the uterine horn and in the middle part of the cervix between D2 and D3. In group ZEN15 (LOAEL dose) (see Table 2), α-ZEL levels in the ovaries and the hypothalamus differed significantly between D1 and D2. Significant differences in this parameter were found in the ovaries and in the ovarian section of the uterine horn between D1 and D3. In the ovarian section of the uterine horn, significant differences in α-ZEL concentrations were determined between D2 and D3.

Table 2. The CF and the mean (±) concentrations of α-ZEL (ng/g) in the reproductive system tissues, hypothalamus, and pituitary glands of sexually immature gilts.

Exposure Dates	Feed Intake [kg/day]	Total ZEN Doses in Groups [μg/kg BW]	Tissue	Group ZEN5 [ng/g]	Group ZEN10 [ng/g]	Group ZEN15 [ng/g]
D1	0.8	80.5/161.9/242.7	Ovary	0	0.51 ± 0.34	1.73 ± 0.45
			Uterine horn, ovarian section	0	1.48 ± 0.98	0.94 ± 0.25
			Uterine horn, uterine section	0	0.50 ± 0.28	1.65 ± 0.18
			Middle part of the cervix	0	4.03 ± 0.16	1.77 ± 1.46
			Hypothalamus	0	0.30 ± 0.20	0.94 ± 0.04
			Pituitary gland	0	0	0
D2	1.1	101.01/196.9/298.2	Ovary	1.04 ± 0.10 [xx yy]	2.65 ± 0.55 [aa]	3.00 ± 0.04 [a]
			Uterine horn, ovarian section	1.04 ± 0.42 [yy]	3.02 ± 0.19	1.90 ± 0.87
			Uterine horn, uterine section	0.51 ± 0.22 [xx yy]	2.67 ± 0.42 [aa]	1.95 ± 0.48
			Middle part of the cervix	4.89 ± 0.60 [x]	3.91 ± 0.08	3.48 ± 0.48
			Hypothalamus	0.29 ± 0.20 [x]	0.50 ± 0.03	0.65 ± 0.08 [a]
			Pituitary gland	0	0	0.246
D3	1.6	128.3/481.4/716.7	Ovary	3.16 ± 0.73	3.23 ± 0.38 [aa]	3.38 ± 0.54 [aa]
			Uterine horn, ovarian section	3.61 ± 0.16	3.91 ± 1.66	4.00 ± 0.32 [aa, bb]
			Uterine horn, uterine section	3.83 ± 0.17	4.24 ± 0.47 [aa bb]	3.02 ± 1.80
			Middle part of the cervix	3.13 ± 0.19 [xx yy]	1.83 ± 0.17 [aa bb]	2.81 ± 0.27
			Hypothalamus	0.43 ± 0.29 [x]	0.65 ± 0.08	0.79 ± 0.15
			Pituitary gland	0	0.195	0.245

Abbreviations: D1—exposure day 7; D2—exposure day 21; D3—exposure day 42. Experimental groups: Group ZEN5—5 μg ZEN/kg BW; Group ZEN10—10 μg ZEN/kg BW; Group ZEN15—15 μg ZEN/kg BW. LOD > values below the limit of detection were expressed as 0. In the pituitary gland, α-ZEL concentrations were assayed in aggregate samples. The differences were regarded as statistically significant at [a], [x] $p \leq 0.05$ and [aa], [bb], [xx], [yy] $p \leq 0.01$; [a], [aa] significant difference between exposure date D1 and exposure dates D2 and D3; [b], [bb] significant difference between exposure date D2 and exposure date D3; [x], [xx] significant difference between group ZEN15 and groups ZEN5 and ZEN10; [yy] significant difference between group ZEN5 and group ZEN10.

On D2 (see Table 2), significant differences in α-ZEL levels in the ovaries and the ovarian section of the uterine horn were observed between group ZEN5 and group ZEN15, and in the ovaries and the ovarian and uterine sections of the uterine horn between group ZEN5 and group ZEN10. On D3, significant differences in α-ZEL levels were noted only in the middle part of the cervix between group ZEN5 and groups ZEN10 and ZEN15.

A graphic presentation of the CF values of α-ZEL (see Figure 2) revealed a certain trend: all CF values were inversely proportional to the results presented in Figure 1. The CF values of α-ZEL in the ovaries of group ZEN5 gilts on D1 were the only exception (the results were below the sensitivity of the method, and these CF values were expressed as 0). An analysis of ZEN and α-ZEL concentrations (see Tables 1 and 2, respectively) on the remaining exposure dates in all groups revealed that α-ZEL levels were much lower than ZEN concentrations, and that the highest α-ZEL concentrations were noted in group ZEN5 on the last two exposure dates. The examined ZEN metabolite was present in nearly all hypothalamus samples. In the pituitary gland, the CF values of α-ZEL were very low in group ZEN15 on D2, and in groups ZEN10 and ZEN15 on D3 (see Figure 2), which indicates that α-ZEL was accumulated gradually in the pituitary gland and that its accumulation was inversely proportional to both the dose and exposure date.

Table 3. The CF and the mean (±) concentrations of β-ZEL (ng/g) in the reproductive system tissues, hypothalamus, and pituitary glands of sexually immature gilts.

Exposure Date	Feed Intake [kg/day]	Total ZEN Doses in Groups [µg/kg BW]	Tissue	Group ZEN5 [ng/g]	Group ZEN10 [ng/g]	Group ZEN15 [ng/g]
D1	0.8	80.5/161.9/242.7	Ovary	0	1.07 ± 0.29	0.98 ± 0.12
			Uterine horn, ovarian section	0	0.36 ± 0.07	0.87 ± 0.14
			Uterine horn, uterine section	0	0.41 ± 0.08	0.93 ± 0.03
			Middle part of the cervix	0	0.42 ± 0.04	1.22 ± 0.02
			Hypothalamus	0	0	0
			Pituitary gland	0	0	0
D2	1.1	101.01/196.9/298.2	Ovary	0.92 ± 0.10	1.05 ± 0.53	0.87 ± 0.06 [xx]
			Uterine horn, ovarian section	0.02 ± 0.02	0.12 ± 0.08 [aa]	0.09 ± 0.01 [aa]
			Uterine horn, uterine section	0.01 ± 0.01	0.29 ± 0.57	0.02 ± 0.02 [aa]
			Middle part of the cervix	0.05 ± 0.01	0.04 ± 0.01 [aa]	0.06 ± 0.02 [aa]
			Hypothalamus	0.09 ± 0.13	0.04 ± 0.009	0.006 ± 0.01
			Pituitary gland	0	0.372	0.462
D3	1.6	128.3/481.4/716.7	Ovary	0.11 ± 0.12 [xx,yy]	1.48 ± 0.25	1.49 ± 0.27 [a]
			Uterine horn, ovarian section	0.01 ± 0.005 [xx,yy]	0.01 ± 0.002 [aa]	0.14 ± 0.02 [aa]
			Uterine horn, uterine section	0.03 ± 0.01	0.14 ± 0.18	0.05 ± 0.03 [aa]
			Middle part of the cervix	0.02 ± 0.01 [x,yy]	0.07 ± 0.02 [aa,z]	0.12 ± 0.02 [aa]
			Hypothalamus	0.04 ± 0.03 [yy]	0.04 ± 0.01 [zz]	0.21 ± 0.03
			Pituitary gland	0.253	0.362	0.536

Abbreviations: D1—exposure day 7; D2—exposure day 21; D3—exposure day 42. Experimental groups: Group ZEN5—5 µg ZEN/kg BW; Group ZEN10—10 µg ZEN/kg BW; Group ZEN15—15 µg ZEN/kg BW. LOD > values below the limit of detection were expressed as 0. In the pituitary gland, β-ZEL concentrations were assayed in aggregate samples. The differences were regarded as statistically significant at [a], [x], [z] $p \leq 0.05$ and at [aa], [xx], [yy], [zz] $p \leq 0.01$; [a], [aa] significant difference between exposure date D1 and exposure dates D2 and D3; [x], [xx] significant difference between group ZEN5 and group ZEN10; [yy] significant difference between group ZEN5 and group ZEN15; [z], [zz] significant difference between group ZEN10 and group ZEN15.

A hierarchical visualization of the CF values of α-ZEL in the examined tissues (see Figure S1) revealed several interesting findings. Firstly, α-ZEL was not detected in group ZEN5 on D1 (its levels were below the sensitivity threshold, see Table 2), and its concentrations peaked on D3. Secondly, α-ZEL concentrations in groups ZEN10 and ZEN15 were higher on D2 than on D1 and D3. Thirdly, the highest α-ZEL levels were noted in the middle part of the cervix, the ovaries, and both sections of the uterine horn, and its accumulation was highest (mathematically and hierarchically) in group ZEN5 on D2 and D3 (see Figure 2).

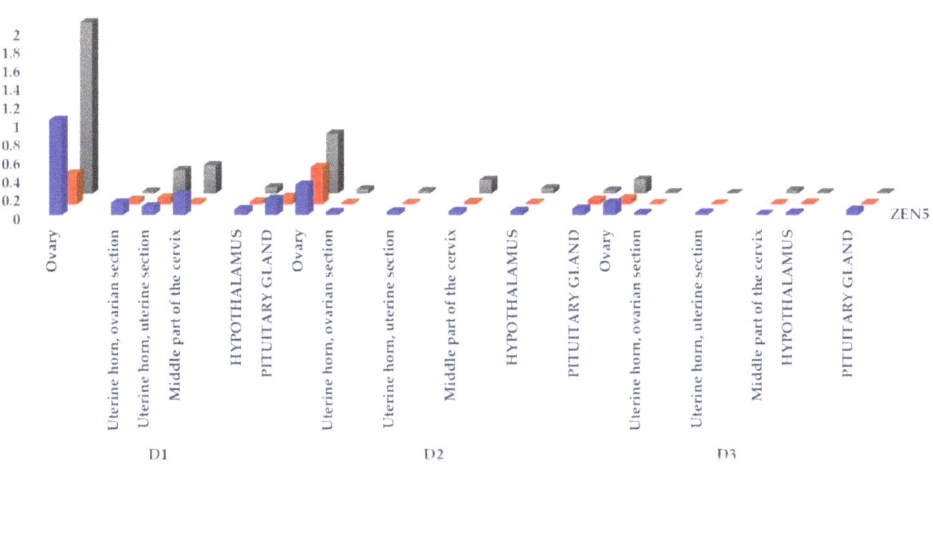

Figure 1. The CF of ZEN in the reproductive system tissues, hypothalamus, and pituitary glands of sexually immature gilts exposed to various ZEN doses. Key: D1—exposure day 7; D2—exposure day 21; D3—exposure day 42. Experimental groups: Group ZEN5—5 µg ZEN/kg BW; Group ZEN10—10 µg ZEN/kg BW; Group ZEN15—15 µg ZEN/kg BW.

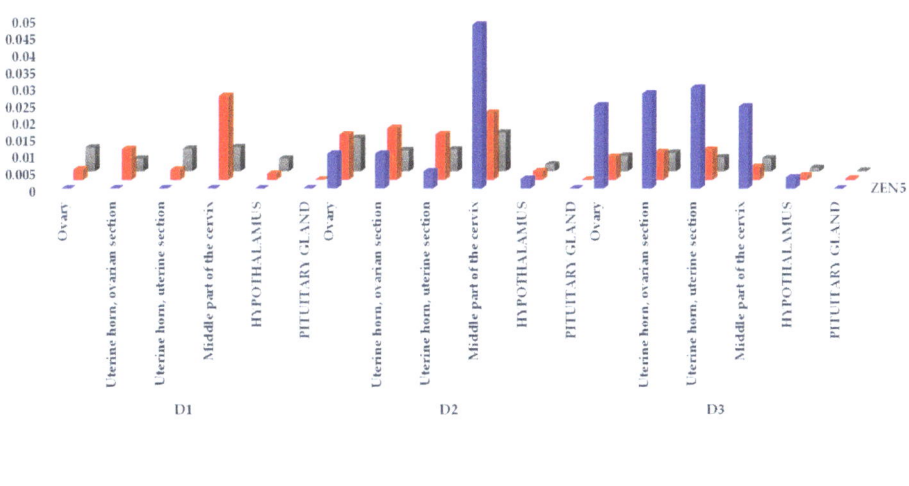

Figure 2. The CF of α-ZEL in the reproductive system tissues, hypothalamus, and pituitary glands of sexually immature gilts exposed to various ZEN doses. Key: D1—exposure day 7; D2—exposure day 21; D3—exposure day 42. Experimental groups: Group ZEN5—5 µg ZEN/kg BW; Group ZEN10—10 µg ZEN/kg BW; Group ZEN15—15 µg ZEN/kg BW.

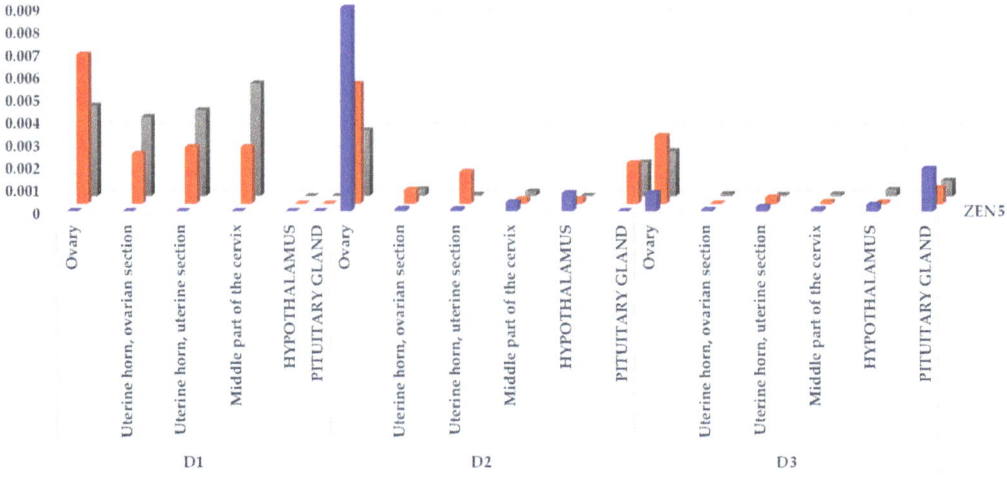

Figure 3. The CF of β-ZEL in the reproductive system tissues, hypothalamus, and pituitary glands of sexually immature gilts exposed to various ZEN doses. Key: D1—exposure day 7; D2—exposure day 21; D3—exposure day 42. Experimental groups: Group ZEN5—5 μg ZEN/kg BW; Group ZEN10—10 μg ZEN/kg BW; Group ZEN15—15 μg ZEN/kg BW.

In group ZEN5, an absence of significant differences in β-ZEL concentrations was noted between tissues on different exposure days (see Table 3). In group ZEN10, clear differences in the studied parameter were found in the ovarian section of the uterine horn and in the middle part of the cervix between samples taken D1 and those taken on D2 and D3. In group ZEN15, differences in β-ZEL levels were noted between the ovaries and the uterine section of the uterine horn, but only on D3.

No significant differences in β-ZEL concentrations were observed between groups on D1 and D2 (see Table 3). On D3, the CF (see Figure 3) values of β-ZEL in the ovaries, the ovarian section of the uterine horn, and the middle part of the cervix were lower in group ZEN5 than in groups ZEN10 and ZEN15. On D3, considerable differences in β-ZEL levels in the hypothalamus were also found between group ZEN5 and group ZEN15. The concentrations of β-ZEL in the middle part of the cervix and the hypothalamus differed significantly between group ZEN10 and group ZEN15.

The graphic presentation of the CF values of β-ZEL (see Figure 3) clearly indicates that the concentrations of this metabolite in the examined tissues were very low. Higher CF values that were proportional to the administered dose were noted only on D1 in groups ZEN10 and ZEN15. The ovaries were the only exception, where saturation with β-ZEL was higher than in the remaining tissues and not always proportional to the administered dose. In the pituitary gland, the CF values of β-ZEL were also higher than in the remaining tissues (excluding on D1), with the exception of the ovaries.

In group ZEN5, β-ZEL was not detected on D1 (see Figure S3) because the values determined in all tissues as below the sensitivity of the method (see Table 3 and Figure 3). In all groups, β-ZEL was not identified in the hypothalamus or pituitary gland on D1. On D2 and D3, the mathematical (see Table 3 and Figure 3) and hierarchical (see Figures S1–S3) values of β-ZEL were generally low and similar. The CF values of β-ZEL were much higher only in the ovaries and the pituitary gland. The hierarchical order of data was not maintained between group ZEN10 and group ZEN15, but it was maintained between exposure dates (D1, D2, and D3).

The parent compound (ZEN) and its two metabolites (α-ZEL and β-ZEL) were deposited in reproductive system tissues, the hypothalamus, and the pituitary gland, even in gilts exposed to very low doses of ZEN (MABEL, NOAEL, and LOAEL). In the analyzed tissues, ZEN accumulation decreased proportionally on successive dates of exposure, and it decreased by ± 50% between D1 and D2, and between D2 and D3.

2.2.2. Blood Concentrations of estradiol and progesterone

Estradiol (E_2) levels were higher in all experimental groups than in group C on all analytical dates (see Figure 4). However, significant differences were noted only on D3 and on successive exposure dates. On these dates, E_2 concentrations were highest in group ZEN5 and lowest in group C (the differences were determined at 6.29 pg/mL on D3, 7.52 pg/mL on D4, 4.53 pg/mL on D5, and 4.96 pg/mL on D6). Estradiol levels were also higher in groups ZEN10 and ZEN15 than in group C on all exposure days, but the observed differences were not significant.

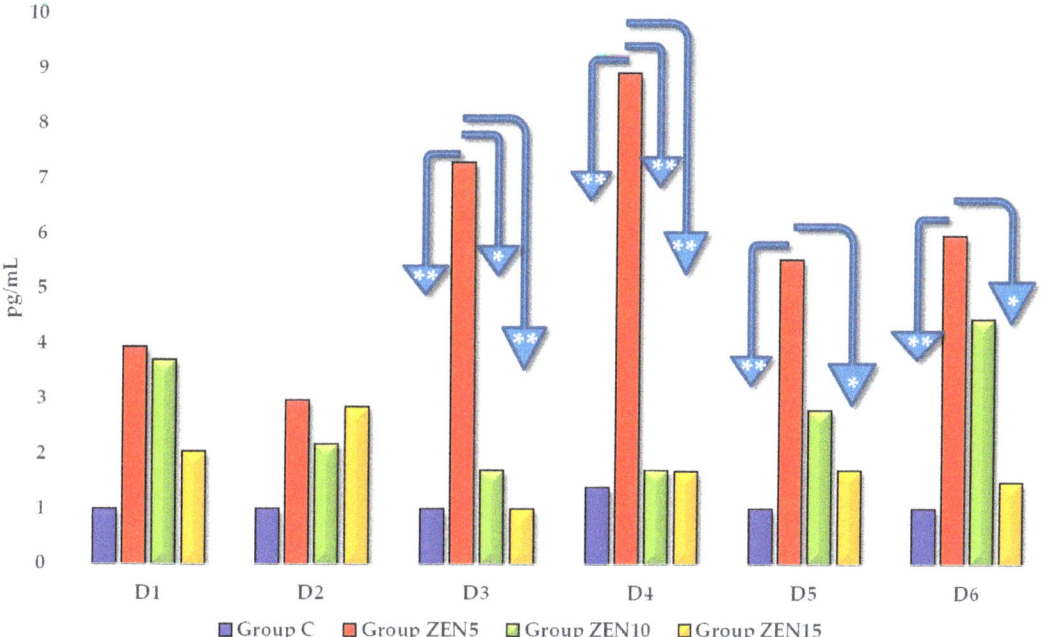

Figure 4. The effect of ZEN on blood E_2 concentrations in pre-pubertal gilts: arithmetic means ($\bar{x}$) of five samples collected on each analytical date (D1–D6) in every group (control [C], ZEN5, ZEN10 and ZEN15). Statistics significant differences were determined at * $p \leq 0.05$ and ** $p \leq 0.01$.

The distribution of P_4 (progesterone) concentrations (see Figure 5) differed throughout the entire experiment. On the first four exposure dates, P_4 levels were highest in group C. On D5 and D6, the analyzed parameter peaked in group ZEN10. Significant differences were observed between group ZEN10 and groups ZEN5 and C (on D5 0.21 ng/mL and D6 0.12 ng/mL).

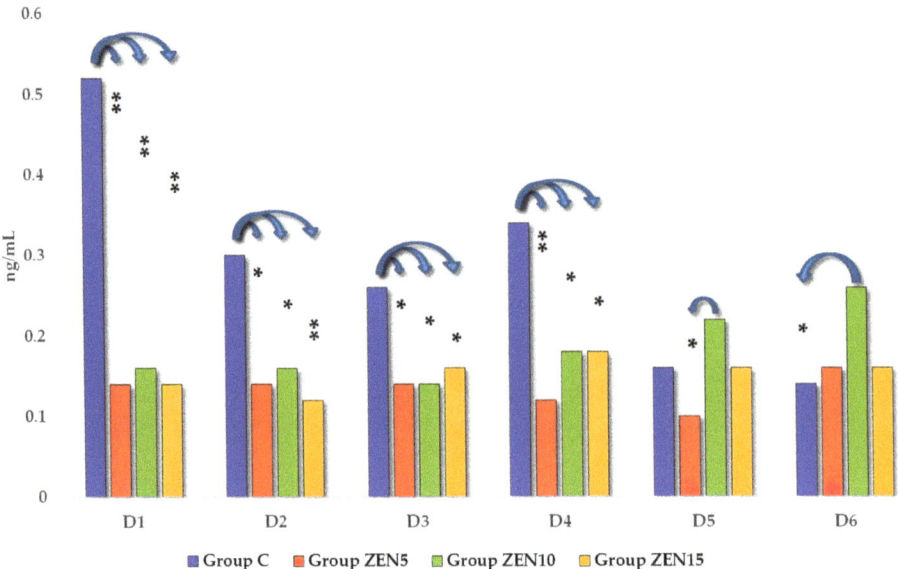

Figure 5. The effect of ZEN on blood P_4 concentrations in pre-pubertal gilts: arithmetic means ($\bar{x}$) of five samples collected on each analytical date (D1–D6) in every group (control [C], ZEN5, ZEN10 and ZEN15). Statistics significant differences were determined at * $p \leq 0.05$ and ** $p \leq 0.01$.

3. Discussion

The results of this quantitative analysis of ZEN, α-ZEL, and β-ZEL levels in selected tissues of the reproductive tract and the HPG axis, and of E_2 and P_4 concentrations in the blood of pre-pubertal gilts may be difficult to interpret because very few studies have addressed this issue.

On exposure date D1, the levels of ZEN and its two metabolites (see Table 1) in the examined tissues can be attributed to ongoing transformation processes in maturing gilts, which do not lead to hyperestrogenism, but merely cater to the physiological demand for endogenous steroids (see Figures 4 and 5) in these animals [37,38]. This observation is problematic because physiologically maturing gilts (during puberty) are naturally deficient in endogenous steroids, and exposure to feed-borne ZEN leads to an increase in steroid levels. The question that arises is: how does this happen? One of the possible explanations is that pre-pubertal gilts adapt to frequent or prolonged exposure to low doses of exogenous steroid-like substances. The results noted for group ZEN5 (MABEL dose) on D1 seem to validate this hypothesis.

We found a lack of both ZEN metabolites in the ZEN5 group at the D1 date (see Tables 2 and 3), probably due to the low supply of endogenous steroid hormones and very low concentrations of exogenous ("free") ZEN [37]. Exogenous ZEN was accumulated in large quantities in the studied tissues, including in the hypothalamus and pituitary gland (see Figure 1). The above could suggest that ZEN biotransformation in the intestines and blood vessels proceeded at a "slower" rate than ZEN binding to steroid hormone receptors, possibly to cater to a very high demand for steroids. This observation is supported by the CF values (see Figure 1) and the hierarchical order of data in the tree maps (see Figure S1), which suggest that ZEN was accumulated mostly in the ovaries and the cervix, followed by the pituitary gland, on D1 in group ZEN5 (MABEL dose) (see Figure S1). This process was accompanied by a marked increase in E_2 concentrations (see Figure 4) in all experimental groups relative to the control group. On D3, E_2 levels differed significantly between the experimental groups and the control group. At the same time, P_4 concentrations (see Figure 5) were much lower in the experimental groups than in group C on all exposure days and remained at a similar level throughout the experiment.

In groups ZEN10 and ZEN15 (NOAEL and LOAEL doses, respectively), ZEN concentrations in the hypothalamus and pituitary gland were inversely proportional to the administered doses, and a shift to other levels in the hierarchy was observed (see Figures S2 and S3, respectively). On D2 (see Figure S2), nervous system tissues ranked second in the data hierarchy. On D3 (see Figure S3), nervous system tissues ranked third in the data hierarchy only in group ZEN5 (MABEL dose). These results could point to the interdependence between the HPG axis and the ovaries, which is very important because ZEN exerts a direct negative effect on the neuroendocrine coordination of reproductive competence [39]. Similar observations were made by Rykaczewska et al. [10,37].

According to other researchers, α-ZEL is the dominant ZEN metabolite in the peripheral blood of pigs [17,40], and the results noted for group ZEN5 (MABEL dose) corroborate this observation. β-ZEL was the dominant ZEN metabolite in only one study [37]. The above could be explained by the host organism's increased demand for compounds characterized by steroid (not only estrogenic) activity, such as α-ZEL and ZEN, but not β-ZEL [41]. These compounds are a source of endogenous steroid hormones which are essential for healthy functioning [42]. It should also be noted that ZEN and α-ZEL form highly stable complexes with albumins that prolong their half-life [7], which is a very important consideration in the interplay of steroid hormones. During exposure to ZEN, adaptive processes, in particular adaptive immunity, end on exposure date D1 [43]. Zearalenone is an endocrine-disrupting chemical (EDC) [44] and a substrate that regulates (inversely) the expression levels of genes encoding hydroxysteroid dehydrogenases (epigenetically [45]), which act as molecular switches and modulate steroid hormone pre-receptors [46]. Zearalenone also slows down proliferative processes in granulosa cells, proportionally to the administered dose, and provokes apoptosis in the ovaries [47]. These processes are accompanied by enterohepatic recirculation which slows down the elimination of mycotoxins [48]. Zearalenone was also found to affect gut microbiota [11] by increasing the log values of specific microbial counts in the distal segment of porcine intestines in the static and dynamic system.

Much like other EDCs [30,44], ZEN can cross the blood-brain barrier, modify hypothalamic and pituitary functions, and exert a negative influence on central and peripheral reproductive tissues. According to He et al. [49], Rykaczewska et al. [37], and Zheng et al. [40], ZEN disrupts biological functions during the release of neurotransmitters which control physiological homeostasis, including levels of the FSH [33]. The discussed mycotoxin also blocks neuroactive ligand-receptor interaction pathways [39] and calcium signaling pathways [50–52] in the mitochondria. The resulting negative feedback initially decreases steroid production [45] and increases steroid synthesis on final dates of exposure. The results of this study could be also explained by the fact that ZEN blocks the activity of the HPG axis, which increases P_4 levels, enhances endometrial receptivity, and induces specific morphometric changes in the reproductive system [37].

These observations suggest that the estrogen-sensitive tissues were saturated with ZEN (already on D1, proportionally to the administered ZEN dose), which leads to changes to the supraphysiological hormonal levels of pre-pubertal gilts, accompanied by an inverse correlation between steroid concentrations [37,38]. In pre-pubertal gilts exposed to ZEN, the strongest response was observed on D1, when hormonal receptors (not only estrogen receptors) were saturated, and neuroactive ligand-receptor interaction pathways were blocked. The accumulation of ZEN decreased considerably on successive dates of exposure, probably because the administered doses were very low, and the gilts' physiological status perpetuated the processes that accompany ZEN mycotoxicosis. Extrapolation of the current findings indicates that ZEN, evaluated quantitatively in the analyzed tissues, affects HPG activity in pre-pubertal gilts in all examined doses due to its promiscuous properties [25].

Analysis of the concentrations (see Tables 1–3) and CF values (see Figures 1–3 and Figures S1–S3) of α-ZEL and β-ZEL based on arithmetic means and hierarchal data revealed certain trends. The concentrations and CF values of ZEN metabolites were inversely proportional to the corresponding values of the parent compound, in all tissues except the ovaries. In the examined nervous system tissues, ZEN metabolites accumulated gradually at concentrations that were inversely proportional to the administered dose (experimental group) and exposure date. This observation indirectly demonstrates that ZEN and α-ZEL (the most prominent mycoestrogens) exerted complementary effects and blocked estrogen receptors in the analyzed reproductive system tissues. However, ZEN probably slowed down the synthesis and release of FSH in the porcine pituitary gland [49]. Inhibited FSH secretion decreased the production of sex steroids, including E_2, P_4, and testosterone [34,37,45,53], and probably enhanced the conversion of steroids into E_2, which increased feed intake and promoted the storage of excess energy in fat cells [10]. Therefore, inhibited pulsatile HPG activation slowed down gonadal development, prolonged sexual maturation, and delayed reproductive maturity.

A comparison of ZEN and α-ZEL concentrations (see Tables 1 and 2) and the CF values of both mycotoxins, presented graphically, leads to another question: why in group ZEN5 (MABEL dose) was ZEN the dominant mycotoxin on D1, whereas α-ZEL was the dominant compound on D3? It could be postulated that "free ZEN" is initially used due to supraphysiological hormonal levels in pre-pubertal gilts [37], whereas biotransformation processes are initiated later, and excess "free" ZEN is metabolically transformed into, for example, α-ZEL which is bound to free estrogen receptors or used to block HPG activity. Therefore, both the parent compound and its metabolite act as epigenetic switches that regulate sexual maturation [45]. In the first week of exposure, only ZEN acts as an epigenetic switch, and on successive dates of exposure, both ZEN and α-ZEL play this role. The role of β-ZEL remains unknown.

4. Summary

The presented quantitative analysis suggests that ZEN and its metabolites can be among the factors that inhibit the somatic development of reproductive system tissues by decreasing the activity of the HPG axis in pre-pubertal gilts [23,34], which exerts a direct negative effect on the neuroendocrine coordination of reproductive competence [37,39]. However, from the breeders' point of view, this is a positive phenomenon because low-dose ZEN mycotoxicosis enables maturing gilts to utilize nutrients for somatic development (most effectively in group ZEN5-MABEL dose) [10] rather than for reproductive development and performance.

5. Materials and Methods

5.1. General Information

This article is a continuation of a previously published study protocol [54].

5.2. Experimental Feed

Analytical samples of ZEN were dissolved in 96 μl of 96% ethanol (SWW 2442-90, Polskie Odczynniki SA, Poland). Gilts were weighed at weekly intervals, and mycotoxin doses were calculated individually based on their BWs [6,11,12]. Gel capsules were saturated with the solution, feed was placed inside the capsules, and they were stored at room temperature to evaporate the alcohol. Throughout the trial, all gilts were given the same feed.

The feed given to all test animals was supplied by the same manufacturer. Friable feed was provided ad libitum twice everyday, at 8:00 a.m. and 5:00 p.m., during the experiment. The composition of the complete diet, as declared by the producer, is presented in Table 4 [6,11,12]. Pigs in the experimental groups received ZEN in gel capsules everyday before morning feeding. Feed was the carrier, and group C gilts received identical gel capsules without ZEN [10,11].

Table 4. Declared composition of the complete diets [37].

Parameters	Composition Declared by The Manufacturer (%)
Soybean meal	16
Wheat	55
Barley	22
Wheat bran	4.0
Limestone	0.3
Zitrosan	0.2
Vitamin-mineral premix [1]	2.5

[1] Composition of the vitamin-mineral premix per kg: vitamin A—500,000 IU; iron—5000 mg; vitamin D3—100,000 IU; zinc—5000 mg; vitamin E (alpha-tocopherol)—2000 mg; manganese—3000 mg; vitamin K—150 mg; copper ($CuSO_4 \cdot 5H_2O$)—500 mg; vitamin B1—100 mg; cobalt—20 mg; vitamin B2—300 mg; iodine—40 mg; vitamin B6—150 mg; selenium—15 mg; vitamin B12—1500 µg; L-lysine—9.4 g; niacin—1200 mg; DL-methionine + cystine—3.7 g; pantothenic acid—600 mg; L-threonine—2.3 g; folic acid—50 mg; tryptophan—1.1 g; biotin—7500 µg; phytase + choline—10 g; ToyoCerin probiotic+calcium—250 g; antioxidant+mineral phosphorus and released phosphorus—60 g; magnesium—5 g; sodium and calcium—51 g.

The approximate chemical composition of the diets fed to pigs in groups C, ZEN5, ZEN10, and ZEN15 was determined using the NIRS™ DS2500 F feed analyzer (FOSS, Hillerød, Denmark), a monochromator-based NIR reflection and transflectance analyzer (FOSS, Hillerød, Denmark) with a scanning range of 850–2500 nm [54].

Toxicological Analysis of Feed

Feed was analyzed for the presence of mycotoxins and their metabolites: ZEN, α-ZEL, and deoxynivalenol (DON). The level of the analyzed mycotoxins in feed samples were determined in accordance with the study protocol described previously [54]. Chromatographic methods were validated at the Department of Veterinary Prevention and Feed Hygiene, Faculty of Veterinary Medicine, University of Warmia and Mazury in Olsztyn, Olsztyn, Poland [55].

5.3. Experimental Animals

An in vivo experiment was performed at the Department of Veterinary Prevention and Feed Hygiene of the Faculty of Veterinary Medicine of the University of Warmia and Mazury in Olsztyn, Poland. The experiment involved 60 clinically healthy pre-pubertal gilts with an initial BW of 14.5 ± 2 kg [10,54]. During the experiment, the animals were housed in pens, fed identical diets, and had ad libitum access to water. The gilts were randomly divided into a control group (group C; $n = 15$) and 3 experimental groups (ZEN5, ZEN10, and ZEN15; $n = 15$ each). Groups ZEN5, ZEN10, and ZEN15 were administered ZEN (Sigma-Aldrich Z2125-26MG, St. Louis, MO, USA) per os at 5 µg/kg BW (MABEL dose), 10 µg/kg BW (NOAEL dose), and 15 µg/kg BW (LOAEL dose), respectively. Each experimental group was maintained in a separate pen in the same building. Each pen had an area of 25 m^2, which complies with the applicable cross-compliance regulations (Regulation (EU) No 1306/2013 of the European Parliament and of the Council Brussels, Belgium of 17 December 2013).

5.4. Toxicological Studies of Reproductive, Hypothalamic, and Pituitary Gland Tissues

5.4.1. Tissue Samples

Five prepubertal gilts from every group were euthanized on analytical date 1 (D1—exposure day 7), date 2 (D2—exposure day 21), and date 3 (D3—exposure day 42). Initially, general sedation was performed by intravenous administration of pentobarbital sodium (Fatro, Ozzano Emilia BO, Italy) and bleeding. Immediately after cardiac arrest, tissue samples (approximately 1×1.5 cm) were collected from the following segments: entire left ovary; left uterine horn (from the ovarian and uterine sections); middle part of the cervix; the entire hypothalamus; and the pituitary gland. The samples were rinsed with phosphate buffer and prepared for analyses. The collected samples were stored at a temperature of −20 °C.

5.4.2. Extraction Procedure

The presence of ZEN, α-ZEL, and β-ZEL in tissue samples was determined in accordance with the with the study protocol described previously [54].

5.4.3. Chromatographic Quantification of Zearalenone and Its Metabolites

Zearalenone and its metabolites were quantified at the Institute of Dairy Industry Innovation in Mrągowo, Poland. The biological activity of ZEN, α-ZEL, and β-ZEL in the tissues was determined in accordance with the study protocol described previously [54].

Mycotoxin concentrations were determined with an external standard and were expressed in ng/mL. Matrix-matched calibration standards were applied in the quantification process to eliminate matrix effects that can reduce sensitivity. Calibration standards were dissolved in matrix samples based on the procedure that was used to prepare the remaining samples. The material for the calibration standards was free of undesirable substances. The limits of detection (LOD) for ZEN, α-ZEL, and β-ZEL were determined as the concentration at which the signal-to-noise proportion decreased to 3. The concentrations of ZEN, alfa-ZEL and beta-ZEL were determined in each group and on 3 analytical dates (see Table 1).

5.4.4. Mass Spectrometry Conditions

The electrospray ionization (ESI) mass spectrometer was operated in the negative ion operation. MS/MS parameters were optimized for every compound. Linearity was tested with a calibration curve including 6 levels. The optimal analytical conditions for the tested mycotoxins are presented in Table 5.

Table 5. Optimized conditions for the tested mycotoxins [15].

Analyte	Precursor	Quantification Ion	Confirmation Ion	LOD (ng mL^{-1})	LOQ (ng mL^{-1})	Linearity (%R^2)
ZEN	317.1	273.3	187.1	0.03	0.1	0.999
α-ZEL	319.2	275.2	160.1	0.3	0.9	0.997
β-ZEL	319.2	275.2	160.1	0.3	1	0.993

5.4.5. CF

Carry-over toxicity takes place when an organism is able to survive under exposure to low doses of mycotoxins. Mycotoxins can exert a negative effect on tissues or organ function [56] and modify their activity [10,37]. The carry-over was determined in the examined tissues when the daily dose of zearalenone (5, 10, or 15 μg ZEN/kg BW) administered to each animal was equivalent to 560-32251.5 μg zearalenone/kg of the complete diet, depending on daily feed consumption. Mycotoxin contents in tissues were expressed in terms of the dry matter content of the samples.

The CF was calculated as follows:

$$CF = \text{toxin concentration in tissue [ng/g]/toxin concentration in diet [ng/g]}$$

5.4.6. Statistical Analysis

Data were processed statistically at the Department of Discrete Mathematics and Theoretical Computer Science, of the Faculty of Mathematics and Computer Science of the University of Warmia and Mazury in Olsztyn, Poland, as described previously [37].

5.5. Toxicological Studies of Blood

Blood samples collection

Blood was sampled in vivo from 5 gilts from every group on each analytical date. The first analytical date was exposure day 7 (D1); the second analytical date was exposure day 14 (D2); the third analytical date was exposure day 21 (D3); the fourth analytical date was exposure day 28 (D4); the fifth analytical date was exposure day 35 (D5), and the sixth analytical date was exposure day 42 (D6). Blood samples of 20 mL each were collected from all gilts (blood was sampled within 20 seconds after immobilization [57]) directly before slaughter by jugular venipuncture with a syringe containing 0.5 mL of heparin solution. The collected blood was centrifuged at 3000 rpm for 20 minutes at 4 °C. The obtained plasma samples were stored at −18 °C until estradiol (E_2) and progesterone (P_4) concentration analyses were performed.

5.6. Determination of Plasma Hormone Concentrations

5.6.1. Estradiol

Estradiol concentrations in the blood plasma of gilts were analyzed at the Institute of Animal Reproduction and Food Research of the Polish Academy of Sciences in Olsztyn, Poland, as described previously [37]. Plasma E_2 levels were determined by the radioimmunoassay (RIA) method with a commercial kit (ESTR-US-CT, CIS BIO ASSAYS) as described previously [58]. Estradiol concentrations were determined in accordance with the method described previously [37].

5.6.2. Progesterone

Progesterone was quantified at the Analytical Laboratory of the Municipal Hospital with Polyclinic in Olsztyn, Poland, by the ECLIA electrochemiluminescence assay with the use of Elecsys Progesterone II and Cobas c 6000 analyzers (Hitachi, Tokyo, Japan). Progesterone concentrations were determined in accordance with the method described previously [37].

5.6.3. Statistical Analysis

Data were processed statistically at the Department of Discrete Mathematics and Theoretical Computer Science, of the Faculty of Mathematics and Computer Science of the University of Warmia and Mazury in Olsztyn, Poland, as described previously [37].

Supplementary Materials: The following supporting information can be downloaded at: https://www.mdpi.com/article/10.3390/toxins14110790/s1, Figure S1. Tree map of ZEN, α-ZEL, and β-ZEL concentrations in reproductive system, hypothalamic, and pituitary gland tissues in Group ZEN5 gilts (5 μg ZEN/kg BW). Key: D1—exposure day 7; D2—exposure day 21; D3—exposure day 42.; Figure S2. Tree map of ZEN, α-ZEL, and β-ZEL concentrations in reproductive system, hypothalamic, and pituitary gland tissues in Group ZEN10 gilts (10 μg ZEN/kg BW). Key: D1—exposure day 7; D2—exposure day 21; D3 – exposure day 42; Figure S3. Tree map of ZEN, α-ZEL, and β-ZEL concentrations in reproductive system, hypothalamic, and pituitary gland tissues in Group ZEN15 gilts (15 μg ZEN/kg BW). Key: D1—exposure day 7; D2—exposure day 21; D3—exposure day 42.

Author Contributions: The experiments were conceived and designed by M.G. and M.T.G. The experiments were performed by M.G., Ł.Z. and A.B. Data were analyzed and interpreted by M.G., Ł.Z. and A.B. The manuscript was drafted by M.G., and critically edited by Ł.Z. and M.T.G. All authors have read and agreed to the published version of the manuscript.

Funding: The study was supported by the Polish Ministry of Science and Higher Education as part of Project No. 12-0080-10/2010. Project financially supported by the Minister of Education and Science under the program entitled "Regional Initiative of Excellence" for the years 2019–2023, Project No. 010/RID/2018/19, amount of funding 12.000.000 PLN.

Institutional Review Board Statement: All experimental procedures involving animals were carried out in compliance with Polish regulations setting forth the terms and conditions of animal experimentation (Opinions No. 12/2016 and 45/2016/DLZ of the Local Ethics Committee for Animal Experimentation of 27 April 2016 and 30 November 2016). All investigators are authorized to perform experiments on animals.

Informed Consent Statement: Not applicable.

Data Availability Statement: Not applicable.

Conflicts of Interest: The authors declare no conflict of interest.

References

1. Thielecke, F.; Nugent, A.P. Contaminants in Grain—A Major Risk for Whole Grain Safety? *Nutrients* **2018**, *10*, 1213. [CrossRef] [PubMed]
2. Fleetwood, J.; Rahman, S.; Holland, D.; Millson, D.; Thomson, L.; Poppy, G. As clean as they look? Food hygiene inspection scores, microbiological contamination, and foodborne illness. *Food Control* **2019**, *96*, 76–86. [CrossRef]
3. Alassane-Kpembi, I.; Pinton, P.; Oswald, I.P. Effects of Mycotoxins on the Intestine. *Toxins* **2019**, *11*, 159. [CrossRef] [PubMed]
4. Piotrowska, M.; Sliżewska, K.; Nowak, A.; Zielonka, Ł.; Żakowska, Z.; Gajęcka, M.; Gajęcki, M. The effect of experimental fusarium mycotoxicosis on microbiota diversity in porcine ascending colon contents. *Toxins* **2014**, *6*, 2064–2081. [CrossRef] [PubMed]
5. Zachariasova, M.; Dzumana, Z.; Veprikova, Z.; Hajkovaa, K.; Jiru, M.; Vaclavikova, M.; Zachariasova, A.; Pospichalova, M.; Florian, M.; Hajslova, J. Occurrence of multiple mycotoxins in European feeding stuffs, assessment of dietary intake by farm animals. *Anim. Feed Sci. Technol.* **2014**, *193*, 124–140. [CrossRef]
6. Knutsen, H.-K.; Alexander, J.; Barregård, L.; Bignami, M.; Brüschweiler, B.; Ceccatelli, S.; Cottrill, B.; Dinovi, M.; Edler, L.; Grasl-Kraupp, B.; et al. Risks for animal health related to the presence of zearalenone and its modified forms in feed. *EFSA J.* **2017**, *15*, 4851. [CrossRef]
7. Faisal, Z.; Vörös, V.; Fliszár-Nyúl, E.; Lemli, B.; Kunsági-Máté, S.; Poór, M. Interactions of zearalanone, α-zearalanol, β-zearalanol, zearalenone-14-sulfate, and zearalenone-14-glucoside with serum albumin. *Mycotoxin Res.* **2020**, *36*, 389–397. [CrossRef]
8. Calabrese, E.J. Hormesis: Path and Progression to Significance. *Int. J. Mol. Sci.* **2018**, *19*, 2871. [CrossRef]
9. Freire, L.; Sant'Ana, A.S. Modified mycotoxins: An updated review on their formation, detection, occurrence, and toxic effects. *Food Chem. Toxicol.* **2018**, *111*, 189–205. [CrossRef]
10. Rykaczewska, A.; Gajęcka, M.; Dąbrowski, M.; Wiśniewska, A.; Szcześniewska, J.; Gajęcki, M.T.; Zielonka, Ł. Growth performance, selected blood biochemical parameters and body weight of pre-pubertal gilts fed diets supplemented with different doses of zearalenone (ZEN). *Toxicon* **2018**, *152*, 84–94. [CrossRef]
11. Cieplińska, K.; Gajęcka, M.; Dąbrowski, M.; Rykaczewska, A.; Zielonka, Ł.; Lisieska-Żołnierczyk, S.; Bulińska, M.; Gajęcki, M.T. Time-dependent changes in the intestinal microbiome of gilts exposed to low zearalenone doses. *Toxins* **2019**, *11*, 296. [CrossRef] [PubMed]
12. Cieplińska, K.; Gajęcka, M.; Nowak, A.; Dąbrowski, M.; Zielonka, Ł.; Gajęcki, M.T. The genotoxicity of caecal water in gilts exposed to low doses of zearalenone. *Toxins* **2018**, *10*, 350. [CrossRef] [PubMed]
13. Gajęcka, M.; Majewski, M.S.; Zielonka, Ł.; Grzegorzewski, W.; Onyszek, E.; Lisieska-Zołnierczyk, S.; Juśkiewicz, J.; Babuchowski, A.; Gajęcki, M.T. Concentration of Zearalenone, Alpha-Zearalenol and Beta-Zearalenol in the Myocardium and the Results of Isometric Analyses of the Coronary Artery in Prepubertal Gilts. *Toxins* **2021**, *13*, 396. [CrossRef]
14. Mróz, M.; Gajęcka, M.; Przybyłowicz, K.E.; Sawicki, T.; Lisieska-Żołnierczyk, S.; Zielonk, Ł.; Gajęcki, M.T. The Effect of Low Doses of Zearalenone (ZEN) on the Bone Marrow Microenvironment and Haematological Parameters of Blood Plasma in Pre-Pubertal Gilts. *Toxins* **2022**, *14*, 105. [CrossRef] [PubMed]
15. Mróz, M.; Gajęcka, M.; Brzuzan, P.; Lisieska-Żołnierczyk, S.; Leski, D.; Zielonka, Ł.; Gajęcki, M.T. Carry-Over of Zearalenone and Its Metabolites to Intestinal Tissues and the Expression of CYP1A1 and GSTπ1 in the Colon of Gilts before Puberty. *Toxins* **2022**, *14*, 354. [CrossRef]
16. Zhou, J.; Zhao, L.; Huang, S.; Liu, Q.; Ao, X.; Lei, Y.; Ji, C.; Ma, Q. Zearalenone toxicosis on reproduction as estrogen receptor selective modulator and alleviation of zearalenone biodegradative agent in pregnant sows. *J. Anim. Sci. Biotechnol.* **2022**, *13*, 36. [CrossRef] [PubMed]
17. Gajęcka, M.; Zielonka, Ł.; Gajęcki, M. Activity of zearalenone in the porcine intestinal tract. *Molecules* **2017**, *22*, 18. [CrossRef] [PubMed]
18. Celi, P.; Verlhac, V.; Pérez, C.E.; Schmeisser, J.; Kluenter, A.M. Biomarkers of gastrointestinal functionality in animal nutrition and health. *Anim. Feed Sci. Technol.* **2019**, *250*, 9–31. [CrossRef]
19. Dąbrowski, M.; Obremski, K.; Gajęcka, M.; Gajęcki, M.; Zielonka, Ł. Changes in the subpopulations of porcine peripheral blood lymphocytes induced by exposure to low doses of zearalenone (ZEN) and deoxynivalenol (DON). *Molecules* **2016**, *21*, 557. [CrossRef]
20. Bryden, W.L. Mycotoxin contamination of the feed supply chain: Implications for animal productivity and feed security. *Anim. Feed Sci. Technol.* **2012**, *173*, 134–158. [CrossRef]
21. Llorens, P.; Herrera, M.; Juan-García, A.; Payá, J.J.; Moltó, J.C.; Ariño, A.; Juan, C. Biomarkers of Exposure to Zearalenone in In Vivo and In Vitro Studies. *Toxins* **2022**, *14*, 291. [CrossRef] [PubMed]
22. Szeliga, A.; Meczekalski, B. Kisspeptin Modulation of Reproductive Function. *Endocrines* **2022**, *3*, 367–374. [CrossRef]
23. Wan, B.; Yuan, X.; Yang, W.; Jiao, N.; Li, Y.; Liu, F.; Liu, M.; Yang, Z.; Huang, L.; Jiang, S. The Effects of Zearalenone on the Localization and Expression of Reproductive Hormones in the Ovaries of Weaned Gilts. *Toxins* **2021**, *13*, 626. [CrossRef]

24. Grenier, B.; Applegate, T.J. Modulation of intestinal functions following mycotoxin ingestion: Meta-analysis of published experiments in animals. *Toxins* **2013**, *5*, 396–430. [CrossRef] [PubMed]
25. Lathe, R.; Kotelevtsev, Y. Steroid signaling: Ligand-binding promiscuity molecular symmetry, and the need for gating. *Steroids* **2014**, *82*, 14–22. [CrossRef]
26. Kramer, H.J.; van den Ham, W.A.; Slob, W.; Pieters, M.N. Conversion Factors Estimating Indicative Chronic No-Observed-Adverse-Effect Levels from Short-Term Toxicity Data. *Regul. Toxicol. Pharm.* **1996**, *23*, 249–255. [CrossRef]
27. Pastoor, T.P.; Bachman, A.N.; Bell, D.R.; Cohen, S.M.; Dellarco, M.; Dewhurst, I.C.; Doe, J.E.; Doerrer, N.G.; Embry, M.R.; Hines, R.N.; et al. A 21st century roadmap for human health risk assessment. *Crit. Rev. Toxicol.* **2014**, *44*, 1–5. [CrossRef] [PubMed]
28. Suh, H.Y.; Peck, C.C.; Yu, K.S.; Lee, H. Determination of the starting dose in the first-in-human clinical trials with monoclonal antibodies: A systematic review of papers published between 1990 and 2013. *Drug Des. Dev. Ther.* **2016**, *10*, 4005–4016. [CrossRef]
29. Vandenberg, L.N.; Colborn, T.; Hayes, T.B.; Heindel, J.J.; Jacobs, D.R.; Lee, D.-H.; Shioda, T.; Soto, A.M.; vom Saal, F.S.; Welshons, W.V.; et al. Hormones and endocrine-disrupting chemicals: Low-dose effects and nonmonotonic dose responses. *Endocr. Rev.* **2012**, *33*, 378–455. [CrossRef]
30. Gonkowski, S.; Gajęcka, M.; Makowska, K. Mycotoxins and the Enteric Nervous system. *Toxins* **2020**, *12*, 461. [CrossRef]
31. Lephart, E.D.; Thompson, J.M.; Setchell, K.D.; Adlercreutz, H.; Weber, K.S. Phytoestrogens decrease brain calcium-binding proteins but do not alter hypothalamic androgen metabolizing enzymes in adult male rats. *Brain Res.* **2000**, *859*, 123–131. [CrossRef]
32. Venkataramana, M.; Chandra Nayaka, S.; Anand, T.; Rajesh, R.; Aiyaz, M.; Divakara, S.T.; Murali, H.S.; Prakash, H.S.; Lakshmana Rao, P.V. Zearalenone induced toxicity in SHSY-5Y cells: The role of oxidative stress evidenced by N-acetyl cysteine. *Food Chem. Toxicol.* **2014**, *65*, 335–342. [CrossRef] [PubMed]
33. Zhao, S.; Guo, Z.; Xiang, W.; Wang, P. The neuroendocrine pathways and mechanisms for the control of the reproduction in female pigs. *Anim. Reprod.* **2021**, *18*, e20210063. [CrossRef] [PubMed]
34. Genchi, V.A.; Rossi, E.; Lauriola, C.; D'Oria, R.; Palma, G.; Borrelli, A.; Caccioppoli, C.; Giorgino, F.; Cignarelli, A. Adipose Tissue Dysfunction and Obesity-Related Male Hypogonadism. *Int. J. Mol. Sci.* **2022**, *23*, 8194. [CrossRef] [PubMed]
35. Marín-García, P.J.; Llobat, L. How does protein nutrition affect the epigenetic changes in pig? A review. *Animals* **2021**, *11*, 544. [CrossRef]
36. Muro, B.B.D.; Leal, D.F.; Carnevale, R.F.; Torres, M.A.; Mendonça, M.V.; Nakasone, D.H.; Martinez, C.H.G.; Ravagnani, G.M.; Monteiro, M.S.; Poor, A.P.; et al. Altrenogest during early pregnancy modulates uterine glandular epithelium and endometrial growth factor expression at the time implantation in pigs. *Anim. Reprod.* **2021**, *18*, e20200431. [CrossRef]
37. Rykaczewska, A.; Gajęcka, M.; Onyszek, E.; Cieplińska, K.; Dąbrowski, M.; Lisieska-Żołnierczyk, S.; Bulińska, M.; Babuchowski, A.; Gajęcki, M.T.; Zielonka, Ł. Imbalance in the Blood Concentrations of Selected Steroids in Prepubertal Gilts Depending on the Time of Exposure to Low Doses of Zearalenone. *Toxins* **2019**, *11*, 561. [CrossRef]
38. Lawrenz, B.; Melado, L.; Fatemi, H. Premature progesterone rise in ART-cycles. *Reprod. Biol.* **2018**, *18*, 1–4. [CrossRef]
39. Li, X.; Lin, B.; Zhang, X.; Shen, X.; Ouyang, H.; Wu, Z.; Tian, Y.; Fang, L.; Huang, Y. Comparative transcriptomics in the hypothalamic-pituitary-gonad axis of mammals and poultry. *Genomics* **2022**, *114*, 110396. [CrossRef]
40. Zheng, W.; Feng, N.; Wang, Y.; Noll, L.; Xu, S.; Liu, X.; Lu, N.; Zou, H.; Gu, J.; Yuan, Y.; et al. Effects of zearalenone and its derivatives on the synthesis and secretion of mammalian sex steroid hormones: A review. *Food Chem. Toxicol.* **2019**, *126*, 262–276. [CrossRef]
41. Yang, D.; Jiang, T.; Lin, P.; Chen, H.; Wang, L.; Wang, N.; Zhao, F.; Tang, K.; Zhou, D.; Wang, A.; et al. Apoptosis inducing factor gene depletion inhibits zearalenone-induced cell death in a goat Leydig cell line. *Reprod. Toxicol.* **2017**, *67*, 129–139. [CrossRef] [PubMed]
42. Kowalska, K.; Habrowska-Górczyńska, D.E.; Piastowska-Ciesielska, A. Zearalenone as an endocrine disruptor in humans. *Environ. Toxicol. Pharmacol.* **2016**, *48*, 141–149. [CrossRef] [PubMed]
43. Benagiano, M.; Bianchi, P.; D'Elios, M.M.; Brosens, I.; Benagiano, G. Autoimmune diseases: Role of steroid hormones. *Best Pract. Res. Clin. Obstet. Gynaecol.* **2019**, *60*, 24–34. [CrossRef] [PubMed]
44. Kiss, D.S.; Ioja, E.; Toth, I.; Barany, Z.; Jocsak, G.; Bartha, T.; Horvath, T.L.; Zsarnovszky, A. Comparative Analysis of Zearalenone Effects on Thyroid Receptor Alpha (TRα) and Beta (TRβ) Expression in Rat Primary Cerebellar Cell Cultures. *Int. J. Mol. Sci.* **2018**, *19*, 1440. [CrossRef]
45. Mucci, A.; Clemente, E. The Role of Genetics in Central Precocious Puberty: Confirmed and Potential Neuroendocrine Genetic and Epigenetic Contributors and Their Interactions with Endocrine Disrupting Chemicals (EDCs). *Endocrines* **2022**, *3*, 433–451. [CrossRef]
46. Gajęcka, M.; Otrocka-Domagała, I. Immunocytochemical expression of 3β- and 17β-hydroxysteroid dehydrogenase in bitch ovaries exposed to low doses of zearalenone. *Pol. J. Vet. Sci.* **2013**, *16*, 55–62. [CrossRef]
47. Liu, X.L.; Wu, R.Y.; Sun, X.F.; Cheng, S.F.; Zhang, R.Q.; Zhang, T.T.; Zhang, X.F.; Zhao, Y.; Shen, W.; Li, L. Mycotoxin zearalenone exposure impairs genomic stability of swine follicular granulosa cells in vitro. *Int. J. Biol. Sci.* **2018**, *14*, 294–305. [CrossRef]
48. Hennig-Pauka, I.; Koch, F.J.; Schaumberger, S.; Woechtl, B.; Novak, J.; Sulyok, M.; Nagl, V. Current challenges in the diagnosis of zearalenone toxicosis as illustrated by a field case of hyperestrogenism in suckling piglets. *Porc. Health Manag.* **2018**, *4*, 1–9. [CrossRef]

49. He, J.; Wei, C.; Li, Y.; Liu, Y.; Wang, Y.; Pan, J.; Liu, J.; Wu, Y.; Cui, S. Zearalenone and alpha-zearalenol inhibit the synthesis and secretion of pig follicle stimulating hormone via the non-classical estrogen membrane receptor GPR30. *Mol. Cell. Endocrinol.* **2018**, *461*, 43–54. [CrossRef]
50. Gellerich, F.N.; Gizatullina, Z.; Trumbeckaite, S.; Nguyen, H.P.; Pallas, T.; Arandarcikaite, O.; Vielhaber, S.; Seppet, E.; Striggow, F. The regulation of OXPHOS by extramitochondrial calcium. *Biochim. Biophys. Acta (BBA)-Bioenerg.* **2010**, *1797*, 1018–1027. [CrossRef]
51. Gajęcka, M.; Przybylska-Gornowicz, B. The low doses effect of experimental zearalenone (ZEN) intoxication on the presence of Ca^{2+} in selected ovarian cells from pre-pubertal bitches. *Pol. J. Vet. Sci.* **2012**, *15*, 711–720. [CrossRef]
52. Gajęcka, M.; Zielonka, Ł.; Gajęcki, M. The Effect of Low Monotonic Doses of Zearalenone on Selected Reproductive Tissues in Pre-Pubertal Female Dogs—A Review. *Molecules* **2015**, *20*, 20669–20687. [CrossRef] [PubMed]
53. Romejko, K.; Rymarz, A.; Sadownik, H.; Niemczyk, S. Testosterone Deficiency as One of the Major Endocrine Disorders in Chronic Kidney Disease. *Nutrients* **2022**, *14*, 3438. [CrossRef] [PubMed]
54. Gajęcka, M.; Mróz, M.; Brzuzan, P.; Onyszek, E.; Zielonka, Ł.; Lipczyńska-Ilczuk, K.; Przybyłowicz, K.E.; Babuchowski, A.; Gajęcki, M.T. Correlations between Low Doses of Zearalenone, Its Carryover Factor and Estrogen Receptor Expression in Different Segments of the Intestines in Pre-Pubertal Gilts—A Study Protocol. *Toxins* **2021**, *13*, 379. [CrossRef] [PubMed]
55. Zielonka, Ł.; Waśkiewicz, A.; Beszterda, M.; Kostecki, M.; Dąbrowski, M.; Obremski, K.; Goliński, P.; Gajęcki, M. Zearalenone in the Intestinal Tissues of Immature Gilts Exposed *per os* to Mycotoxins. *Toxins* **2015**, *7*, 3210–3223. [CrossRef]
56. Meerpoel, C.; Vidal, A.; Tangni, E.K.; Huybrechts, B.; Couck, L.; De Rycke, R.; De Bels, L.; De Saeger, S.; Van den Broeck, W.; Devreese, M.; et al. A Study of Carry-Over and Histopathological Effects after Chronic Dietary Intake of Citrinin in Pigs, Broiler Chickens and Laying Hens. *Toxins* **2020**, *12*, 719. [CrossRef]
57. Kowalski, A.; Kaleczyc, J.; Gajęcki, M.; Zieliński, H. Adrenaline, noradrenaline and cortisol levels in pigs during blood collection. *Med. Weter.* **1996**, *52*, 716–718. (In Polish)
58. Stanczyk, F.Z.; Xu, X.; Sluss, P.M.; Brinton, L.A.; McGlynn, K.A. Do metabolites account for higher serum steroid hormone levels measured by RIA compared to mass spectrometry? *Clin. Chim. Acta* **2018**, *484*, 223–225. [CrossRef]

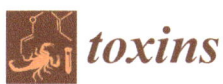

Article

Does Deoxynivalenol Affect Amoxicillin and Doxycycline Absorption in the Gastrointestinal Tract? Ex Vivo Study on Swine Jejunum Mucosa Explants

Marta Mendel [1,*], Wojciech Karlik [1], Urszula Latek [1], Magdalena Chłopecka [1], Ewelina Nowacka-Kozak [2], Katarzyna Pietruszka [2] and Piotr Jedziniak [2]

1. Institute of Veterinary Medicine, Warsaw University of Life Sciences, Nowoursynowka St. 166, 02-786 Warsaw, Poland
2. Department of Pharmacology and Toxicology, National Veterinary Research Institute, Partyzantów 57, 24-100 Puławy, Poland
* Correspondence: marta_mendel@sggw.edu.pl; Tel.: +48-22-5936065

Abstract: The presence of deoxynivalenol (DON) in feed may increase intestinal barrier permeability. Disturbance of the intestinal barrier integrity may affect the absorption of antibiotics used in animals. Since the bioavailability of orally administered antibiotics significantly affects their efficacy and safety, it was decided to evaluate how DON influences the absorption of the most commonly used antibiotics in pigs, i.e., amoxicillin (AMX) and doxycycline (DOX). The studies were conducted using jejunal explants from adult pigs. Explants were incubated in Ussing chambers, in which a buffer containing DON (30 μg/mL), AMX (50 μg/mL), DOX (30 μg/mL), a combination of AMX + DON, or a combination of DOX + DON was used. Changes in transepithelial electrical resistance (TEER), the flux of transcellular and intracellular transport markers, and the flux of antibiotics across explants were measured. DON increased the permeability of small intestine explants, expressed by a reduction in TEER and an intensification of transcellular marker transport. DON did not affect AMX transport, but it accelerated DOX transport by approximately five times. The results suggest that DON inhibits the efflux transport of DOX to the intestinal lumen, and thus significantly changes its absorption from the gastrointestinal tract.

Keywords: deoxynivalenol; amoxicillin; doxycycline; Ussing chamber; swine jejunum mucosa explants

Key Contribution: DON does not affect AMX transport but inhibits the efflux transport of DOX to the intestinal lumen, and thus significantly changes the kinetics of DOX absorption from the gastrointestinal tract.

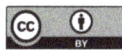

1. Introduction

Foodstuffs and feed contamination, including simultaneous contamination of agricultural products with numerous mycotoxins and modified mycotoxins, is a frequent and widely recognised worldwide problem [1–4]. These unavoidable toxins are secondary metabolites produced by different genera of filamentous fungi. They occur on dietary staple foods and fodder, especially cereals, along the whole production chain, including under pre- and post-harvest conditions. In Europe, the most frequently reported mycotoxins and secondary metabolites in feed include deoxynivalenol (DON), zearalenone, ochratoxin A, fumonisin B1, fumonisin B2, and T2/HT2 toxin [3]. Considering pigs' diet, cereals, including maize and cereal-based products, are probably the most commonly used constituents in feed, supplying most of the animal's nutrients. Nevertheless, there are mycotoxins in maize called trichothecenes, most importantly zearalenone and DON [2,3,5,6].

Deoxynivalenol is a type B trichothecene produced by Fusarium species. It is believed to be one of the least acutely toxic trichothecenes, but it is highly incident and relevant in animal husbandry [4]. Chronic exposure to low doses of this mycotoxin heavily suppresses the immune response and intestinal functions, induces anorexia, reduces weight gain, and causes neuroendocrine changes [7–10]. There is sufficient evidence revealing the impairing effect of DON on gut barrier permeability and integrity. The mycotoxin induces the activity of mitogen-activated protein kinases (MAPKs) and decreases the expression of tight junction proteins [11].

Consequently, bacteria and antigens translocation from the lumen of the gut might be intensified [11,12]. Despite the knowledge of DON's potency to change intestine permeability, little interest has been paid so far to its possible effects on the absorption rate of other xenobiotics at the time of combined exposure [13–16]. In addition to nutrients, the spectrum of chemicals which might be found in the lumen of the gut due to conscious administration of feed and environmental contaminations include veterinary medicinal products (VMPs), feed additives, fertilisers, plant protection products, air pollutants, and others.

In the case of VMPs, a group of special considerations are antimicrobials. Their use in modern pig production remains one of the elements in maintaining animal health. However, under some conditions, the hazards related to their use could negate their benefits due to the potential risks, including exposure to antimicrobial residues in food or the environment [17,18]. Using antimicrobials might provoke antimicrobial resistance in animal- and human-related bacteria, and thus, compromise animal and human health [19].

Amoxycillin (AMX) and doxycycline (DOX) represent two commonly used antimicrobials for oral application in pigs. Their recommended doses guarantee effectiveness against pathogens and safety of use. Dosing antibiotics (as with all drugs) is based on pharmacokinetic parameters, of which oral bioavailability is one of the key parameters. In the case of orally administered antibiotics in food-producing animals, the level of absorption of the medicine from the gastrointestinal tract affects not only its antibacterial efficacy but also is essential for the safety of food consumers and the environment. In the event of a disturbance in the functioning of the intestinal barrier, the bioavailability of an orally administered antibiotic may change, which in turn may affect the effectiveness and safety of its action. To the best of our knowledge, there is hardly any evidence of the interaction of mycotoxins with antimicrobials within the gastrointestinal tract. An in-depth literature search revealed only one study by Goossens et al. [13] on DON–DOX interaction at the stage of absorption in pigs. Therefore, this study aimed to verify the impact of DON on two antibiotics' (AMX and DOX) absorption in the intestine isolated from clinically healthy pigs.

2. Results

2.1. The Effect of Deoxynivalenol on the Viability, Integrity, and Permeability of Jejunum Mucosa Explants

The application of DON at the concentration of 30 µg/mL to the luminal compartment of the Ussing chamber, and incubation of mucosa explants in its presence for 90 min resulted in a significant drop of the transepithelial electrical resistance (TEER) value. It reached only 52.4 ± 0.7 Ohm·cm^2 at the end of exposure, whereas the control incubation with no mycotoxin resulted in a TEER measurement of 77.1 ± 1.2 Ohm·cm^2 (Figure 1).

DON caused a remarkable increase in paracellular permeability measured indirectly by the penetration rate of paracellular transport markers. Both Lucifer Yellow (LY) and mannitol (MAN), administered at concentrations of 100 µg/mL, underwent more intense transportation across mucosa explants in intestine specimens treated with DON than in the control chambers (Figures 2 and 3).

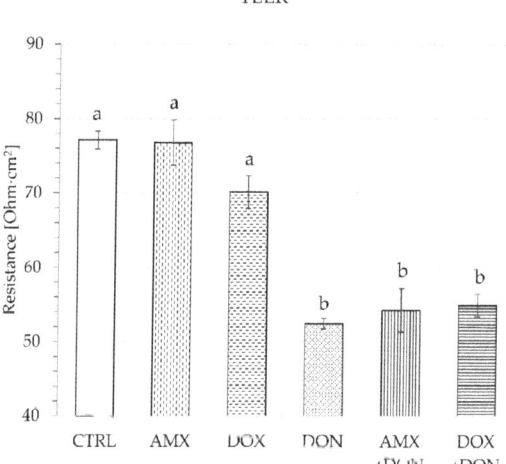

Figure 1. TEER of intestine explants measured after 90 min incubation in buffer supplemented with: amoxicillin—AMX, doxycycline—DOX, deoxynivalenol—DON, and combination AMX + DON or DOX + DON, or CTRL—control condition without antibiotics and DON. Bars show the mean of the 6 replicates ± SEM (standard errors of the mean). Different letters above the bars indicate a statistically significant difference at p-value < 0.05.

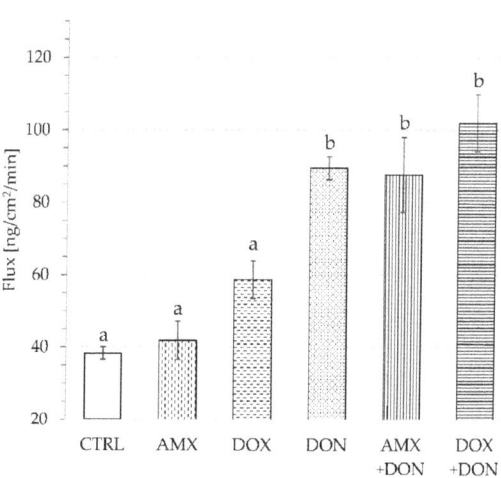

Figure 2. Lucifer Yellow transport through intestine explants during 90 min of incubation in buffer supplemented with: amoxicillin—AMX, doxycycline—DOX, deoxynivalenol—DON, combination AMX + DON or DOX + DON, or CTRL—control condition without antibiotics and DON. Bars show the mean of the 6 replicates ± SEM (standard errors of the mean). Different letters above the bars indicate a statistically significant difference at p-value < 0.05.

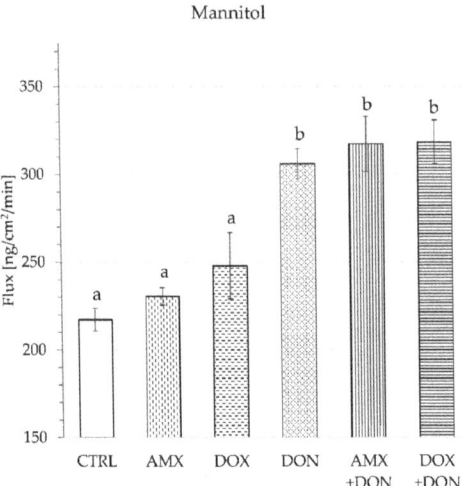

Figure 3. Mannitol transport through intestine explants during 90 min incubation in buffer supplemented with: amoxicillin—AMX, doxycycline—DOX, deoxynivalenol—DON, combination AMX + DON or DOX + DON, or CTRL—control condition without antibiotics and DON. Bars show the mean of the 6 replicates ± SEM (standard errors of the mean). Different letters above the bars indicate a statistically significant difference at p-value < 0.05.

The flux of LY and MAN amounted to 89.5 ± 3.2 and 306.0 ± 8.6 ng/min/cm^2, respectively, in the presence of DON, and to 38.3 ± 1.7 and 217.3 ± 6.5 ng/min/cm^2, respectively, in the absence of the mycotoxin. The flux of the transcellular transport marker (caffeine—CAF) did not change when mucosa explants were incubated in a DON-containing buffer. The addition of mycotoxin caused CAF penetration through intestine explants at the level of 2.9 ± 0.2 µg/min/cm^2, whereas in the control trial, the flux came to 2.6 ± 0.1 µg/min/cm^2 (Figure 4).

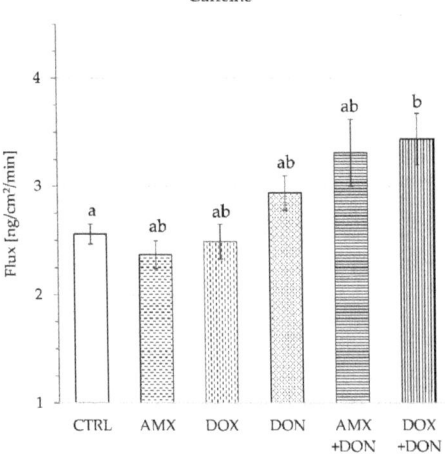

Figure 4. Caffeine transport through intestine explants during 90 min incubation in buffer supplemented with: amoxicillin—AMX, doxycycline—DOX, deoxynivalenol—DON, combination AMX + DON or DOX + DON, or CTRL—control condition without antibiotics and DON. Bars show the mean of the 6 replicates ± SEM (standard errors of the mean). Different letters above the bars indicate a statistically significant difference at p-value < 0.05.

Moreover, the use of DON did not provoke any cytotoxicity measured by LDH leakage. The activity of LDH detected in the buffer amounted to 4.9 ± 0.2% and 4.7 ± 0.2% of total LDH activity in the presence and absence of the mycotoxin, respectively (Figure 5).

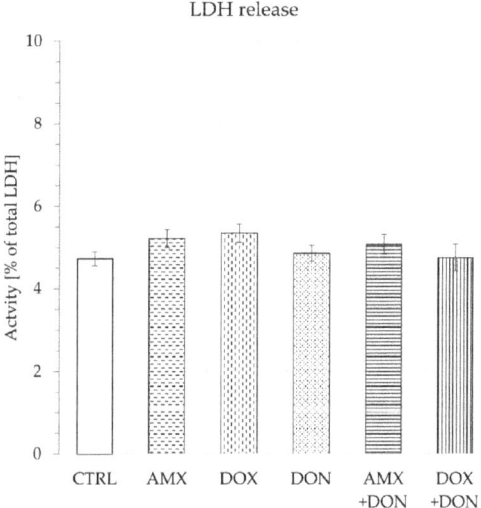

Figure 5. Relative LDH activity in the luminal compartment of intestine explants at 90 min of incubation in buffer supplemented with: amoxicillin—AMX, doxycycline—DOX, deoxynivalenol—DON, combination AMX + DON or DOX + DON, or CTRL—control condition without antibiotics and DON. The LDH activity measured after explant homogenisation was taken to be 100%. Bars show the mean of the 6 replicates ± SEM (standard errors of the mean).

2.2. The Effect of Amoxicillin and Doxycycline on the Viability, Integrity, and Permeability of Jejunum Mucosa Explants

The single exposure of mucosa explants to either AMX (50 μg/mL) or DOX (30 μg/mL) did not provoke a significant change in TEER values during 90 min of incubation. The final measurement of TEER indicated 76.8 ± 3.1 and 70.1 ± 2.2 Ohm·cm^2 for AMX- and DOX-treated jejunum tissues, respectively. In contrast, no addition of antibiotics caused a TEER reading of 77.1 ± 1.2 Ohm·cm^2 (Figure 1). The use of AMX did not provoke any significant change in the penetration of paracellular transport markers because the flux of LY and MAN amounted to 41.8 ± 5.3 and 230.6 ± 5.0 ng/min/cm^2, respectively (Figures 2 and 3). Similarly, AMX did not affect the penetration rate of the transcellular transport marker. The flux of CAF was measured as 2.4 ± 0.1 μg/min/cm^2 in the presence of this antibiotic and 2.6 ± 0.1 μg/min/cm^2 when the explants were incubated in AMX-free medium (Figure 4). Likewise, the addition of DOX did not modify the intensity of CAF penetration across mucosa explants. DOX revealed the tendency to increase the intensity of transportation of paracellular transport markers. The flux of LY and MAN reached 58.7 ± 5.15 and 247.8 ± 18.9 ng/min/cm^2, respectively (Figures 2 and 3). Additionally, none of the tested antibiotics increased the release of LDH compared to the control conditions. The enzyme activity in the KRB amounted to 5.2 ± 0.2 and 5.4 ± 0.2% of total LDH activity for AMX and DOX, respectively (Figure 5).

2.3. The Effect of Combined Exposure to Deoxynivalenol and Amoxicillin or Doxycycline on the Viability, Integrity, and Permeability of Jejunum Mucosa Explants

The combined exposure of mucosa explants to DON and one of the antibiotics did not provoke a more profound alteration in intestine integrity and permeability than the mycotoxin used solely. Simultaneous exposure to AMX + DON or DOX + DON did not alter the magnitude of the TEER drop compared to the effect of DON alone. TEER readings were at the same level and amounted to 54.2 ± 2.9, 54.9 ± 1.5, and 52.4 ± 0.7 Ohm·cm^2 for AMX + DON, DOX + DON, and DON, respectively (Figure 1). In the case of the penetration of paracellular and transcellular transport markers through mucosa explants, there were no remarkable differences between tissue samples incubated only in the presence of DON and those incubated in a cocktail of DON and one of the antibiotics. The flux of LY came to 87.7 ± 10.6, 101.9 ± 7.8, and 89.5 ± 13.2 ng/min/cm^2 for AMX + DON, DOX + DON, and DON, respectively (Figure 2). The penetration of MAN ranked at 317.3 ± 15.7, 318.4 ± 12.6, and 306.0 ± 8.6 ng/min/cm^2, respectively, for AMX + DON, DOX + DON, and DON-containing KRB, respectively (Figure 3). Similarly, the extra addition of AMX or DOX did not cause any significant change in CAF penetration across jejunum mucosa in comparison to the effect of DON (Figure 4). However, the rate of CAF penetration was significantly higher in the presence of DOX + DON when compared to the control trial. The cytotoxicity measured in the LDH leakage test was at the same level for explants incubated in DON-containing incubation medium with and without antibiotics (Figure 5).

2.4. The Effect of Deoxynivalenol on Amoxicillin and Doxycycline Penetration across Swine Jejunum Explants

The penetration rate of AMX across jejunum mucosa explants amounted to 18.8 ± 2.5 ng/min/cm^2. The intensity of AMX transportation did not change in the presence of DON because antibiotic flux remained very similar, i.e., at the level of 16.6 ± 1.2 ng/min/cm^2 (Figure 6A). In the case of DOX, the basic penetration rate (in the absence of the toxin) was 0.7 ± 0.1 ng/min/cm^2. The combined exposure to DOX and DON caused a 5-fold increase in the antibiotic penetration rate, which finally came to 3.8 ± 0.5 ng/min/cm^2 (Figure 6B).

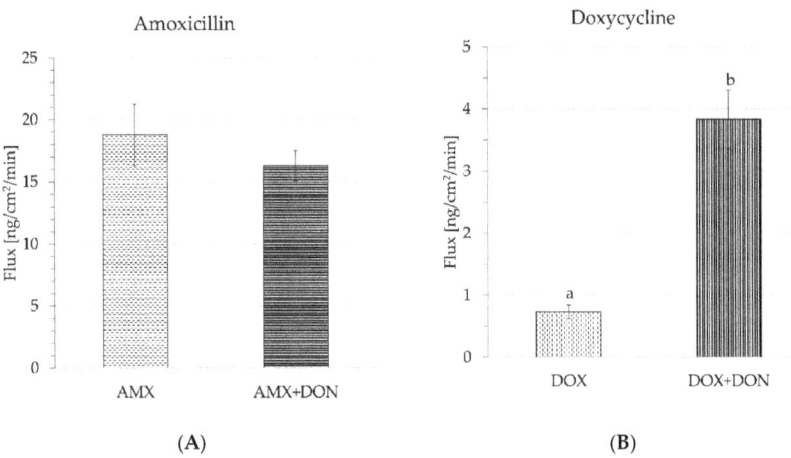

Figure 6. Effect of DON on the transport of antibiotics through intestine explants during 90 min of incubation. (**A**) Transport of AMX used alone (AMX) and in the presence of DON (AMX + DON); (**B**) Transport of DOX used alone (DOX) and in the presence of DON (DOX + DON). Bars show the mean of the 6 replicates ± SEM (standard errors of the mean). Different letters above the bars indicate a statistically significant difference at p-value < 0.05.

3. Discussion

Due to their ubiquitous presence, mycotoxins affect the health of humans and animals consuming plant-based food and feeds. Financial losses caused by mycotoxins occur because of decreased crop yields, loss of crop value, effects on domestic animal productivity, and human health impacts. In the framework of the presented study, the toxic effect of DON on pig jejunum was confirmed. The results obtained with the alternative model of jejunum mucosa explants isolated from routinely slaughtered, clinically healthy adult pigs delivered evidence of DON potency to decrease mucosa barrier integrity and increase its permeability. A significant drop of TEER values over the time of tissue incubation in the presence of the mycotoxin proved progressively declining integrity of intestine explants (Figure 1), which confirms previous observations from cell- and tissue-based experiments [11,20,21]. Modification of TEER values indicate disturbances in epithelial barrier function or the transcellular permeability of ions [11]. Since the rate of caffeine, a transcellular transport marker, translocation remained unaffected in the presence of DON (Figure 4), it is concluded that the toxin does not affect this transportation pathway. Our finding of increased paracellular permeability measured by enhanced penetration of LY and MAN, two markers of paracellular transport, from luminal to contraluminal compartment (Figures 2 and 3) is in line with remarks of others [11,20,22]. A significant difference between the results generated herein and data collected by others is the relatively high dose of DON engaged by us. However, the differences in sample collection, especially the use of adult pigs as explant donors, seem to justify the discrepancies, as discussed previously [23]. Nevertheless, presented data confirm the potency of DON to increase intestine permeability and affect the absorption rate of chemicals and other antigens present in the lumen of the gut at the same time as the mycotoxin.

Most of the toxicological data refers to the effects of chemical contaminants when present alone; however, animals are usually exposed to cocktails of numerous compounds, which might impact their health [14]. In animal production, concurrent oral exposure to mycotoxins and veterinary medicinal products cannot be ruled out. The One Health strategy turns attention to the consequences of the combined presence of antimicrobials and intestine-affecting mycotoxins, in particular DON. To understand the interactions between DON and antimicrobials, we have selected two popular antibiotics used to control infectious diseases in pigs, i.e., amoxicillin and doxycycline. First-line antibiotics are among the most commonly used antibiotics in food-producing animals, including pigs.

Moreover, these antibiotics are often used orally after mixing with feed or dissolved in drinking water. According to the new AMEG categorisation, both amoxicillin and doxycycline belong to Category D "Prudence", meaning the risk to public health associated with the use in veterinary medicine of substances included in this category is considered low [24]. To maintain the usefulness of AMX and DOX, it is crucial to keep their dosing adequate for effectiveness and, simultaneously, to cause no risk of remaining residues in animal-origin products. For both studies, antibiotics have a potency of augmented absorption under favourable conditions like those induced by gut barrier permeability enhancers, including DON. Enhanced absorption of antibiotics from the gastrointestinal tract might influence their pharmacokinetic parameters. Consequently, their pharmacodynamic activity might pose the risk of prolonged presence of antibiotics in animal bodies, contributing to the development of bacterial resistance, environmental persistence, and ecotoxicity.

According to the results presented herein, none of the tested antibiotics possesses the ability to influence intestine integrity and permeability, and they also do not contract the disturbances induced by DON (Figures 1–5). Intestine disturbances provoked by DON did not affect the intensity of AMX penetration across mucosa explants under proposed experimental conditions (Figure 6A), but increased DOX transport by about five times (Figure 6B).

To the best of our knowledge, there is no other trial analysing AMX or other aminopenicillins' representative absorption intensity in the presence of mycotoxins in pigs. Regarding DOX, Goossens et al. [13] observed that the plasma concentration of DOX was remarkably higher in the pigs that received DON-contaminated feed supplemented with the mycotoxin binder. In pigs exposed solely to DON, there was only a small, statistically insignificant, increase of mean plasma DOX concentration compared to control animals [13]. The possible explanation for the discrepancies between quoted data and our results is using different experimental conditions and doses of the mycotoxin in both studies. In our study, we observe a clear effect of DON on the transport of DOX under conditions controlled for the presence of all substances that may affect the absorption process. Goossens points out in his research, that feed ingredients other than DON can influence the absorption of DOX [13].

Based on the obtained results, it is impossible to define the mechanism of the observed interactions between DON and DOX. The analysis of markers flux in the presence of both DON and DOX, indicating that the intensification of paracellular transport is more probable than the enhancement of transcellular absorption. However, it is possible to hypothesise that DOX and DON compete against access to glycoprotein P (GPP).

Studies in the field of pharmacokinetics indicate that DOX, applied in therapeutic doses, absorbs from swine gut according to the first-order kinetics [25–28]. This means that the intensity of DOX absorption depends only on the concentration of the antibiotic, and there is no need to consider other mechanisms involved in the transportation process. Even if an additional transport mechanism for DOX is recognised (efflux involving GPP) and happens in pigs during the absorption phase in the gut, its impact on total DOX transportation is not limited by the accessibility of transport mechanism (the presence of such mechanism does not need to be included in the kinetic equation for DOX absorption).

The observations and conclusions from pharmacokinetic studies align with our experiment's conditions because the concentrations of DOX and AMX in the mucosal chamber are similar to those measured in vivo in the intestine. The concentrations of the antibiotics applied in the study presented herein, i.e., AMX = 50 µg/mL, DOX = 30 µg/mL, represent the preliminary concentrations of those drugs in the gut lumen when administered orally with drinking water in pigs. The recommended dose of AMX in pigs is 10–20 mg/kg b.w. every 12 h [29]. Moreover, the recommended dose of DOX amounts to 10 mg/kg b.w. every 12 h [30]. Assuming treated pigs' average daily water intake comes to 0.1 L/kg b.w., AMX and DOX should be applied at the concentration of 150 µg and 100 µL per 1 mL of drinking water, respectively. When an antibiotic is drunk once by a pig, it gets diluted 2–4 fold by the content of the stomach and intestine before it gets absorbed. Hence, the expected concentration of selected antibiotics at the beginning of the jejunum absorption phase amounts to 50 and 30 µg/mL for AMX and DOX, respectively.

Our observation of increased intensity of DOX transportation across mucosa explant in the presence of DON suggests the involvement of a mechanism which amplifies the penetration of DOX from mucosal to serosal chamber. These findings cannot be explained only as a consequence of increased mucosa barrier permeability (induced by DON) and subsequent enhancement of the paracellular transport of DOX because the first-order absorption kinetic of DOX (observed in pharmacokinetic studies) means that only the concentration of DOX determines absorption. In other words, the assumptions of first-order kinetics result in unlimited DOX penetration by paracellular transport, which already occurs under control conditions (DON-free medium). Another possibility includes the switching out of a transport mechanism, which is in opposition to the absorption of DOX and which, in the presence of DON, occurs as an important component determining the penetration of DOX across the mucosa barrier. Therefore, it is speculated that in the presence of DON, the mechanism of efflux transport of DOX is revealed as a significant factor influencing the intensity of DOX absorption from the gut. The increase of DOX transportation in the presence of DON possibly depends on transport by GPP. There is evidence that GPP transports DON, and acting on GPP may affect the transport of other drugs [31–33]. Martinez et al. (2013) observed that concurrent exposure of IPEC-J2 cells to fosfomycin (580 µg/mL) and DON (1 µg/mL) resulted in a remarkably higher intracellular concentration of the antibiotic in the enterocytes, confirming the potency of DON to enhance drug penetration from the lumen of the gut [16]. DOX is also transported via GPP [34,35]. GPP is responsible for the transport of DOX from the enterocytes' cytoplasm to the gastrointestinal tract's lumen (efflux transport).

The results presented herein demonstrate that there is a possible competition between DON and DOX against GPP. The mycotoxin, as a compound of higher affinity to GPP, might block the efflux of DOX if the efflux mechanism of DOX is switched out. The transportation of the antibiotic increases what is indicated by the enhanced flux of DOX across the intestine.

Regardless of the mechanism of DON's impact on DOX absorption, and bearing in mind the assumptions of pharmacokinetic model describing DOX absorption from the gut, the first-order kinetic must be ruled out at the co-occurrence of DOX and DON.

4. Conclusions

In summary, DON intensifies the transportation of DOX across the porcine gut wall but displays no impact on AMX absorption. The increase of DOX penetration might result from reduced availability of the GGP efflux transport system for the antibiotic. Such an effect of DON can cause remarkable changes in DOX pharmacokinetics and affect the pharmacodynamic properties and safety of DOX in pigs.

The results presented herein justify further in vivo research on DON's impact on DOX absorption, bioavailability, and excretion to realise consumer exposure, environmental persistence, and ecotoxicity.

Bearing in mind that climate change globally, the fungal population and mycotoxin patterns in different regions and crops are changing [36]. Their impact on animal health and the potency of inducing interaction with other xenobiotics, including antimicrobials, should not be underestimated and requires more in-depth investigation.

5. Materials and Methods

5.1. Chemicals

Caffeine (CAF), Cytotoxicity Detection Kit (LDH) Roche, D-mannitol (MAN), D-Mannitol Colorimetric Assay Kit, disodium fumarate, deoxynivalenol (DON), L-glutamate, lucifer yellow (LY), and sodium pyruvate were obtained from Sigma Aldrich (St. Louis, MO, USA). All inorganic salts required for preparing Krebs Bicarbonate Buffer (KRB), ethanol, and glucose were purchased from Avantor (Gliwice, Poland). Amoxicillin trihydrate (AMX) and doxycycline hyclate (DOX) were generously donated by the pharmaceutical company Biofaktor Sp. z o.o. (Skierniewice, Poland) The quality of antibiotics was consistent with the monographs of the European Pharmacopoeia and corresponded to the quality of active substances used in the production of veterinary drugs.

Tissue transportation, preparation, and incubation were performed in Krebs Bicarbonate Buffer (KRB) containing 108 mM NaCl, 4.7 mM KCl, 1.8 mM Na_2HPO_4, 0.4 mM KH_2PO_4, 15 mM $NaHCO_3$, 1.2 mM $MgSO_4$, 1.25 mM $CaCl_2$, 11.5 mM glucose, 4.9 mM L-glutamate, 5.4 mM disodium furmate, and 4.9 mM sodium pyruvate at pH 7.4, and saturated with oxygen using a 95%/5% O_2/CO_2 mixture by gassing for 60 min [37].

For HPLC and LC-MS/MS analysis, acetonitrile, methanol, and formic acid (HPLC grade) were obtained from Avantor Chemicals (Radnor, PA, USA), trichloracetic acid and heptafluorobutyric acid were obtained from Sigma Aldrich (St. Louis, MO, USA).

5.2. Tissue Preparation

Healthy female and male (60%:40%) adult landrace and large white pigs of approx. 100 kg body weight subjected to routine slaughtering were used for the collection of intestinal tissue. In total 18 animals were used as tissue donors. Segments of the jejunum (approx. 150 cm aboral to pylorus) were obtained and handled as described in other research [21–23,38–40],. Briefly, jejunum pieces of approx. 50 cm in length were gently incised immediately after stunning and flushed to remove intestine content. Next, the samples were immersed in ice-cold KRB and brought to the laboratory where they were subjected to the preparation. Firstly, they were cut into pieces of 10–20 cm and opened longitudinally. Secondly, the serosa and muscular layers were carefully stripped from the mucosa using forceps. Eventually, four mucosa explants were gained from each animal. Each resulting sheet of mucosa with attached submucosa was mounted separately between two Ussing-type half chambers (1.54 cm^2 tissue exposure area). Jejunum sheets were bathed on luminal (mucosal) and contraluminal (serosal) surfaces in 10 mL of KRB, maintained at pH 7.4 and 37 °C. Mucosa explants were continuously oxygenated on luminal and contraluminal surfaces with a 95%/5% O_2/CO_2 mixture delivered by gas lift. The complete system was firstly preincubated for 10 min for the equilibration of the tissue. Afterwards, the incubation medium was replaced by fresh KRB in the serosal chamber, and KRB supplemented with LY in concentration 100 µg/mL, mannitol 100 µg/mL, and caffeine 100 µg/mL (KRB + LY + MAN + CAF) in the mucosal chamber.

5.3. Measurement of the Viability, Integrity, and Permeability of Mucosa Explants

The viability of the swine jejunal mucosa sheet was analysed by measuring several markers directly after preincubation (time 0), and 30, 60 and 90 min afterward. The integrity of mucosa explants was controlled by measuring transepithelial electrical resistance (TEER) using a Millicell ERS-2 Epithelial Volt-Ohm Meter (Merck GA, Darmstadt, Germany). The prerequisite of TEER readings greater than 70 $\Omega \cdot cm^2$ at time 0 was settled to verify jejunum preparations' usefulness for other parts of the experiment. Additionally, the integrity and viability of the explants were verified by measuring the flux of LY, MAN, and CAF over time from the luminal to the contraluminal compartment. To assess the possible tissue damage caused by the presence of active proteases or experiment duration, the leakage of lactate dehydrogenase (LDH) to both the mucosal and serosal compartments was recorded.

5.4. Ex Vivo Exposure of Swine Jejunum to Deoxynivalenol and Antibiotics

Four explants of jejunum mucosa were prepared from each pig and fixed separately in Ussing-type chambers. All explants underwent 10-min preincubation followed by 90-min incubation in KRB (serosal chamber). In the mucosal chamber, pure KRB was replaced by: (i) KRB + LY + MAN + CAF with neither addition of DON nor AMX nor DOX (control condition), (ii) KRB + LY + MAN + CAF supplemented with DON (30 µg/mL), (iii) KRB + LY + MAN + CAF containing DON (30 µg/mL) and AMX (50 µg/mL) or DOX (30 µg/mL), (iv) KRB + LY + MAN + CAF containing AMX or DOX (50 and 30 µg/mL, respectively). After the KRB exchange in the luminal compartment, the incubation was continued for another 90 min. TEER measurement and sample collection (800 µL) for later LY, MAN, CAF, LDH, DON, and AMX or DOX assays were carried out at times 0, 30, 60 and 90 min after the onset of incubation.

5.5. Analyses

LY was analysed directly in samples using an FLx800 Microplate fluorescence reader (BioTek Instruments, Inc., Winooski, VT, USA) at excitation wavelength 485 nm and emission wavelength 530 nm. According to the manufacturer's instructions, MAN concentration and LDH activity were determined using a D-Mannitol Colorimetric Assay Kit and Cytotoxicity Detection Kit (LDH) Roche.

CAF concentration was analysed by the HPLC-UV method as follows. The sample was centrifuged, and the supernatant was filtered through a 0.22 µm filter. Next, 20 µL of filtered samples were injected into the HP 1100 HPLC system consisting of a quaternary pump, thermostatic autosampler, sample thermostat, column thermostat, and diode array detector. The system was fitted with a Nucleosil® 120-5C18 HPLC (250 mm × 4.6 mm, 5 µm) column (Supelco, Bellefonte, PA, USA). The mobile phase was methanol. The flow rate was 1 mL/min. Detection was performed at a wavelength of 254 nm (ref. 360 nm). The analytes were identified with retention times of pure reference standards. The reference standards were also used to prepare a standard solution to establish calibration curves. Chromatographic peak areas of the analytes were measured using the integrator software for the HPLC system (Agilent ChemStation Rev. A.06.01 [403] Hewlett Packard Company, Palo Alto, CA, USA).

For the extraction of DOX and AMX, 100 µL of cell fluid collected from the serosal chamber was placed into a 1.5 mL microcentrifuge tube, then 20 µL of IS and 100 µL of 5% trichloracetic acid (DOX)/0.1% formic acid (AMX) were added, mixed, diluted, and centrifuged at 14,500× g for 5 min. The supernatant was filtered through a 0.22 µm PVDF syringe filter into an LC vial for UHPLC-MS/MS analysis.

The analysis of antibiotics was performed using ultra-high-performance liquid chromatography with detection by triple quadrupole mass spectrometry (UHPLC-MS/MS: Shimadzu Nexera X2, Kyoto, Japan coupled with QTRAP 4500, AB Sciex, Framingham, MA, USA.). The following parameters were used: temperature—450 °C; curtain gas (N_2)—20; nebuliser gas (N_2)—60; collision gas (N_2)—medium; auxiliary gas—65; ion spray voltage—4500 V (Table 1).

Table 1. Detailed MS/MS conditions of doxycycline and amoxicillin analysis.

Analyte	Parent Ion M + H$^+$ [m/z]	Daughter Ions [m/z]	DP [V]	CE [eV]	Dwell Time [ms]
Doxycycline (444.4 g/mol)	445.4	428.0; 154.0	60	24; 41	250
Amoxicillin (365.4 g/mol)	366.1	349.0; 208.0	45	12; 18	250

The chromatographic separation assay was performed using an Agilent InfinityLab Poroshell 120 EC-C18 (150 mm × 2.1 mm, 2.7 μm) column (Agilent, St. Clara, CA, USA) with an octadecyl guard column (2 × 4 mm) maintained at 35 °C. The mobile phase consisted of 0.025% heptafluorobutyric acid (A) and acetonitrile (B) at a flow rate of 0.3 mL/min, with an injection volume of 5 μL. Gradient elution for AMX was conducted as follows: 0–1 min 95% A, 5–8 min 20% A, 8–8.01 min 50% A, and finally from 8.01 to 10 min back to 95% A; for DOX 0–5 min 50% A, 5–6 min 10% A, 6–8 min 10% A, and finally from 8.01 to 10 min back to 95% A The total run time in both cases was 10 min.

The method has been validated. LOQ values (DOX 0.01 ng/L, AMX 0.02 ng/L), linearity, reproducibility (CV: DOX 5.6–8.7%, AMX 7.7–10.0%), and recovery (DOX 85–105%, AMX 90–97%) were determined.

The results of LY, MAN, CAF, AMX, and DOX penetration across intestine mucosa explants are expressed as mass flux. The amount of LDH leakage into the incubation media is expressed as a percentage of total LDH, which was analysed after explants homogenisation in ice-cold KRB with a Potter S Homogenizer (B. Braun Biotech International, Berlin, Germany) for 2 min at 1000 rpm.

5.6. Statistical Analysis

The experimental result is expressed as means ± SEM. Differences between groups were statistically determined using one-way ANOVA followed by Tukey's multiple comparisons test or t-test if only two groups were compared. Results were considered statistically significant when $p < 0.05$.

Analyses were performed using GraphPad Prism version 8.0.0 for Windows, GraphPad Software, San Diego, CA, USA, www.graphpad.com.

Author Contributions: Conceptualization, M.M. and P.J.; Data curation, W.K.; Formal analysis, M.M., W.K., M.C. and E.N.-K.; Funding acquisition, P.J.; Investigation, M.M., W.K., U.L., M.C., E.N.-K. and K.P.; Methodology, M.M. and P.J.; Project administration, P.J.; Software, W.K. and E.N.-K.; Writing—original draft, M.M., U.L., M.C., E.N.-K. and K.P.; Writing—review and editing, M.M., W.K. and P.J. All authors have read and agreed to the published version of the manuscript.

Funding: This research was funded by the National Science Centre Poland, grant number UMO-2016/23/B/N27/02273.

Institutional Review Board Statement: Not applicable.

Informed Consent Statement: Not applicable.

Data Availability Statement: Not applicable.

Conflicts of Interest: The authors declare no conflict of interest.

References

1. Gruber-Dorninger, C.; Jenkins, T.; Schatzmayr, G. Global Mycotoxin Occurrence in Feed: A Ten-Year Survey. *Toxins* **2019**, *11*, 375. [CrossRef] [PubMed]
2. Khodaei, D.; Javanmardi, F.; Khaneghah, A.M. The global overview of the occurrence of mycotoxins in cereals: A three-year survey. *Curr. Opin. Food Sci.* **2021**, *39*, 36–42. [CrossRef]
3. Palumbo, R.; Crisci, A.; Venâncio, A.; Cortiñas Abrahantes, J.; Dorne, J.-L.; Battilani, P.; Toscano, P. Occurrence and Co-Occurrence of Mycotoxins in Cereal-Based Feed and Food. *Microorganisms* **2020**, *8*, 74. [CrossRef] [PubMed]
4. Santos Pereira, C.; Cunha, C.S.; Fernandes, J.O. Prevalent Mycotoxins in Animal Feed: Occurrence and Analytical Methods. *Toxins* **2019**, *11*, 290. [CrossRef]
5. Munkvold, G.P.; Arias, S.; Taschl, I.; Gruber-Dorninger, C. Mycotoxins in Corn: Occurrence, Impacts, and Management. In *Corn. Chemistry and Technology*, 3rd ed.; Serna-Saldivar, S.O., Ed.; Elsevier Inc. in Cooperation with AACC International: Duxford, UK, 2019; pp. 235–287. [CrossRef]
6. Panasiuk, L.; Jedziniak, P.; Pietruszka, K.; Piatkowska, M.; Bocian, L. Frequency and levels of regulated and emerging mycotoxins in silage in Poland. *Mycotoxin Res.* **2019**, *35*, 17–25. [CrossRef]
7. Cheng, Y.H.; Weng, C.F.; Chen, B.J.; Chang, M.H. Toxicity of different Fusarium mycotoxins on growth performance, immune responses and efficacy of a mycotoxin degrading enzyme in pigs. *Anim Res.* **2006**, *55*, 579–590. [CrossRef]
8. Martínez, G.; Diéguez, S.N.; Fernández Paggi, M.B.; Riccio, M.B.; Pérez Gaudio, D.S.; Rodríguez, E.; Amanto, F.A.; Tapia, M.O.; Soraci, A.L. Effect of fosfomycin, Cynara scolymus extract, deoxynivalenol and their combinations on intestinal health of weaned piglets. *Animal Nutr.* **2019**, *5*, 386–395. [CrossRef]
9. Pinton, P.; Accensi, F.; Beauchamp, E.; Cossalter, A.M.; Callu, P.; Grosjean, F.; Oswald, I.P. Ingestion of deoxynivalenol (DON) contaminated feed alters the pig vaccinal immune responses. *Toxicol. Lett.* **2008**, *177*, 215–222. [CrossRef]
10. Rotter, B.A. Toxicology of deoxynivalenol (vomitoxin). *J. Toxicol. Environ. Health* **1996**, *48*, 1–34. [CrossRef]
11. Pinton, P.; Nougayrede, J.P.; del Rio, J.C.; Moreno, C.; Marin, D.; Ferrier, L.; Barcarense, A.P.; Kolf-Clauw, M.; Oswald, I.P. The food contaminant, deoxynivalenol, decreases intestinal barrier function and reduces claudin expression. *Toxicol. Appl. Pharmacol.* **2009**, *237*, 41–48. [CrossRef]
12. Pestka, J.J.; Zhou, H.R.; Moon, Y.; Chung, Y.J. Cellular and molecular mechanisms for immune modulation by deoxynivalenol and other trichothecenes: Unraveling a paradox. *Toxicol. Lett.* **2004**, *153*, 61–73. [CrossRef] [PubMed]
13. Goossens, J.; Vandenbroucke, V.; Pasmans, F.; De Baere, S.; Devreese, M.; Ossclaere, A.; Verbrugghe, E.; Haesebrouck, F.; De Saeger, S.; Eeckhout, M.; et al. Influence of Mycotoxins and a Mycotoxin Adsorbing Agent on the Oral Bioavailability of Commonly Used Antibiotics in Pigs. *Toxins* **2012**, *4*, 281–295. [CrossRef] [PubMed]
14. Le, T.H.; Alassane-Kpembi, I.; Oswald, I.P.; Pinton, P. Analysis of the interactions between environmental and food contaminants, cadmium and deoxynivalenol, in different target organs. *Sci. Total Environ.* **2018**, *622–623*, 841–848. [CrossRef] [PubMed]
15. Maresca, M.; Mahfoud, R.; Garmy, N.; Fantini, J. The mycotoxin deoxynivalenol affects nutrient absorption in human intestinal epithelial cells. *J. Nutr.* **2002**, *132*, 2723–2731. [CrossRef] [PubMed]
16. Martinez, G.; Perez, D.S.; Soraci, A.L.; Tapia, M.O. Penetration of Fosfomycin into IPEC-J2 Cells in the Presence or Absence of Deoxynivalenol. *PLoS ONE* **2013**, *8*, e75068. [CrossRef]
17. Leung, E.; Weil, D.E.; Raviglionea MNakatania, H. World Health Organization World Health Day Antimicrobial Resistance Technical Working Group. The WHO policy package to combat antimicrobial resistance. *Bull. World Health Organ.* **2011**, *89*, 390–392. [CrossRef]
18. Wei, R.; Ge, F.; Huang, S.; Chen, M.; Wang, R. Occurrence of veterinary antibiotics in animal wastewater and surface water around farms in Jiangsu Province, China. *Chemosphere* **2011**, *82*, 1408–1414. [CrossRef]
19. Ungemach, F.R.; Muller-Bahrdt, D.; Abraham, G. Guidelines for prudent use of antimicrobials and their implications on antibiotic usage in veterinary medicine. *Int. J. Med. Microbiol.* **2006**, *296* (Suppl. S41), 33–38. [CrossRef]
20. Akbari, P.; Braber, S.; Alizadeh, A.; Verheijden, K.A.T.; Schoterman, M.H.C.; Kraneveld, A.D.; Garssen, J.; Fink-Gremmels, J. Galacto-oligosaccharides protect the Intestinal Barrier by Maintaining the Tight Junction Network and Modulating the Inflammatory Responses after a Challenge with the Mycotoxin Deoxynivalenol in Human Caco-2 Cell Monolayers and B6C3F1 Mice. *J. Nutr.* **2015**, *145*, 1604–1613. [CrossRef]
21. Halawa, A.; Dänicke, S.; Kersten, S.; Breves, G. Effects of deoxynivalenol and lipopolysaccharide on electrophysiological parameters in growing pigs. *Mycotoxin Res.* **2012**, *28*, 243–252. [CrossRef]
22. García, G.R.; Payros, D.; Pinton, P.; Dogi, C.A.; Laffitte, J.; Neves, M.; González Pereyra, M.L.; Cavaglieri, L.R.; Oswald, I.P. Intestinal toxicity of deoxynivalenol is limited by Lactobacillus rhamnosus RC007 in pig jejunum explants. *Arch. Toxicol.* **2018**, *92*, 983–993. [CrossRef] [PubMed]
23. Mendel, M.; Karlik, W.; Chłopecka, M. The impact of chlorophyllin on deoxynivalenol transport across jejunum mucosa explants obtained from adult pigs. *Mycotoxin Res.* **2019**, *35*, 187–196. [CrossRef] [PubMed]
24. EMA/CVMP/CHMP/682198/2017; Categorisation of Antibiotics in the European Union. European Medicinces Agency: Amsterdam, The Netherlands, 12 December 2019.
25. Baert, K.; Croubels, S.; Gasthuys, F.; de Busser, J.; de Backer, P. Pharmacokinetics and oral bioavailability of a doxycycline formulation (DOXYCYCLINE 75%) in nonfasted young pigs. *J. Vet. Pharmacol. Ther.* **2000**, *23*, 45–48. [CrossRef] [PubMed]
26. Bousquet, E.; Nouws, J.; Terlouw, P.; de Kleyne, S. Pharmacokinetics of doxycycline in pigs following oral administration in feed. *Vet. Res. BioMed. Cent.* **1998**, *29*, 475–485. Available online: https://hal.archives-ouvertes.fr/hal-00902540 (accessed on 1 October 2022).

27. Prats, C.; El Korchi, G.; Giralt, M.; Cristofol, C.; Pena, J.; Zorrilla, I.; Saborit, J.; Perez, B. PK and PK/PD of doxycycline in drinking water after therapeutic use in pigs. *J. Vet. Pharmacol. Ther.* **2005**, *28*, 525–530. [CrossRef] [PubMed]
28. Sanders, P.; Gicquel, M.; Hurtaud, D.; Chapel, A.M.; Gaudiche, C.; Bousquet, E. Absolute bioavailability of doxycycline after oral administration in medicated feed to pigs. In Proceedings of the International Pig Veterinary Society 14th Congress, Bologna, Italy, 7–10 July 1996; p. 663.
29. Papaich, M.G.; Rivere, J.E. β-lactam antibiotics: Penicillins, cephalosporins, and related drugs. In *Veterinary Pharmacology and Therapeutics*, 9th ed.; Riviere, J.E., Papich, M.G., Adams, H.R., Eds.; Wiley-Blackwell: Oxford, UK, 2009; pp. 865–893.
30. Papaich, M.G.; Rivere, J.E. Tetracycline Antibiotics. In *Veterinary Pharmacology and Therapeutics*, 9th ed.; Riviere, J.E., Papich, M.G., Adams, H.R., Eds.; Wiley-Blackwell: Oxford, UK, 2009; pp. 895–913.
31. Ivanova, L.; Fæste, C.K.; Solhaug, A. Role of P-glycoprotein in deoxynivalenol-mediated in vitro toxicity. *Toxicol. Lett.* **2018**, *284*, 21–28. [CrossRef]
32. Li, X.; Mu, P.; Wen, J.; Deng, Y. Carrier-Mediated and Energy-Dependent Uptake and Efflux of Deoxynivalenol in Mammalian Cells. *Sci. Rep.* **2017**, *7*, 5889. [CrossRef]
33. Videmann, B.; Tep, J.; Cavret, S.; Lecoeur, S. Epithelial transport of deoxynivalenol: Involvement of human P-glycoprotein (ABCB1) and multidrug resistance-associated protein 2 (ABCC2). *Food Chem. Toxicol.* **2007**, *45*, 1938–1947. [CrossRef]
34. Mealey, K.L.; Barhoumi, R.; Burghardt, R.C.; Safe, S.; Kochevar, D.T. Doxycycline induces expression of P glycoprotein in MCF-7 breast carcinoma cells. *Antimicrob. Agents Chemother.* **2002**, *46*, 755–761. [CrossRef]
35. Agbedanu, P.N.; Anderson, K.L.; Brewer, M.T.; Carlson, S.A. Doxycycline as an inhibitor of p-glycoprotein in the alpaca for the purpose of maintaining avermectins in the CNS during treatment for parelaphostrongylosis. *Vet. Parasitol.* **2015**, *212*, 303–307. [CrossRef]
36. Eskola, M.; Kos, G.; Elliott, C.T.; Hajšlová, J.; Mayar, S.; Krska, R. Worldwide contamination of food-crops with mycotoxins: Validity of the widely cited 'FAO estimate' of 25. *Crit. Rev. Food Sci. Nutr.* **2020**, *60*, 2773–2789. [CrossRef] [PubMed]
37. Ungell, A.L.; Andreasson, A.; Lundin, K.; Utter, L. Effects of enzymatic inhibition and increased paracellular shunting on transport of vasopressin analogues in the rat. *J. Pharm. Sci.* **1992**, *87*, 640–645. [CrossRef] [PubMed]
38. Lucioli, J.; Pinton, P.; Callu, P.; Laffitte, J.; Grosjean, F.; Kolf-Clauw, M.; Oswald, I.P.; Bracarense, A.P. The food contaminant deoxynivalenol activates the mitogen activated protein kinases in the intestine: Interest of ex vivo models as an alternative to in vivo experiments. *Toxicon* **2013**, *66*, 31–36. [CrossRef] [PubMed]
39. Westerhout, J.; van de Steeg, E.; Grossouw, D.; Zeijdner, E.E.; Krul, C.A.M.; Verwei, M.; Wortelboer, H.M. A new approach to predict human intestinal absorption using porcine intestinal tissue and biorelevant matrices. *Eur. J. Parmac. Sci.* **2014**, *63*, 167–177. [CrossRef] [PubMed]
40. Sjöberg, Å.; Lutz, M.; Tannergren, C.; Wingolf, C.; Borde, A.; Ungell, A.L. Comprehensive study on regional human intestinal permeability and prediction of fraction absorbed of drugs using the Ussing chamber technique. *Eur. J. Pharm. Sci.* **2013**, *48*, 166–180. [CrossRef]

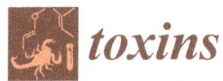

Article

Carry-Over of Zearalenone and Its Metabolites to Intestinal Tissues and the Expression of CYP1A1 and GSTπ1 in the Colon of Gilts before Puberty

Magdalena Mróz [1], Magdalena Gajęcka [1,*], Paweł Brzuzan [2], Sylwia Lisieska-Żołnierczyk [3], Dawid Leski [4], Łukasz Zielonka [1] and Maciej T. Gajęcki [1]

[1] Department of Veterinary Prevention and Feed Hygiene, Faculty of Veterinary Medicine, University of Warmia and Mazury in Olsztyn, Oczapowskiego 13/29, 10-718 Olsztyn, Poland; magdalena.mroz@uwm.edu.pl (M.M.); lukaszz@uwm.edu.pl (Ł.Z.); gajecki@uwm.edu.pl (M.T.G.)
[2] Department of Environmental Biotechnology, Faculty of Environmental Sciences and Fisheries, University of Warmia and Mazury in Olsztyn, Słoneczna 45G, 10-719 Olsztyn, Poland; brzuzan@uwm.edu.pl
[3] Independent Public Health Care Centre of the Ministry of the Interior and Administration, and the Warmia and Mazury Oncology Centre in Olsztyn, Wojska Polskiego 37, 10-228 Olsztyn, Poland; lisieska@wp.pl
[4] Research and Development Department, Wipasz S.A., Wadąg 9, 10-373 Wadąg, Poland; dawid.leski@wipasz.pl
* Correspondence: mgaja@uwm.edu.pl; Tel.: +48-89-523-3773; Fax: +48-89-523-3618

Abstract: The objective of this study was to evaluate whether low doses of zearalenone (ZEN) affect the carry-over of ZEN and its metabolites to intestinal tissues and the expression of CYP1A1 and GSTπ1 in the large intestine. Prepubertal gilts (with a BW of up to 14.5 kg) were exposed in group ZEN to daily ZEN5 doses of 5 μg/kg BW ($n = 15$); in group ZEN10, 10 μg/kg BW ($n = 15$); in group ZEN15, 15 μg/kg BW ($n = 15$); or were administered a placebo (group C, $n = 15$) throughout the experiment. After euthanasia, tissues were sampled on exposure days 7, 21, and 42 (D1, D2, and D3, respectively). The results confirmed that the administered ZEN doses (LOAEL, NOAEL, and MABEL) were appropriate to reliably assess the carry-over of ZEN. Based on the observations made during 42 days of exposure to pure ZEN, it can be hypothesized that all mycotoxins (ZEN, α-zearalenol, and β-zearalenol) contribute to a balance between intestinal cells and the expression of selected genes encoding enzymes that participate in biotransformation processes in the large intestine; modulate feminization processes in prepubertal gilts; and elicit flexible, adaptive responses of the macroorganism to mycotoxin exposure at the analyzed doses.

Keywords: zearalenone; low dose; intestines; carry-over; CYP1A1 and GSTπ1; prepubertal gilts

Key Contribution: Zearalenone mycotoxicosis in a dose of MABEL plays a beneficial role in the processes of somatic development of prepubertal gilts, which is important for breeders. The question arises—should one perform ZEN detoxification in doses of MABEL in feed materials or animal feed?

Citation: Mróz, M.; Gajęcka, M.; Brzuzan, P.; Lisieska-Żołnierczyk, S.; Leski, D.; Zielonka, Ł.; Gajęcki, M.T. Carry-Over of Zearalenone and Its Metabolites to Intestinal Tissues and the Expression of CYP1A1 and GSTπ1 in the Colon of Gilts before Puberty. *Toxins* **2022**, *14*, 354. https://doi.org/10.3390/toxins14050354

Received: 20 April 2022
Accepted: 17 May 2022
Published: 18 May 2022

Publisher's Note: MDPI stays neutral with regard to jurisdictional claims in published maps and institutional affiliations.

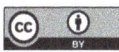

Copyright: © 2022 by the authors. Licensee MDPI, Basel, Switzerland. This article is an open access article distributed under the terms and conditions of the Creative Commons Attribution (CC BY) license (https://creativecommons.org/licenses/by/4.0/).

1. Introduction

Zearalenone is an undesirable substance that is widely encountered in cereal kernels and cereal products [1]. It is produced mainly by *Fusarium graminearum* as a metabolite with estrogenic properties. Pure ZEN is a white crystalline compound with the chemical formula $C_{18}H_{22}O_5$, a molecular mass of 318.36 g/mol, and a melting temperature range of 161–163 °C. Zearalenone is not soluble in water, but it dissolves easily in alkaline solutions, ether, benzene, methanol, and ethanol. This mycotoxin can be metabolized by various organisms during phase I and II biotransformation processes [2]. Feeds contain modified forms of ZEN (ZELs), including phase I biotransformation products such as α-zearalenol, β-zearalenol, α-zearalanol, β-zearalanol, and zearalanon, as well as phase II biotransformation products conjugated with glucose, sulfate, and glucuronic acid. The presence of ZEN in the food chain can pose a health threat to humans and livestock [3]. This promiscuous compound induces the expression of estrogen receptors [4], contributes to reproductive disorders, and can even lead to changes in reproductive organs. Zearalenone also disrupts the hormonal balance [2,5,6], metabolic profile [7], and gut microbiota [8]. It exerts hepatotoxic [9,10], immunotoxic [11], hematotoxic [12], and genotoxic effects [13].

In humans and animals, ingested ZEN initially interacts with the gastrointestinal system [14]. Two research problems can be formulated in this stage. Firstly, ZEN's influence on intestinal health [15,16] and its carry-over from the intestinal digesta to intestinal tissues [16] has attracted considerable research interest in recent years. Secondly, in line with the hormesis paradigm [17], efforts are being made to evaluate the macroorganism's response to low mycotoxin doses that are frequently encountered in feed materials. Researchers have also attempted to determine tissue and cell dysfunctions in mammals exposed to the pure parent compound without metabolites or modified mycotoxins [4,18]. In view of our previous findings [5,7,8,13], potential clinical symptoms of ZEN mycotoxicosis of varying severity were taken into account. Therefore, three ZEN doses were considered in the interpretation of our previous results and the findings of other authors: the lowest adverse effect observed level (LOAEL, >10 μg ZEN/kg BW) [19–21] that causes clinical symptoms [22]; (ii) the no adverse effect observed level (NOAEL, 10 μg ZEN/kg BW) as the highest dose that does not cause clinical symptoms (sub-clinical states) [23]; and (iii) the minimal anticipated biological effect level (MABEL, <10 ZEN/kg BW) as the lowest dose that can be measured in tissues, entering into positive interactions with the host at various stages in life [24,25].

The observation that mycotoxins modulate the expression of enzymes that participate in phase I and II biotransformation processes [26] was taken into consideration in the current experiment. The biotransformation of undesirable substances, including ZEN and its metabolites, is affected by two types of enzymes in cells. During phase I biotransformation, enzymes such as CYP P450 trigger chemical reactions (hydroxylation) to remove undesirable substances that can act as enzyme substrates [27]. These enzymes exhibit maximum activity in the liver and the small intestine, which are responsible for detoxication. They are also involved in the biosynthesis of steroid hormones [28] and fatty acid metabolism, as well as the activation/inactivation of drugs and other exogenous compounds in the body [29,30]. During phase II biotransformation, metabolic rates can be measured based on the activity of glutathione S-transferase (GST). The rate of biotransformation and the rate at which undesirable feed-borne substances are excreted from the body affect the response of the intestinal mucosal immune system to toxins. The π isoform of glutathione transferase (GSTπ1) codes for various proteins involved in these processes. Glutathione S-transferase reduces the biological activity of various (not only exogenous) substances by creating conjugates of glutathione with electrophilic drugs and other exogenous toxins. These conjugates protect the body against the adverse effects of oxidative stress and prevent damage to lipids and nucleic acids. It is worth noting that conjugates can break down again in the lumen of the gut, thus increasing the concentration of mycotoxins and theoretically increasing the activity of enzymes such as CYP1A1 and GSTπ1 [26,30].

The objective of this study was to determine how in vivo low doses of ZEN (MABEL (5 μg/kg BW), the greatest values of NOAEL (10 μg/kg BW), and LOAEL (15 μg/kg BW)) administered orally for 42 days influence the level of ZEN and selected ZELs in intestinal wall tissues on different dates of exposure and contribute to the expression of genes encoding selected enzymes (CYP1A1 and GSTπ1) in the colon in prepubertal gilts.

2. Results

The present results confirmed that ZEN is biotransformed in the initial stage of the carry-over process when this mycotoxin and its metabolites are transported from the lumen of the gut to the intestinal wall. Parent mycotoxin and its two most widely investigated metabolites (α-ZEL and β-ZEL) are accumulated in this stage.

The above observation was confirmed by the mean concentrations of ZEN and its metabolites in the intestinal wall on different exposure days (see Figure 1). The percentage share of each substance in the total pool was consistent with the anticipated values for pigs, but the carry-over factor (CF) was much lower, which cannot be attributed solely to low-dose ZEN mycotoxicosis.

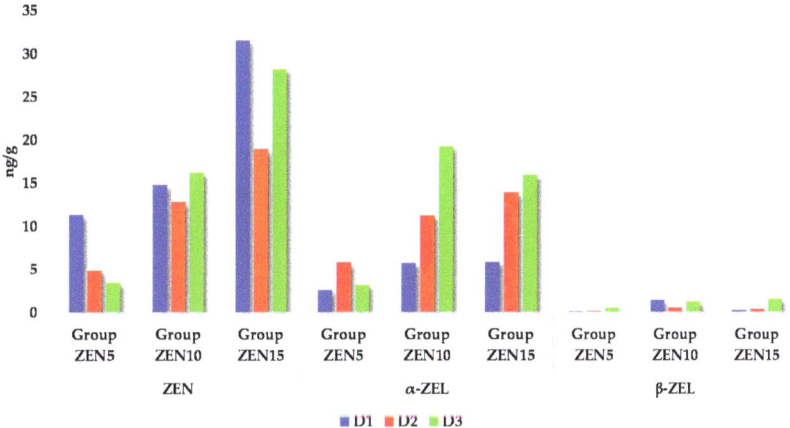

Figure 1. Mean values of ZEN and its metabolites (ng/g) in the intestinal wall in all experimental groups and on each exposure date. Key: D1—exposure day 7; D2—exposure day 21; D3—exposure day 42. Experimental groups: group ZEN5—5 μg ZEN/kg BW; group ZEN10—10 μg ZEN/kg BW; group ZEN15—15 μg ZEN/kg BW.

2.1. Experimental Feed

The analyzed feed did not contain mycotoxins, or its mycotoxin content was below the sensitivity of the method (VBS). The concentrations of masked mycotoxins were not analyzed.

2.2. Clinical Observations

The results presented in this paper were acquired during a large-scale experiment where clinical signs of ZEN mycotoxicosis were not observed. However, changes in specific tissues or cells were frequently noted in analyses of selected serum biochemical parameters, hematological parameters, the heart muscle, the bone marrow microenvironment, coronary artery, the genotoxicity of cecal water, selected steroid concentrations, gut microbiota parameters, and weight gains. Samples for laboratory analyses were collected from the same prepubertal gilts. The results of these analyses were presented in our previous studies [5,7,8,12,13,31,32].

2.3. Concentrations of Zearalenone and Its Metabolites in the Intestinal Tract of Prepubertal Gilts

Significant differences in ZEN levels between exposure date D1 and exposure dates D2 and D3 (see Table 1) were observed in the ascending colon centrifugal gyrus and the ascending colon centripetal gyrus in group ZEN5. In group ZEN10, significant differences were found in the transverse colon between D3 vs. D1 and D2. In group ZEN15, no significant differences were noted between exposure dates.

A comparison of ZEN concentrations in the examined segments of the intestinal tract (see Table 1) on the analyzed exposure dates in group ZEN5 revealed that: (i) in nearly all intestinal segments (excluding the ileum), ZEN concentrations were highest on D1; (ii) ZEN concentrations were highest in both gyri of the ascending colon, the jejunum, and cecum; (iii) ZEN concentrations were low and similar on all exposure dates only in the ileum (3.13, 3.26, and 4.10 ng/g, respectively); (iv) interestingly, ZEN concentrations tended to decrease over time in all intestinal segments.

Table 1. The transfer coefficient and mean (±) concentration of ZEN (ng/g) in the intestines of gilts before puberty.

Exposure Dates	Feed Intake (kg/day)	Total ZEN Doses in Groups (µg/kg BW)	Tissues	Group ZEN5 (ng/g)	Carry-Over Factor	Group ZEN10 (ng/g)	Carry-Over Factor	Group ZEN15 (ng/g)	Carry-Over Factor
D1	0.8	80.5/161.9/242.7	Duodenum	12.81 ± 8.49	1×10^{-4}	64.36 ± 71.16	3×10^{-4}	48.35 ± 43.92	1×10^{-4}
			Jejunum	15.59 ± 20.40	1×10^{-6}	15.24 ± 13.65	9×10^{-5}	13.31 ± 4.92	5×10^{-5}
			Ileum	3.13 ± 0.69	3×10^{-5}	4.67 ± 4.50	2×10^{-5}	18.36 ± 13.81 [c]	7×10^{-5}
			Cecum	15.07 ± 8.14	1×10^{-4}	6.84 ± 4.18	4×10^{-5}	47.99 ± 34.30 [d]	1×10^{-4}
			CFG	14.74 ± 7.59	1×10^{-4}	8.63 ± 5.09	5×10^{-5}	33.13 ± 48.53	1×10^{-4}
			CPG	18.24 ± 12.39	2×10^{-4}	9.67 ± 4.95	5×10^{-5}	28.48 ± 17.20	1×10^{-4}
			Transverse colon	4.59 ± 2.74	5×10^{-5}	4.30 ± 2.99	2×10^{-5}	31.13 ± 20.40 [c,d]	1×10^{-4}
			Descending colon	6.11 ± 3.67	7×10^{-5}	4.50 ± 2.68	2×10^{-5}	31.69 ± 38.52	1×10^{-4}
D2	1.1	101.01/196.9/298.2	Duodenum	7.67 ± 4.56	7×10^{-5}	46.41 ± 33.57 [c]	2×10^{-4}	8.23 ± 10.24 [d]	2×10^{-5}
			Jejunum	6.81 ± 5.80	6×10^{-5}	4.95 ± 1.94	2×10^{-5}	5.56 ± 5.97	1×10^{-5}
			Ileum	3.26 ± 2.32	3×10^{-5}	3.30 ± 2.07	1×10^{-5}	11.66 ± 5.46 [cc,dd]	3×10^{-5}
			Cecum	8.52 ± 6.13	8×10^{-5}	12.56 ± 10.45	6×10^{-5}	38.11 ± 38.07	1×10^{-4}
			CFG	3.68 ± 1.06 [aa]	3×10^{-5}	12.13 ± 9.63	6×10^{-5}	35.15 ± 37.92	1×10^{-4}
			CPG	4.73 ± 1.76 [a]	4×10^{-5}	8.22 ± 8.53	4×10^{-5}	24.82 ± 19.84	8×10^{-5}
			Transverse colon	2.19 ± 1.31	2×10^{-5}	7.64 ± 3.91	3×10^{-5}	9.39 ± 8.98	3×10^{-5}
			Descending colon	2.23 ± 1.18	2×10^{-5}	7.31 ± 4.09	3×10^{-5}	18.35 ± 13.56 [c]	6×10^{-5}
D3	1.6	128.3/481.4/716.7	Duodenum	8.84 ± 4.20	6×10^{-5}	39.84 ± 2.22 [cc]	8×10^{-5}	57.34 ± 8.98 [cc,dd]	8×10^{-5}
			Jejunum	2.83 ± 4.26	2×10^{-5}	3.02 ± 3.76	6×10^{-6}	8.03 ± 0.98	1×10^{-5}
			Ileum	4.10 ± 2.87	3×10^{-5}	8.34 ± 0.94 [c]	1×10^{-5}	15.11 ± 0.66 [cc,dd]	2×10^{-5}
			Cecum	4.46 ± 4.73	3×10^{-5}	17.17 ± 20.89	3×10^{-5}	39.86 ± 2.30 [cc]	5×10^{-5}
			CFG	1.76 ± 2.07 [aa]	1×10^{-5}	16.73 ± 22.78	3×10^{-5}	18.10 ± 2.50 [cc,d]	6×10^{-5}
			CPG	2.21 ± 1.56 [a]	1×10^{-5}	8.91 ± 2.80 [cc]	1×10^{-5}	18.17 ± 2.78 [cc,dd]	2×10^{-5}
			Transverse colon	1.10 ± 1.15	8×10^{-6}	22.70 ± 12.87 [a,b,c]	4×10^{-5}	20.19 ± 1.30 [c]	2×10^{-5}
			Descending colon	2.30 ± 1.35	1×10^{-5}	13.26 ± 16.42	2×10^{-5}	18.94 ± 2.11	2×10^{-5}

Key: CFG—Ascending colon centrifugal gyrus; CPG—Ascending colon centripetal gyrus; exposure dates: D1—exposure day 7; D2—exposure day 21; D3—exposure day 42. Experimental groups: group ZEN5—5 µg ZEN/kg BW; group ZEN10—10 µg ZEN/kg BW; group ZEN15—15 µg ZEN/kg BW. The statistically notable differences were determined at [a], [b], [c], [d] $p \leq 0.05$ and [aa], [cc], [dd] $p \leq 0.01$; [a], [aa] notable difference between exposure date D1 and exposure dates D2 and D3; [b] notable difference between exposure date D2 and exposure date D3; [c], [cc] notable difference between group ZEN5 and groups ZEN10 and ZEN15; [d], [dd] notable difference between group ZEN10 and group ZEN15.

The concentrations of ZEN differed in the ZEN10 group (see Table 1). In the duodenum, ZEN concentrations were very high and similar on all exposure dates (D1–D3) (64.36, 46.41, and 39.84 ng/g, respectively). In the remaining intestinal segments, ZEN concentrations were very low (3–20 ng/g) on D2 and D3, with a rising trend on successive dates of exposure.

In group ZEN15, ZEN concentrations were relatively high on D1 compared with the remaining dates of exposure (see Table 1). On D2, ZEN concentrations decreased in almost all sections of the intestine (excluding the ascending colon centrifugal gyrus—35.15 ng/g). On the last exposure date, ZEN concentrations increased in nearly all intestinal segments (excluding the centripetal gyri of the ascending colon—8.17 ng/g). The observed changes in ZEN values were relatively low in all intestinal segments, excluding the duodenum and the transverse colon.

In group ZEN5, significant differences in αZEL concentrations (see Table 2) were observed between D3 and D2 and between D2 and D1. In both cases, these differences were noted in the cecum and the centrifugal gyri of the ascending colon. In group ZEN10, significant differences were found in the cecum between D3 and D1, between D3 and D2, and in the centripetal gyri of the ascending colon between D3 and D1. In group ZEN 15, significant differences were noted in the duodenum, jejunum, cecum, and the centrifugal gyri of the ascending colon between D3 vs. D2 and D1 and between D2 and D1.

On D1 (see Table 2), significant differences in αZEL concentrations between groups ZEN10 and ZEN15 vs. group ZEN5 were found only in the cecum. On D2, the analyzed parameter differed significantly between group ZEN5 and group ZEN15 only in the centripetal gyri of the ascending colon and the transverse colon. On D3, significant differences between group ZEN5 and group ZEN15 were noted in the jejunum, cecum, and the centrifugal gyri of the ascending colon.

An analysis of αZEL concentrations (see Table 2) in different intestinal segments revealed that in group ZEN5, they were very low and similar (0.78 to 3.98 ng/g) on D1 and D3, whereas a wider range of values (1.07 ng/g on D1 to 6.69 ng/g on D3) was observed only in the ileum. On D2, αZEL levels were two or even three times higher than on D1 and D3, ranging from 7.00 ng/g in the descending colon to 49.47 ng/g in the cecum.

In group ZEN10, αZEL concentrations (see Table 2) were proportional to the time of exposure. However, on D2, αZEL concentrations in the ileum were below the values noted on D1 (difference of 2.00 ng/g) and D3 (difference of 4.03 ng/g).

In group ZEN15, αZEL concentrations were proportional in each intestinal segment. However, the analyzed parameter decreased in some segments (ileum) and increased rapidly in other parts of the intestinal tract (cecum). Alpha-ZEL levels were very low on exposure day 42, e.g., in the descending colon.

It should be noted that significant differences in β-ZEL concentrations were very rarely observed on exposure dates D1 and D2, and the highest number of significant differences was noted on D3 (see Table 3), in particular in group ZEN15. In group ZEN5, highly significant differences in β-ZEL concentrations were found only between D3 and D1 in the duodenum, jejunum, and cecum, and between D3 and D2 in the duodenum and jejunum. In group ZEN10, significant differences in the analyzed parameter were observed between D3 vs. D1 and D2 in the centrifugal gyri of the ascending colon. In group ZEN15, significant differences were noted between D3 and D1 in nearly all intestinal segments, excluding the ileum and the centripetal gyri of the ascending colon; significant differences were also noted between D3 and D2 in the jejunum, centripetal gyri of the ascending colon, transverse colon, and descending colon. Additionally, significant differences in β-ZEL levels were noted between D2 and D1 in the duodenum, jejunum, and cecum.

An analysis of β-ZEL concentrations (see Table 3) on different exposure dates revealed significant differences on D1 between group ZEN5 vs. groups ZEN10 and ZEN15 in the cecum and between group ZEN10 and group ZEN15 in the cecum. On D2, significant differences in β-ZEL concentrations were observed between group ZEN5 vs. groups ZEN10 and ZEN15 in the jejunum and cross member and between group ZEN10 and group ZEN15 in the jejunum. On D3, differences in the studied parameter were noted between group ZEN5 vs. groups ZEN10 and ZEN15 in the centrifugal gyri of the ascending colon and between group ZEN5 and group ZEN15 in the duodenum and descending colon.

Table 2. The transfer coefficient and mean (±) concentration of αZEL (ng/g) in the intestines of gilts before puberty.

Exposure Date	Tissues	Group ZEN5 (ng/g)	Carry-Over Factor	Group ZEN10 (ng/g)	Carry-Over Factor	Group ZEN15 (ng/g)	Carry-Over Factor
D1	Duodenum	3.72 ± 1.68	4×10^{-5}	6.25 ± 2.57	3×10^{-5}	6.66 ± 6.32	2×10^{-5}
	Jejunum	2.85 ± 2.78	3×10^{-5}	5.24 ± 3.95	3×10^{-5}	9.62 ± 1.66	3×10^{-5}
	Ileum	1.07 ± 0.21	1×10^{-5}	6.46 ± 7.25	3×10^{-5}	2.88 ± 3.21	1×10^{-5}
	Cecum	3.45 ± 1.05	4×10^{-5}	12.01 ± 4.36 [cc]	7×10^{-5}	11.85 ± 2.04 [cc]	4×10^{-5}
	CFG	3.15 ± 0.49	3×10^{-5}	5.58 ± 1.83	3×10^{-5}	4.59 ± 2.78	1×10^{-5}
	CPG	3.98 ± 2.43	4×10^{-5}	6.88 ± 2.65	4×10^{-5}	6.41 ± 4.58	2×10^{-5}
	Transverse colon	1.07 ± 0.95	1×10^{-5}	2.26 ± 1.74	1×10^{-5}	2.05 ± 0.99	8×10^{-6}
	Descending colon	1.48 ± 0.60	1×10^{-5}	1.47 ± 0.80	9×10^{-6}	2.68 ± 3.04	1×10^{-5}
D2	Duodenum	6.43 ± 2.36	6×10^{-5}	9.12 ± 8.11	4×10^{-5}	6.97 ± 0.31	2×10^{-5}
	Jejunum	5.36 ± 3.87	5×10^{-5}	22.37 ± 20.81	1×10^{-4}	14.28 ± 1.92 [a]	4×10^{-5}
	Ileum	6.58 ± 7.01	6×10^{-5}	4.46 ± 2.99	2×10^{-5}	8.49 ± 2.52	2×10^{-5}
	Cecum	11.23 ± 4.47 [aa]	1×10^{-4}	22.74 ± 17.44	1×10^{-4}	35.59 ± 14.60 [a]	1×10^{-4}
	CFG	6.01 ± 2.01 [a]	5×10^{-5}	10.80 ± 10.41	5×10^{-5}	10.88 ± 1.74 [aa]	3×10^{-5}
	CPG	7.01 ± 2.76	6×10^{-5}	11.86 ± 4.88	6×10^{-5}	27.08 ± 15.25 [c]	9×10^{-5}
	Transverse colon	2.42 ± 1.59	2×10^{-5}	5.86 ± 2.61	2×10^{-5}	6.65 ± 1.55 [c]	2×10^{-5}
	Descending colon	1.51 ± 0.88	1×10^{-5}	2.75 ± 1.74	1×10^{-5}	1.07 ± 0.40	3×10^{-6}
D3	Duodenum	3.72 ± 1.68	2×10^{-5}	30.00 ± 22.55 [c]	6×10^{-5}	20.12 ± 4.65 [aa,bb]	2×10^{-5}
	Jejunum	2.85 ± 2.78	2×10^{-5}	16.42 ± 5.54 [cc]	3×10^{-5}	19.64 ± 1.82 [aa,b,cc]	2×10^{-5}
	Ileum	6.69 ± 1.68	5×10^{-5}	4.60 ± 4.00	9×10^{-6}	7.32 ± 4.10	1×10^{-5}
	Cecum	3.45 ± 1.05 [bb]	2×10^{-5}	49.47 ± 9.75 [aa,bb,cc]	1×10^{-4}	37.04 ± 5.08 [a,cc]	5×10^{-5}
	CFG	3.15 ± 0.49 [b]	2×10^{-5}	12.67 ± 8.59 [c]	2×10^{-5}	15.56 ± 1.34 [aa,b,c]	2×10^{-5}
	CPG	3.98 ± 2.43	3×10^{-5}	25.84 ± 10.70 [a,c]	5×10^{-5}	16.13 ± 11.21	2×10^{-5}
	Transverse colon	0.80 ± 0.94	6×10^{-6}	8.08 ± 7.40	1×10^{-5}	5.91 ± 6.88	8×10^{-6}
	Descending colon	0.78 ± 0.74	6×10^{-6}	7.00 ± 5.59	1×10^{-5}	5.53 ± 3.86	4×10^{-6}

Key: CFG—Ascending colon Centrifugal gyrus; CPG—Ascending colon Centripetal gyrus; Exposure dates: D1—exposure day 7; D2—exposure day 21; D3—exposure day 42. Experimental groups: group ZEN5—5 μg ZEN/kg BW; group ZEN10—10 μg ZEN/kg BW; group ZEN15—15 μg ZEN/kg BW. LOD > values below the limit of detection were expressed as 0. The statistically notable differences were determined at [a], [b], [c] $p \leq 0.05$ and [aa], [bb], [cc] $p \leq 0.01$; [a], [aa] notable difference between exposure date D1 and exposure date D2 and D3; [b], [bb] notable difference between exposure date D2 and exposure date D3; [c], [cc] notable difference between group ZEN5 and groups ZEN10 and ZEN15.

2.4. Carry-Over Factor (CF)

Natural contamination of cereals and feeds with mycotoxins is frequently reported. Mycotoxins ingested by livestock with feed are carried over to food products of animal origin [16]. Undesirable substances are transferred from contaminated feed to animal tissues. The CF and the resulting health risks remain insufficiently investigated in vivo, in particular during low-dose mycotoxicosis, which is why they were analyzed in this study.

The carry-over rate of ZEN from the intestinal lumen to the intestinal wall was affected by the dose and time of exposure in each group (see Table 1). The highest CF values were noted on D1 in groups ZEN5 (centrifugal gyri of the ascending colon) and ZEN10 (duodenum). In group ZEN15, the highest CF values were observed in six of the eight investigated intestinal segments (excluding the jejunum and ileum). In turn, the lowest CF values were noted on D3 in all groups: in the transverse colon in group ZEN5 (8×10^{-6}), in the jejunum in group ZEN10 (6×10^{-6}), and in the jejunum in group ZEN15 (3×10^{-6}).

The CF of αZEL in the intestinal tract ranged from 10^{-4} to 10^{-6} (see Table 2). The lowest values of this parameter (10^{-6}) were noted in group ZEN5 on D3 in the transverse colon and the descending colon; in group ZEN10 on D1 in the descending colon and on D3 in the transverse colon and the descending colon; in group ZEN15 on D1 in the ileum, centripetal gyri of the ascending colon, transverse colon, and descending colon; on D2 in all intestinal segments, excluding the cecum; and on D3 in the ileum, transverse colon, and descending colon. Interestingly, CF values were lowest in the descending colon on all days of exposure. In turn, the highest values of CF (10^{-4}) were found in group ZEN5 on D2 in the cecum; in group ZEN10 on D2 and D3 in the jejunum and cecum; and in group ZEN15 on D2 in the cecum. In 80% of the cases, the highest CF values were noted in the cecum.

Table 3. The transfer coefficient and mean (±) concentration of βZEL (ng/g) in the intestines of gilts before puberty.

Exposure Date	Tissue	Group ZEN5 (ng/g)	Carry-Over Factor	Group ZEN10 (ng/g)	Carry-over Factor	Group ZEN15 (ng/g)	Carry-Over Factor
D1	Duodenum	0.16 ± 0.09	1×10^{-6}	3.49 ± 6.14	2×10^{-5}	0.29 ± 0.07	1×10^{-6}
	Jejunum	0.07 ± 0.08	8×10^{-7}	2.17 ± 3.61	1×10^{-5}	0.12 ± 0.02	4×10^{-7}
	Ileum	0	0	0.64 ± 0.77	3×10^{-6}	0.02 ± 0.03	8×10^{-8}
	Cecum	0.14 ± 0.04	1×10^{-6}	1.19 ± 0.20 [cc]	7×10^{-6}	0.54 ± 0.10 [cc,dd]	2×10^{-6}
	CFG	0.13 ± 0.07	1×10^{-6}	0.44 ± 0.28	2×10^{-6}	0.30 ± 0.02	1×10^{-6}
	CPG	0.18 ± 0.10	2×10^{-6}	2.37 ± 3.66	1×10^{-5}	0.27 ± 0.09	1×10^{-6}
	Transverse colon	0.12 ± 0.18	1×10^{-6}	0.77 ± 1.10	4×10^{-6}	0.09 ± 0.06	3×10^{-7}
	Descending colon	0.02 ± 0.01	2×10^{-7}	0.22 ± 0.17	1×10^{-6}	0.05 ± 0.01	2×10^{-7}
D2	Duodenum	0.08 ± 0.10	7×10^{-7}	0.26 ± 0.17	1×10^{-6}	0.08 ± 0.09 [aa]	2×10^{-7}
	Jejunum	0.07 ± 0.10	6×10^{-7}	1.11 ± 0.11 [cc]	5×10^{-6}	0.69 ± 0.11 [aa,cc,dd]	2×10^{-6}
	Ileum	0.14 ± 0.11	1×10^{-6}	0.27 ± 0.18	1×10^{-6}	0.05 ± 0.06	1×10^{-7}
	Cecum	0.30 ± 0.19	2×10^{-6}	1.07 ± 1.00	5×10^{-6}	1.10 ± 0.26 [a]	3×10^{-6}
	CFG	0.17 ± 0.13	7×10^{-7}	0.45 ± 0.29	2×10^{-6}	0.24 ± 0.16	8×10^{-7}
	CPG	0.13 ± 0.11	1×10^{-6}	0.41 ± 0.12	2×10^{-6}	0.46 ± 0.53	1×10^{-6}
	Transverse colon	0.03 ± 0.03	1×10^{-7}	0.27 ± 0.09 [cc]	1×10^{-6}	0.25 ± 0.05 [cc]	8×10^{-7}
	Descending colon	0.03 ± 0.02	1×10^{-7}	0.23 ± 0.27	1×10^{-6}	0.08 ± 0.04	2×10^{-7}
D3	Duodenum	1.11 ± 0.67 [aa,bb]	8×10^{-6}	2.21 ± 0.73	5×10^{-6}	3.06 ± 0.17 [aa,cc]	4×10^{-6}
	Jejunum	0.91 ± 0.45 [aa,bb]	7×10^{-6}	2.46 ± 1.51	5×10^{-6}	3.08 ± 0.16 [aa,bb]	4×10^{-6}
	Ileum	0.21 ± 0.28	1×10^{-6}	0.89 ± 1.32	1×10^{-6}	0.61 ± 0.52	8×10^{-7}
	Cecum	0.63 ± 0.24 [aa]	4×10^{-6}	1.18 ± 0.38	2×10^{-6}	1.15 ± 0.19 [a]	1×10^{-6}
	CFG	0.48 ± 0.34	3×10^{-6}	1.37 ± 0.18 [a,b,cc]	2×10^{-6}	1.66 ± 0.21 [a,b,cc]	2×10^{-6}
	CPG	0.47 ± 0.41	3×10^{-6}	0.27 ± 0.20	5×10^{-7}	0.80 ± 0.13	1×10^{-6}
	Transverse colon	0.20 ± 0.14	1×10^{-6}	0.76 ± 0.59	1×10^{-6}	1.06 ± 0.20 [aa,bb]	1×10^{-6}
	Descending colon	0.16 ± 0.16	1×10^{-6}	0.53 ± 0.19	1×10^{-6}	0.79 ± 0.11 [aa,bb,c]	1×10^{-6}

Key: CFG—ascending colon centrifugal gyrus; CPG—ascending colon centripetal gyrus; exposure dates: D1—exposure day 7; D2—exposure day 21; D3—exposure day 42. Experimental groups: group ZEN5—5 μg ZEN/kg BW; group ZEN10—10 μg ZEN/kg BW; group ZEN15—15 μg ZEN/kg BW. LOD > values below the limit of detection were expressed as 0. The statistically notable differences were determined at [a],[b],[c] $p \leq 0.05$ and [aa],[bb],[cc],[dd] $p \leq 0.01$; [a],[aa] notable difference between exposure date D1 and exposure dates D2 and D3; [b],[bb] notable difference between exposure date D2 and exposure date D3; [c],[cc] notable difference between group ZEN5 and groups ZEN10 and ZEN15; [dd] notable difference between group ZEN10 and group ZEN15.

The carry-over rates of β-ZEL (see Table 3) in different segments of the intestinal tract were determined within a narrower range of values (10^{-5} to 10^{-8}) than the carry-over rates of ZEN and α-ZEL. The highest CF values were noted on D1 in group ZEN10 in the duodenum, jejunum, and centripetal gyri of the ascending colon; on D2 in group ZEN10 in the jejunum and cecum; and on D3 in group ZEN5 in the duodenum and jejunum. In group ZEN15, the highest CF values were observed on D3 in the ileum. The CF factor was calculated in 72 cases, and it reached 10^{-8} in 1 case (ileum, group ZEN15, D1), 10^{-7} in 17 cases, 10^{-6} in 50 cases, 10^{-5} in 3 cases, and 0 in 1 case (ileum, group ZEN5, D1).

2.5. Expression of CYP1A1 and GSTP1 Genes

Cytochrome P450 1A1 (CYP1A1) participates in the phase I metabolism of xenobiotics and drugs. It can exert protective effects on DNA and does not contribute to potentially cancerogenic DNA modifications, which could be attributed to the fact that CYP1A1 is highly active in the intestinal mucosa and prevents xenobiotics and carcinogens from reaching the circulatory system [33]. In this experiment, the *CYP1A1 m*RNA gene was generally silenced in both segments of the large intestine in all groups (see Figure 2). In the ascending colon, on D1 and D3, *CYP1A1 m*RNA expression was most strongly silenced in group C in comparison with the experimental groups. Similar results were reported by

Sun et al. [6] in Leydig cells exposed in vitro to ZEN. In the ascending colon, on D1 and D3, *CYP1A1 mRNA* expression was most strongly silenced in group C (1.226 and 0.623, respectively). In contrast, on D2, *CYP1A1 mRNA* expression was more silenced in the experimental groups (1.103, 0.983, and 0.929, respectively) than in group C (1.313). The reverse was noted in the descending colon, where *CYP1A1 mRNA* expression was more silenced in the experimental groups on D1 (0.952, 0.613, and 0.676, respectively) and D3 (0.542, 0.480, and 0.462, respectively). On D2, *CYP1A1 mRNA* expression was most strongly silenced in groups C and ZEN5 (0.536 and 0.588, respectively).

Glutathione S-transferases (GSTs) are detoxification enzymes that catalyze conjugation reactions between endogenous glutathione and electrophilic metabolites produced during phase I biotransformation [34]. These enzymes protect cells against the harmful effects of electrophilic chemical compounds and oxidation products. Glutathione S-transferases are a family of dimeric enzymes responsible for the conjugation of exogenous and endogenous compounds with glutathione. Glutathione protects DNA against damage by binding toxic compounds in the cytoplasm and preventing them from interacting with nucleic acid [35].

In the present study, the expression of the GSTπ1 gene was silenced [34,36] as a result of low-dose zearalenone mycotoxicosis (see Figure 3). The suppression of gene expression was directly proportional to the zearalenone dose in the experimental groups. The expression of GSTP1 mRNA in both intestinal segments was highest in group C on all dates of exposure. In the ascending colon, significant differences were found between group C vs. groups ZEN10 and ZEN15 on all exposure dates (difference of 0.187 and 0.404 on D1; difference of 0.302 and 0.405 on D2; difference of 0.331 and 0.351 on D3, respectively). In group ZEN5, GSTP1 mRNA expression was also more strongly silenced than in group C, but the difference was not statistically notable. In the descending colon, notable differences were not observed on D1 and D2, whereas on D3, a significant difference (0.303) was noted between group C and group ZEN15.

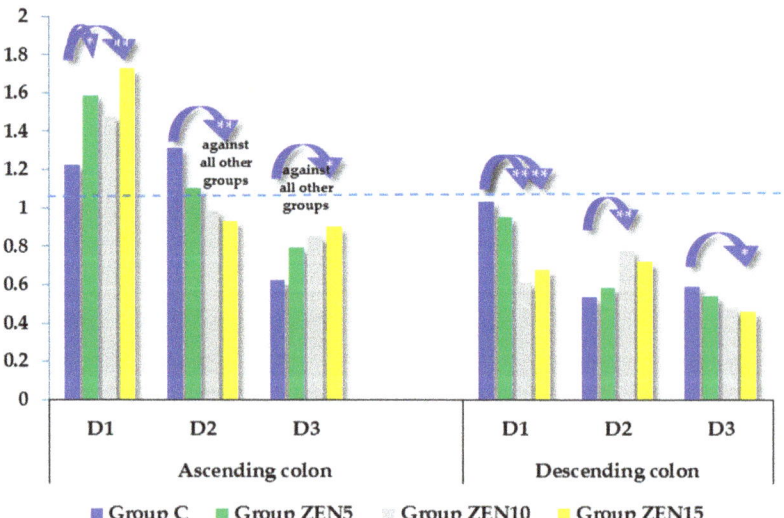

Figure 2. The expression of CYP1A1 in the ascending colon and descending colon at different dates of exposure. Bars represent the mean values (n = 5) of enzyme gene expression ratios ($\pm$) relative to the control sample at the beginning of the experiment (ER = 1.00; dashed line). Asterisks (*) denote experimental groups (group ZEN5—5 µg ZEN/kg BW; group ZEN10—10 µg ZEN/kg BW; group ZEN15—15 µg ZEN/kg BW), which differed significantly in mRNA levels compared to the corresponding control (C) groups (* $p \leq 0.05$, ** $p \leq 0.01$).

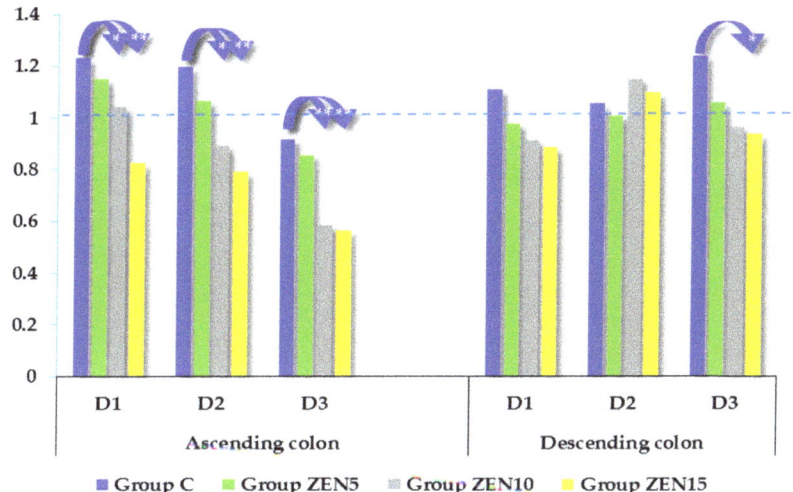

Figure 3. The expression of GSTπ1 in the ascending colon and descending colon at different dates of exposure. Bars represent the mean values (*n* = 5) of enzyme gene expression ratios (±) relative to the control sample at the beginning of the experiment (ER = 1.00; dashed line). Asterisks (*) denote experimental groups (group ZEN5—5 µg ZEN/kg BW; group ZEN10—10 µg ZEN/kg BW; group ZEN15—15 µg ZEN/kg BW), which differed significantly in mRNA levels compared to the corresponding control (C) groups (* $p \leq 0.05$, ** $p \leq 0.01$).

3. Discussion

This study demonstrated that the absorption and biotransformation of ZEN and its metabolites in prepubertal gilts were highly individualized (see Tables 1–3). A comparison between the current and previous studies indicates that long-term exposure to low ZEN doses stimulates proliferation processes and migration on all dates of exposure [5,7,8,12,13,20,31,37]. The question that remains to be answered is why ZEN metabolites were detected in intestinal tissues if their concentrations were considerably lower in the blood [5] and the heart muscle [31] and if they were completely absent in the bone marrow microenvironment [12].

3.1. Zearalenone and its Metabolites

3.1.1. Zearalenone Concentrations

An analysis of ZEN concentrations in gut tissue (see Table 1) revealed the highest values in the duodenum on exposure date D1 (ZEN levels were not always proportional to the ingested dose) in group ZEN10. This observation can be explained by the fact that in the initial stages of intestinal absorption, ZEN is most effectively absorbed in the duodenum, where it is hydroxylated to α-ZEL and β-ZEL [3]. This is because the duodenum and jejunum have firmly adherent mucus and polysaccharide layers [38], and prepubertal gilts have high requirements for estrogen and estrogenic compounds [5] due to supr;aphysiological hormonal levels [39]. In groups ZEN10 and ZEN15, higher ZEN concentrations could also be attributed to the presence of "free ZEN", which contributes to: (i) the inhibition of steroidogenesis [6]; (ii) the conversion of testosterone (ZEN suppresses testosterone levels) to estradiol (which inhibits maturation processes in prepubertal gilts, [40]); and (iii) increased feed intake and the accumulation of energy [7], supporting homeostasis and, at later procreation of the organism, reproduction in prepubertal gilts [41]. It should also be noted that the period of adaptation to an ongoing mycotoxicosis ends after seven dates of exposure (i.e., on D1) [42].

On D2 and D3, ZEN levels in intestinal tissues increased (see Figure 1) in all groups, but values recorded in groups ZEN10 and ZEN15 (excluding the centrifugal gyri of the ascending colon) were proportionally lower than in group ZEN5. This is because the intestinal tract constitutes the first line of defense against the harmful effects of mycotoxins [14,43]. The intestines are covered by a layer of mucus and polysaccharides that adhere loosely or firmly to the intestinal wall [38] and determine the rate of absorption processes. Mycotoxins, including ZEN, exert negative effects mainly during prolonged exposure to high doses [14]. Zearalenone stimulated the proliferation of colonic cells in vitro [3]. Therefore, intestinal responses are determined mainly by the ZEN dose. Low doses promote proliferation and migration [44], while high doses have cytotoxic effects and inhibit biotransformation processes [3], which probably occurred in group ZEN15 in the early stages of exposure.

In view of the above, the present results suggest that the administered ZEN doses (LOAEL, NOAEL, and MABEL) were appropriate to reliably assess the carry-over of ZEN in the digestive tract of prepubertal gilts.

3.1.2. Concentrations of ZEN and Its Metabolites

The levels of ZEN metabolites (α-ZEL and β-ZEL; see Tables 2 and 3, Figure 1) in intestinal tissues were proportional to the administered doses and time of exposure. The proportions of α-ZEL and β-ZEL were similar to those noted in other studies [3], which is natural in our opinion [5,45]. The bioavailability of ZEN metabolites in intestinal tissues was influenced by biotransformation processes during pubescence. The distribution of concentration values in intestinal tissues preceded the values obtained in blood [5]. Zearalenone metabolites were not found in the blood of ZEN5 animals on D1 due to a very low supply of endogenous steroid hormones [5] (supraphysiological hormonal levels [39]). Mycoestrogens supplementation [46] can modify the levels of estrogen hormones [7,37] and the anti-Müllerian hormone [47].

The following arguments should be also considered: (i) adaptive processes end on D1 [42]; and (ii) ZEN metabolites can be used as substrates that regulate the expression levels of genes encoding hydroxysteroid dehydrogenases [20] that act as molecular switches and allow for the modulation of steroid hormone pre-receptors. In this study, these processes were particularly noticeable in group ZEN5, where ZEN concentrations decreased and α-ZEL concentrations increased on successive dates of exposure (see Table 2). The above indicates that in prepubertal gilts, even the smallest amounts of estrogenic compounds are used by the body [48] to make up for the deficiency of endogenous estrogen [5]. In the remaining groups, metabolite levels increased proportionally to the ingested ZEN dose.

Based on previous research findings [49,50] and extrapolation, the above observations could be attributed to the activity of transport proteins in the intestinal wall. The activity of the antiporter plays a very important role in the initial stage stages of mycotoxin biotransformation. Processes with the participation of antiport proteins are influenced by the availability of energy compounds (which were depleted) [7], which affect active ion pumps that transport ZEN from and to the intestinal lumen, thus stabilizing ZEN concentrations inside cells [51]. In enterocytes, numerous detoxification enzymes are localized near the cell wall. When mycotoxins and their metabolites do not undergo further biotransformation, they reach the cytosol and, consequently, the circulatory system. To prevent this from happening, active ion pumps remove mycotoxins and their metabolites from cells. These toxins return to the intestinal lumen and are subsequently recirculated to enterocytes. The described mechanisms restore energy reserves in cells, and mycotoxins can be metabolized again before they reach the cytosol and cause pathological states. Antiporter activity in the intestines is also determined by phase I enzymes, including the cytochrome P450 3A4 isoenzyme, which plays a key role in detoxification [15] and energy supply [7].

These observations could suggest that α-ZEL contributes to the modulation of life processes by participating in feminization processes in prepubertal gilts.

3.1.3. Carry-Over Factor

One of the main objectives of risk management in the food processing industry is to protect public health through the effective identification and control of known threats and selecting the most appropriate strategies for mitigating these risks. The significance of the CF has to be understood before a given strategy is selected and implemented [1]. The CF is the concentration ratio of the undesirable substances (mycotoxin) in contaminated digesta to the concentrations of ZEN and its metabolites in gut tissues, which marks the beginning of biotransformation processes. Our previous research demonstrated that even MABEL doses can induce specific changes in homeostasis [52], metabolic processes [7], endocrine processes [5,6], and gut microbiota [8] in prepubertal gilts.

The CF values noted in the current study suggest that the accumulation of the parent compound in the intestinal wall was low and stable on the first two dates of exposure (D1 and D2). A different trend was noted in group ZEN10 in the duodenum, where ZEN is most easily and rapidly absorbed [38]. These values were sufficient to induce considerable disruptions in metabolic processes [18] and, most importantly, steroidogenesis [6,20,53,54] via estrogen receptors [4,52]. These findings confirm that the effects exerted by mycotoxins applied at low doses have not been fully elucidated in prepubertal females. However, on D3, the CF values were higher in the ZEN15 group than in the other groups, which may suggest the rate of biotransformation processes decreases over time. These observations are difficult to interpret because little is known about the rate and course of biological processes in sexually immature pigs. It can only be speculated that estrogen supply and estrogen demand reach equilibrium and that the steroid hormone profile is modified when testosterone is converted to estradiol [5,42] or when detoxification processes begin to dominate [55].

The CF values of both ZEN metabolites were characterized by different trends (Tables 2 and 3). In general, this parameter was highest in group ZEN10 on all exposure dates, with a decreasing trend in the colon. On D3, the CF of α-ZEL in the ZEN10 group increased in all sections of the small intestine. The CF of β-ZEL was highest in group ZEN5 and also in the small intestine. Interestingly, a comparison of the CF values of both ZEN metabolites on all exposure dates revealed average values on D3. These observations suggest that after 21 days of exposure to the pure parent compound, life processes in prepubertal gilts are stabilized, and biotransformation processes are shifted towards detoxification [55,56]. This indicates that the macroorganism has developed tolerance to low ZEN doses due to the availability of "free ZEN" [20], its suppressive effects on testosterone and progesterone levels [6], and the negative feedback effect on FSH synthesis and secretion [5,57]. These effects could be ascribed to the fact that prepubertal gilts were fed a balanced diet [7,58], and the amount of gut microbiota was higher in the distal part of the intestinal tract [8], where mycotoxin concentrations were lower.

Contrary to the observations made in vitro by Alvarez-Ortega et al. [59], the present study did not provide any evidence to prove that exposure to low doses of ZEN, the determined concentrations of ZEN and its metabolites, and CF values enhanced proliferation processes in the analyzed tissues. It can be concluded that the noted CF values indicate that the tested ZEN doses did not exert harmful effects and that the macroorganism relatively easily adapted to these doses.

3.2. Expression of CYP1A1 and GSTπ1 Genes

The biotransformation of xenobiotics, including ZEN, often alters the biological activity and chemical properties of these compounds. Phase I metabolic processes usually enhance the functionality of their molecules, while phase II is often considered the detoxification stage. However, the nature and extent of these processes are highly compound-specific and can vary between individuals [2]. During the biotransformation process, ZEN is not only eliminated from the body, but the parent compound is inactivated, and the products of phase I biotransformation are activated. Various types of enzymes participate in these processes, including cytochrome P450 isoenzymes and CYP1A family enzymes in phase

I, in particular in intestinal tissues. Microsomal GST enzymes are involved in successive phases of biotransformation [3].

The cytochrome P450 1A1 enzyme adds hydroxyl groups in the phase I metabolism of xenobiotics. Hydroxyl groups increase the polarity of xenobiotics, thus facilitating their excretion via urine, and they also act as sites for further modification in phase II biotransformation processes. As a result of enzymatic modifications, ZEN is partly transformed to more active forms (such as α-ZEL; it should be noted that pure ZEN was administered per os in this study) [2] that more easily interact with the molecular targets in cells (such as estrogen receptors) [60] and effectively participate in phase II biotransformation. These processes occur in two mutually opposing directions.

Analysis of the expression of the CYP1A1 gene in the ascending and descending colon (Figure 2) on dates D1 and D2 showed that the absorption and accumulation of ZEN and its metabolites in the gut tissues of prepubertal gilts (Figure 1) corresponded to the CF values in the analyzed intestinal segments (see Table 1). The above could be attributed to physiological estrogen deficiency [6,39] as well as the fact that the parent compound (ZEN) absorbed in intestinal tissues was biotransformed to a more active form (α-ZEL). These processes promote effective modulation of molecular targets in cells, facilitate steroidogenesis [5], and induce cross-talk between the receptors activated by undesirable substances (the estrogen receptor and the aryl hydrocarbon receptor). The interactions between these receptors increase the expression of the respective target genes [60].

It should also be noted that various substrates can stimulate or inhibit the activity of proteins, which significantly influences the biotransformation of ZEN catalyzed by these enzymes. In addition to protein polymorphism, the induction of biotransforming enzymes is also responsible for differences in the susceptibility to ZEN and the mycotoxin's impact on gilts before puberty. Mean concentrations of ZEN and its metabolites in the intestinal wall (Figure 1) were inversely related to the expression of the CYP1A1 gene in two sections of the colon (see Figure 2), and these differences were more pronounced on successive dates of exposure [6]. The above can be attributed to the increasing accumulation of mycotoxins in the intestinal wall on day 42 of exposure (D3). In an in silico study, all mycotoxins (ZEN, α-ZEL, and β-ZEL) acted as substrates, inducers, and inhibitors ranging from 60% to 90%, 21% to 38%, and 23% to 32%, respectively, for the CYP1A1 isoform [15], which was not confirmed in vivo in this study. These observations could suggest that these mycotoxins suppress the expression of the CYP1A1 gene.

Glutathione S-transferases (GSTs) are a family of dimeric enzymes that conjugate exogenous and endogenous substances with glutathione. Glutathione prevents DNA damage by binding toxic compounds in the cytoplasm and preventing their interactions with nucleic acid. It should be noted that GSTs are a part of the unified cellular defense system [61]. In the GST family, the GSTπ1 subclass predominates in the colon [62]. The substrates for GSTs, in particular for the GSTπ1 subclass, include active metabolites of cyclophosphamide, platinum derivatives, and xenobiotics. GSTπ1 plays a special role in the conjugation of reactive cyclophosphamide metabolites with glutathione [63]. In the present study, a minor increase (non-significant) in GSTπ1 expression in the descending colon was noted only on D2 in groups ZEN10 and ZEN15 (Figure 3), which suggests that proliferation processes are somewhat dominant in enterocytes [64,65]. These results are difficult to interpret due to the scarcity of published data for comparisons. In most experimental weeks, GSTπ1 expression tended to be higher in the ascending colon and lower in the descending colon. Increased GSTπ1 expression in the ascending colon is attributable to hyperestrogenism in prepubertal gilts. Lower levels of GSTπ1 expression in the descending colon were also reported by Hokaiwado et al. [66], who concluded that GSTπ1 silencing decreases cell proliferation, promotes apoptosis, and contributes to controlled proliferation. According to other authors, GSTπ1 can be silenced in response to chemical stress [28,34], including exposure to ZEN. However, there are no published data that can be directly compared with our findings. Our previous studies revealed that both ZEN and deoxynivalenol (DON) could silence GSTπ1 expression [4,36].

As a result, long-term exposure to ZEN applied at low doses induced functional changes in the distal gastrointestinal tract in gilts before puberty. However, GSTπ1 expression in the descending colon was higher in group C on D2. This observation could be attributed to: (i) the balanced supply and demand (homeostasis) of GSTπ1 for the maintenance of cytoprotective and detoxification functions in phase II biotransformation processes; (ii) excess intracellular levels of GSTπ1 in the ascending and descending colon in response to high GSTπ1 expression [63]; or (iii) intensified apoptosis [66].

Exposure to low mycotoxin doses led to controlled silencing of GSTπ1 expression, thus promoting a balance between intestinal cells, the degree of exposure to toxic compounds, and the detoxifying effect.

4. Summary and Conclusions

The gut tissues are the first line of defense against any substances that enter the body. A healthy intestinal barrier guarantees homeostasis in the body. On the basis of the presented research, it could be hypothesized that the obtained results confirm the correctness of the adopted nomenclature of doses (LOAEL, NOAEL, and MABEL) used in the experience. Based on the observations made during 42 days of exposure to pure ZEN, it can be hypothesized that all mycotoxins (ZEN, α-ZEL, and β-ZEL) contribute to a balance between gut cells and the expression of genes that encode enzymes that participate in biotransformation processes in the large intestine, modulate feminization processes in prepubertal gilts, and elicit flexible, adaptive responses of the macroorganism to mycotoxin exposure at the analyzed doses.

5. Materials and Methods

5.1. General Information

All experimental procedures on animals were carried out in accordance with the Polish regulations specifying the conditions for conducting experiments on animals (Opinions No. 12/2016 and 45/2016/DLZ issued by the Local Ethics Committee for Animal Experimentation of the University of Warmia and Mazury in Olsztyn, Poland, on 30 November 2016). This article is a continuation of the previously published study protocol [32].

5.2. Experimental Feed

ZEN analytical samples were dissolved in 96 μL of 96% ethanol (SWW 2442-90, Polskie Odczynniki SA, Poland) in doses appropriate for various body weights (BWs). The food was placed in gel capsules saturated with the solution and kept at room temperature until the alcohol was evaporated. All groups of gilts received the same feed throughout the trial. The animals were weighed at weekly intervals, and the results were used to adjust the individual mycotoxin doses [8,13,67].

The feed given to all test animals was supplied by the same producer. The brittle feed was administered ad libitum twice a day at 8:00 a.m. and 5:00 p.m. throughout the experiment. The composition of the complete diet declared by the producer is presented in Table 4 [8,13,67]. Zearalenone analytical samples were dissolved in 96 μL of 96% ethanol (SWW 2442-90, Polskie Odczynniki SA, Poland) in appropriate weight doses. The feeds containing various amounts of ZEN in the alcoholic solution were placed in gel capsules. Prior to administration, the capsules were stored at room temperature until the alcohol evaporated. Pigs in the experimental groups received ZEN in gel capsules daily before morning feeding. The animals were weighed at weekly intervals to adjust the individual mycotoxin doses. The carrier was feed, and the gilts from group C received identical gel capsules without ZEN [7,8]. The feeds were supplied by the same manufacturer. During the experiment, the gilts were fed brittle fodder ad libitum twice a day (at 8:00 a.m. and 5:00 p.m.). The composition of the complete diets was specified by the producer, and it is presented in Table 4.

Table 4. Declared composition of the complete diet [12].

Parameters	Composition Declared by the Manufacturer (%)
Soybean meal	16
Wheat	55
Barley	22
Wheat bran	4.0
Chalk	0.3
Zitrosan	0.2
Vitamin–mineral premix [1]	2.5

[1] Composition of the vitamin-mineral premix per kg: vitamin A—500.000 IU; iron—5000 mg; vitamin D3—100.000 IU; zinc—5000 mg; vitamin E (alpha-tocopherol)—2000 mg; manganese—3000 mg; vitamin K—150 mg; copper ($CuSO_4 \cdot 5H_2O$)—500 mg; vitamin B1—100 mg; cobalt—20 mg; vitamin B2—300 mg; iodine—40 mg; vitamin B6—150 mg; selenium—15 mg; vitamin B12—1500 μg; L-lysine—9.4 g; niacin—1200 mg; DL—methionine+cystine—3.7 g; pantothenic acid—600 mg; L-threonine—2.3 g; folic acid—50 mg; tryptophan—1.1 g; biotin—7500 μg; phytase + choline—10 g; ToyoCerin probiotic + calcium—250 g; antioxidant + mineral phosphorus and released phosphorus—60 g; magnesium—5 g; sodium and calcium—51 g.

The proximate chemical composition of the diets fed to pigs in groups C, ZEN5, ZEN10, and ZEN15 was determined using the NIRS™ DS2500 F feed analyzer (FOSS, Hillerød, Denmark), a monochromator-based NIR reflectance and transflectance analyzer with a scanning range of 850–2500 nm [32].

Toxicological Analysis of Feed

Feed was analyzed for the presence of mycotoxins and their metabolites: ZEN, α-ZEL, and deoxynivalenol (DON). Mycotoxin concentrations in feed were determined by separation in immunoaffinity columns (Zearala-Test™ Zearalenone Testing System, G1012, VICAM, Watertown, MA, USA; DON-Test™ DON Testing System, VICAM, Watertown, MA, USA). Feed samples were ground in a laboratory mill. Ground samples of 25 g each were eluted with 150 mL of acetonitrile (90%) to extract the mycotoxins. A total of 10 mL of the resulting solution was withdrawn and diluted with 40 mL of water. The obtained solution (10 mL) was collected and passed through the immunoaffinity column (VICAM). The immunoaffinity bed in the column was subsequently washed with demineralized water (Millipore Water Purification System, Millipore S.A., Molsheim, France). The column was eluted with 99.8% methanol (LIChrosolv™, No. 1.06 007, Merck-Hitachi, Germany) to remove the bound mycotoxin. The obtained solutions were analyzed by high-performance liquid chromatography (HPLC system, Hewlett Packard type 1050 and 1100), coupled with a diode array detector (DAD), a fluorescence detector (FLD), and chromatography columns (Atlantis T3 3 μm 3.0 150 mm Column No. 186003723, Waters, AN Etten-Leur, Ireland). Mycotoxins were separated in a mobile phase of acetonitrile:water:methanol (46:46:8, $v/v/v$). The flow rate was 0.4 mL/min. The limit of detection was set at 5 μg/kg of feed for DON and 2 μg/kg of feed for ZEN, based on validation of chromatographic methods for the determination of ZEN and DON levels in feed materials and feeds. Chromatographic methods were validated at the Department of Veterinary Prevention and Feed Hygiene [68]; see File S1 in Supplementary Materials.

5.3. Experimental Animals

An in vivo experiment involving 60 clinically healthy prepubertal gilts with initial BW of 14.5 ± 2 kg was performed at the Department of Veterinary Prevention and Feed Hygiene of the Faculty of Veterinary Medicine at the University of Warmia and Mazury in Olsztyn, Poland [7,32]. During the experiment, the animals were housed in pens, fed identical diets, and provided with ad libitum access to water. The gilts were randomly divided into a control group (group C; n = 15) and three experimental groups (ZEN5, ZEN10, and ZEN15; n = 15 each) [69,70]. Groups ZEN5, ZEN10, and ZEN15 were administered ZEN (Sigma-Aldrich Z2125-26MG, St. Louis, MO, USA) per os at 5 μg/kg BW, 10 μg/kg BW, and 15 μg/kg BW, respectively. Each experimental group was kept in a separate pen in the same building. Pens had an area of 25 m^2 each, which is consistent with the applicable cross-compliance regulations (Regulation (EU) No 1306/2013 of the European Parliament and of the Council of 17 December 2013).

5.3.1. Toxicological Analysis of Intestinal Tissues

Tissues Samples

Five prepubertal gilts from every group were euthanized on analytical date 1 (D1—exposure day 7), date 2 (D2—exposure day 21), and date 3 (D3—exposure day 42) by intravenous administration of pentobarbital sodium (Fatro, Ozzano Emilia BO, Italy) and bleeding. Immediately after cardiac arrest, tissue samples (approximately 1×1.5 cm) were collected from entire intestinal cross-sections, from the following segments of the gastrointestinal tract: duodenum—third part; jejunum and ileum—middle part; cecum—1 cm from the ileocecal valve; colon—middle part of the centrifugal gyri of the ascending colon and centripetal gyri of the ascending colon (ascending colon), transverse colon, and descending colon. The samples were rinsed with phosphate buffer and prepared for analyses. The collected samples were stored at a temperature of -20 °C.

Extraction Procedure

The presence of ZEN, α-ZEL, and β-ZEL in tissue samples was determined with the use of immunoaffinity columns. Tissue samples were transferred to centrifuge tubes and homogenized with 7 mL of methanol (99.8%) for 4 min. The tubes were vortexed 4 times at 5 min intervals, after which they were centrifuged at 5000 rpm for 15 min. Samples of 5 mL were collected from the suspension and combined with 20 mL of deionized water, and 12.5 mL of the resulting solution was used to extract ZEN. The supernatant was carefully collected and passed through immunoaffinity columns (Zearala-TestTM Zearalenone Testing System, G1012, VICAM, Watertown, MA, USA) at a rate of 1–2 drops per second. The immunoaffinity bed in the column was subsequently washed with demineralized water (Millipore Water Purification System, Millipore S.A., Molsheim, France). Isocratic elution was performed with 99.8% methanol (LIChrosolvTM, No. 1.06 007, Merck-Hitachi, Germany) to remove the bound mycotoxin. After extraction, the eluents were placed in a water bath at a temperature of 50 °C and were evaporated in a stream of nitrogen. Dry residues were stored at -20 °C until chromatographic analysis. Next, 0.5 mL of 99.8% acetonitrile (ACN) was added to dry residues to dissolve the mycotoxin. The process was monitored with the use of internal standards (Cayman Chemical 1180 East Ellsworth Road Ann Arbor, Michigan 48108 USA, ZEN-catalog number 11353; Batch 0593470-1; a-ZEN-catalog number 16549; Batch 0585633-2; β-ZEN-catalog number 19460; Batch 0604066-7).

Chromatographic Quantification of ZEN and Its Metabolites

Zearalenone and its metabolites were quantified at the Institute of Dairy Industry Innovation in Mrągowo, Poland. The biological activity of ZEN, α-ZEL, and β-ZEL in the bone marrow microenvironment was determined by combined separation methods involving immunoaffinity columns (Zearala-TestTM Zearalenone Testing System, G1012, VICAM, Watertown, MA, USA), Agilent 1260 liquid chromatography (LC) system, and a mass spectrometry system (MS, Agilent 6470). Samples were analyzed on a chromatographic column (Atlantis T3, 3 µm 3.0×150 mm, column No. 186003723, Waters, AN Etten-Leur, Ireland). The mobile phase was composed of 70% acetonitrile (LiChrosolvTM, No. 984730109, Merck-Hitachi, Mannheim, Germany), 20% methanol (LIChrosolvTM, No. 1.06 007, Merck-Hitachi, Mannheim, Germany), and 10% deionized water (Milipore-Water Purification System, Millipore S.A. Molsheim-France) with the addition of 2 mL of acetic acid per 1 L of the mixture. The flow rate was 0.4 mL/min., and the temperature of the oven column was 40 °C. The chromatographic analysis was completed in 4 min. The column was flushed with 99.8% methanol (LIChrosolvTM, No. 1.06 007, Merck-Hitachi, Mannheim, Germany) to remove the bound mycotoxin. The flow rate was 0.4 mL/min., and the temperature of the oven column was 40 °C. The chromatographic analysis was completed in 4 min.

Mycotoxin concentrations were determined with an external standard and expressed in ppb (ng/mL). Matrix-matched calibration standards were applied in the quantification process to eliminate matrix effects that can decrease sensitivity. Calibration standards were dissolved in matrix samples based on the procedure that was used to prepare the remaining samples. The material for calibration standards was free of mycotoxins. The limits of detection (LOD) for ZEN, α-ZEL, and β-ZEL were determined as the concentration at which the signal-to-noise ratio decreased to 3. The concentrations of ZEN, α-ZEL, and β-ZEL were determined in each group and on three analytical dates (see Table 1).

Mass Spectrometric Conditions

The mass spectrometer was operated with ESI in the negative ion mode. The MS/MS parameters were optimized for each compound. The linearity was tested by a calibration curve including six levels. Table 5 shows the optimized analysis conditions for the mycotoxins tested.

Table 5. Optimized conditions for mycotoxins tested [71].

Analyte	Precursor	Quantification Ion	Confirmation Ion	LOD (ng mL^{-1})	LOQ (ng mL^{-1})	Linearity (%R^2)
ZEN	317.1	273.3	187.1	0.03	0.1	0.999
α-ZEL	319.2	275.2	160.1	0.3	0.9	0.997
β-ZEL	319.2	275.2	160.1	0.3	1	0.993

Carry-Over Factor

Carry-over toxicity occurs when the body is able to survive under the influence of low doses of mycotoxins. Mycotoxins may impair the functions of tissues or organs [72] and modify their biological activity [5,7]. CF was determined in the intestinal tissues when the daily dose of ZEN (5 μg ZEN/kg BW, 10 μg ZEN/kg BW or 15 μg ZEN/kg BW) administered to each animal was equivalent to 560–32251.5 μg ZEN/kg complete diet, depending on the daily feed intake. The concentrations of mycotoxins in the tissues were expressed as the dry matter content of the samples.

The CF was calculated as follows:

$$CF = \text{toxin concentration in tissue [ng/g]} / \text{toxin concentration in diet [ng/g]}$$

Statistical Analysis

The data were statistically processed at the Department of Discrete Mathematics and Theoretical Computer Science, Faculty of Mathematics and Computer Science, University of Warmia and Mazury in Olsztyn. The bioavailability of ZEN and its metabolites in gut tissues was analyzed in group C and three experimental groups on three analytical dates. Results are expressed as means (±) with standard deviation (SD). The following parameters were analyzed: (i) the differences in the mean values for the various doses of ZEN (experimental groups) and the control group on the three analytical dates, and (ii) the differences in the mean values for the individual doses (groups) of ZEN at the three dates. Differences between mean values were determined using one-way ANOVA. If there were significant differences between groups, the differences between the pairs of means were determined using Tukey's multiple comparison test. If all values were below the LOD (mean and variance equal to zero) in either group, values in the remaining groups were analyzed by one-way ANOVA (if the number of remaining groups was greater than two), and the means of these groups were compared with zero on Student's t-test. The differences between the groups were determined by Student's t-test. The results were considered to be highly significant at $p < 0.01$ (**) and significant at $0.01 < p < 0.05$ (*). The data were statistically processed using Statistica v.13 software (TIBCO Software Inc., Silicon Valley, CA, USA, 2017). Dose–response relationships were established using Pearson's correlation analysis. Differences were considered significant at $p \leq 0.05$. Results are presented as the means ± standard error of the mean (SEM).

5.4. Expression of CYP1A1 and GSTπ1

5.4.1. Sampling and Storage for RNA Extraction

Immediately after cardiac arrest, tissue samples were collected from the mid-ascending and descending colon. The samples were stored in RNAlater (Sigma-Aldrich; Taufkirchen, Germany) according to the manufacturer's instructions. Tissue samples were collected at the same time.

5.4.2. Complete RNA Extraction and cDNA Synthesis

Total RNA was extracted from RNAlater-preserved tissues (approx. 20 mg per sample; $n = 5$ in each treatment group) using the Total RNA Mini isolation kit (A&A Biotechnology; Gdansk, Poland) according to the manufacturer's protocol. RNA samples were incubated with RNase-free DNase I (Roche Diagnostics; Mannheim, Germany) to prevent contamination of genomic DNA. The overall RNA quality and purity of all samples were assessed with a BioPhotometer (Eppendorf; Hamburg, Germany), and the results were used for cDNA synthesis with the RevertAid™ First Strand cDNA Synthesis Kit (Fermentas; Burlington, Canada). The cDNA synthesis reaction mixture for each sample contained 1 μg of total RNA and 0.5 μg of oligo (dT) primer, and the reaction was performed according to the manufacturer's protocol. The first synthesized cDNA strand was stored at −20 °C until further analysis.

5.4.3. qPCR

Real-time PCR primers for the CYP1A1 and GSTπ1 mRNAs were designed using the Primer-BLAST tool based on the reference species (Table 6). The real-time PCR test was performed on an ABI 7500 Real-time PCR system thermalcycler (Applied Biosystems; USA) in singleplex mode. Subsequent treatments were applied in accordance with the producents' recommendations.

Table 6. Real-time PCR primers for the proposed study.

Primer		Sequence (5′→3′)	Amplicon Length (bp)	References
CYP1A1	Forward	cagagccgcagcagccaccttg	226	[68]
	Reverse	ggctcttgcccaaggtcagcac		
GSTP1	Forward	acctgcttcggattcaccag	178	[68]
	Reverse	ctccagccacaaagccctta		
β-Actin	Forward	catcaccatcggcaaaga	237	[73]
	Reverse	gcgtagaggtccttcctgatgt		

The quantitative cycle (Cq) values of qPCR were converted to copy number using a standard curve plot (Cq vs. log copy number) according to the methodology developed by [74] and described by Spachmo and Arukwe [75].

The rationale for the use of the standard curve is based on the assumption that the unknown samples have an equal amplification efficiency (usually above 90%), which is checked before extrapolating the unknown standards to the standard curve [75]. To generate standard curves, the purified PCR products of each mRNA were used to prepare a series of 6 10-fold dilutions with known copy number amounts that were used as templates in real-time PCR. The Cq values obtained for each dilution series were plotted against the log copy number and used to extrapolate the unknown samples to the copy number. The mRNA copy numbers of the samples collected from all experimental groups in each exposure date were divided by the averaged numbers from the C group, determined at the beginning of the experiment (control 0d), to obtain relative expression values, which were presented as the expression ratio (R).

5.4.4. Statistical Analysis

The expression of the CYP1A1 and GSTP1 genes in the ascending and descending colon was presented as mean (±) SD values for each sample. The results were analyzed with Statistica software (StatSoft Inc., Tulsa, OK, USA). Mean values in the control and experimental groups were compared by a one-way ANOVA with repeated measures based on the dose of ZEN administered to the gilts before puberty. If differences between the groups were found, a post hoc Tukey test was performed to determine which pairs of mean groups were significantly different. In ANOVA, group samples were taken from normally distributed populations with the same variance. If the above assumptions were not met in all cases, the equality of the mean groups was tested using the Kruskal–Wallis rank test and the multiple-comparisons test in ANOVA. Different pairs of groups were identified by multiple post hoc comparisons of the rank means for all groups.

Supplementary Materials: The following supporting information can be downloaded at: https://www.mdpi.com/article/10.3390/toxins14050354/s1. File S1: "Task 4. Validation of chromatographic determination methods for zearalenone, α-zearalenol, and DON in pig feed".

Author Contributions: The experiments were conceived and designed by M.M., M.G. and M.T.G. The experiments were performed by M.M., P.B., S.L.-Ż., D.L. and M.G. Data were analyzed and interpreted by M.M., P.B. and M.G. The manuscript was drafted by M.M. and M.G. and critically edited by Ł.Z. and M.T.G. All authors have read and agreed to the published version of the manuscript.

Funding: This study was supported by the "Healthy Animal-Safe Food" Scientific Consortium of the Leading National Research Centre (KNOW) pursuant to decision no. 05-1/KNOW2/2015 of the Ministry of Science and Higher Education. The project was financially supported by the Minister of Education and Science under the "Regional Initiative of Excellence" program for 2019–2022, project no. 010/RID/2018/19, amount of funding PLN 12,000,000.

Institutional Review Board Statement: All experimental procedures on animals were carried out in accordance with the Polish regulations specifying the conditions for conducting experiments on animals (opinions no. 12/2016 and 45/2016/DLZ issued by the Local Ethics Committee for Animal Experimentation of the University of Warmia and Mazury in Olsztyn, Poland, on 30 November 2016).

Informed Consent Statement: Not applicable.

Data Availability Statement: The data presented in this study are available in this article and Supplementary Materials.

Conflicts of Interest: The authors declare no conflict of interest.

References

1. Tolosa, J.; Rodríguez-Carrasco, Y.; Ruiz, M.J.; Vila-Donat, P. Multi-mycotoxin occurrence in feed, metabolism and carry-over to animal-derived food products: A review. *Food Chem. Toxicol.* **2021**, *158*, 112661. [CrossRef] [PubMed]
2. Flasch, M.; Bueschl, C.; Del Favero, G.; Adam, G.; Schuhmacher, R.; Marko, D.; Warth, B. Elucidation of xenoestrogen metabolism by non-targeted, stable isotope-assisted mass spectrometry in breast cancer cells. *Environ. Int.* **2022**, *158*, 106940. [CrossRef] [PubMed]
3. Pierzgalski, A.; Bryła, M.; Kanabus, J.; Modrzewska, M.; Podolska, G. Updated Review of the Toxicity of Selected *Fusarium* Toxins and Their Modified Forms. *Toxins* **2021**, *13*, 768. [CrossRef]
4. Gajęcka, M.; Dąbrowski, M.; Otrocka-Domagała, I.; Brzuzan, P.; Rykaczewska, A.; Cieplińska, K.; Barasińska, M.; Gajęcki, M.T.; Zielonka, Ł. Correlation between the exposure of deoxynivalenol and zearalenone and the immunohistochemical expression of estrogen receptors in the intestinal epithelium and *m*RNA of selected colonic enzymes in pre-pubertal gilts. *Toxicon* **2020**, *173*, 75–93. [CrossRef]
5. Rykaczewska, A.; Gajęcka, M.; Onyszek, E.; Cieplińska, K.; Dąbrowski, M.; Lisieska-Żołnierczyk, S.; Bulińska, M.; Babuchowski, A.; Gajęcki, M.T.; Zielonka, Ł. Imbalance in the Blood Concentrations of Selected Steroids in Prepubertal Gilts Depending on the Time of Exposure to Low Doses of Zearalenone. *Toxins* **2019**, *11*, 561. [CrossRef]
6. Sun, L.; Dai, J.; Xu, J.; Yang, J.; Zhang, D. Comparative Cytotoxic Effects and Possible Mechanisms of Deoxynivalenol, Zearalenone and T-2 Toxin Exposure to Porcine Leydig Cells In Vitro. *Toxins* **2022**, *14*, 113. [CrossRef]
7. Rykaczewska, A.; Gajęcka, M.; Dąbrowski, M.; Wiśniewska, A.; Szcześniewska, J.; Gajęcki, M.T.; Zielonka, Ł. Growth performance, selected blood biochemical parameters and body weights of pre-pubertal gilts fed diets supplemented with different doses of zearalenone (ZEN). *Toxicon* **2018**, *152*, 84–94. [CrossRef]

8. Cieplińska, K.; Gajęcka, M.; Dąbrowski, M.; Rykaczewska, A.; Lisieska-Żołnierczyk, S.; Bulińska, M.; Zielonka, Ł.; Gajęcki, M.T. Time-Dependent Changes in the Intestinal Microbiome of Gilts Exposed to Low Zearalenone Doses. *Toxins* **2019**, *11*, 296. [CrossRef]
9. Tanaka, N.; Aoyama, T.; Kimura, S.; Gonzalez, F.J. Targeting nuclear receptors for the treatment of fatty liver disease. *Pharmacol. Therapeut.* **2017**, *179*, 142–157. [CrossRef]
10. Skiepko, N.; Przybylska-Gornowicz, B.; Gajęcka, M.; Gajęcki, M.; Lewczuk, B. Effects of Deoxynivalenol and Zearalenone on the Histology and Ultrastructure of Pig Liver. *Toxins* **2020**, *12*, 463. [CrossRef]
11. Dąbrowski, M.; Obremski, K.; Gajęcka, M.; Gajęcki, M.T.; Zielonka, Ł. Changes in the Subpopulations of Porcine Peripheral Blood Lymphocytes Induced by Exposure to Low Doses of Zearalenone (ZEN) and Deoxynivalenol (DON). *Molecules* **2016**, *21*, 557. [CrossRef] [PubMed]
12. Mróz, M.; Gajęcka, M.; Przybyłowicz, K.E.; Sawicki, T.; Lisieska-Żołnierczyk, S.; Zielonka, Ł.; Gajęcki, M.T. The Effect of Low Doses of Zearalenone (ZEN) on the Bone Marrow Microenvironment and Haematological Parameters of Blood Plasma in Pre-Pubertal Gilts. *Toxins* **2022**, *14*, 105. [CrossRef] [PubMed]
13. Cieplińska, K.; Gajęcka, M.; Nowak, A.; Dąbrowski, M.; Zielonka, Ł.; Gajęcki, M.T. The Genotoxicity of Caecal Water in Gilts Exposed to Low Doses of Zearalenone. *Toxins* **2018**, *10*, 350. [CrossRef] [PubMed]
14. Kozieł, M.J.; Ziaja, M.; Piastowska-Ciesielska, A.W. Intestinal Barrier, Claudins and Mycotoxins. *Toxins* **2021**, *13*, 758. [CrossRef]
15. Agahi, F.; Juan, C.; Font, G.; Juan-García, A. In silico methods for metabolomic and toxicity prediction of zearalenone, α-zearalenone and β-zearalenone. *Food Chem. Toxicol.* **2020**, *146*, 111818. [CrossRef]
16. Pleadin, J.; Lešić, T.; Milićević, D.; Markov, K.; Šarkanj, B.; Vahčić, N.; Kmetič, I.; Zadravec, M. Pathways of Mycotoxin Occurrence in Meat Products: A Review. *Processes* **2021**, *9*, 2122. [CrossRef]
17. Calabrese, E.J. Hormesis: Path and Progression to Significance. *Int. J. Mol. Sci.* **2018**, *19*, 2871. [CrossRef]
18. Freire, L.; Sant'Ana, A.S. Modified mycotoxins: An updated review on their formation, detection, occurrence, and toxic effects. *Food Chem. Toxicol.* **2018**, *111*, 189–205. [CrossRef]
19. Gajęcka, M.; Zielonka, Ł.; Gajęcki, M. The effect of low monotonic doses of zearalenone on selected reproductive tissues in pre-pubertal female dogs—A review. *Molecules* **2015**, *20*, 20669–20687. [CrossRef]
20. Gajęcka, M.; Zielonka, Ł.; Gajęcki, M. Activity of zearalenone in the porcine intestinal tract. *Molecules* **2017**, *22*, 18. [CrossRef]
21. Stopa, E.; Babińska, I.; Zielonka, Ł.; Gajęcki, M.; Gajęcka, M. Immunohistochemical evaluation of apoptosis and proliferation in the mucous membrane of selected uterine regions in pre-pubertal bitches exposed to low doses of zearalenone. *Pol. J. Vet. Sci.* **2016**, *19*, 175–186. [CrossRef] [PubMed]
22. Alassane-Kpembi, I.; Pinton, P.; Oswald, I.P. Effects of Mycotoxins on the Intestine. *Toxins* **2019**, *11*, 159. [CrossRef] [PubMed]
23. Kramer, H.J.; van den Ham, W.A.; Slob, W.; Pieters, M.N. Conversion Factors Estimating Indicative Chronic No-Observed-Adverse-Effect Levels from Short-Term Toxicity Data. *Regul. Toxicol. Pharm.* **1996**, *23*, 249–255. [CrossRef]
24. Pastoor, T.P.; Bachman, A.N.; Bell, D.R.; Cohen, S.M.; Dellarco, M.; Dewhurst, I.C.; Doe, J.E.; Doerrer, N.G.; Embry, M.R.; Hines, R.N.; et al. A 21st century roadmap for human health risk assessment. *Crit. Rev. Toxicol.* **2014**, *44*, 1–5. [CrossRef] [PubMed]
25. Suh, H.Y.; Peck, C.C.; Yu, K.S.; Lee, H. Determination of the starting dose in the first-in-human clinical trials with monoclonal antibodies: A systematic review of papers published between 1990 and 2013. *Drug Des. Dev. Ther.* **2016**, *10*, 4005–4016. [CrossRef]
26. Chang, S.; Su, Y.; Sun, Y.; Meng, X.; Shi, B.; Shan, A. Response of the nuclear receptors PXR and CAR and their target gene mRNA expression in female piglets exposed to zearalenone. *Toxicon* **2018**, *151*, 111–118. [CrossRef]
27. Nandekar, P.P.; Khomane, K.; Chaudhary, V.; Rathod, V.P.; Borkar, R.M.; Bhandi, M.M.; Srinivas, R.; Sangamwar, A.T.; Guchhait, S.K.; Bansal, A.K. Identification of leads for antiproliferative activity on MDA-MB-435 human breast cancer cells through pharmacophore and CYP1A1-mediated metabolism. *Eur. J. Med. Chem.* **2016**, *115*, 82–93. [CrossRef]
28. Kovacevic, Z.; Sahni, S.; Lok, H.; Davies, M.J.; Wink, D.A.; Richardson, D.R. Regulation and control of nitric oxide (NO) in macrophages: Protecting the "professional killer cell" from its own cytotoxic arsenal via MRP1 and GSTP1. *BBA Gen. Subj.* **2017**, *1861*, 995–999. [CrossRef]
29. Billat, P.A.; Roger, E.; Faure, S.; Lagarce, F. Models for drug absorption from the small intestine: Where are we and where are we going? *Drug Discov. Today* **2017**. [CrossRef]
30. Gajęcka, M.; Zielonka, Ł.; Gajęcki, M.T. *A Complementary Analysis of the Effects of Low-Dose Zearalenone Mycotoxicosis on Selected Health Status Indicators in Pre-Pubertal Gilts*; Danielewska, A., Maciąg, K., Eds.; Wydawnictwo Naukowe TYGIEL Sp. Zo.o.: Lublin, Poland, 2020; pp. 41–70. ISBN 979-83-66489-21-9. (In Polish)
31. Gajęcka, M.; Majewski, M.S.; Zielonka, Ł.; Grzegorzewski, W.; Onyszek, E.; Lisieska-Żołnierczyk, S.; Juśkiewicz, J.; Babuchowski, A.; Gajęcki, M.T. Concentration of Zearalenone, Alpha-Zearalenol and Beta-Zearalenol in the Myocardium and the Results of Isometric Analyses of the Coronary Artery in Prepubertal Gilts. *Toxins* **2021**, *13*, 396. [CrossRef]
32. Gajęcka, M.; Mróz, M.; Brzuzan, P.; Onyszek, E.; Zielonka, Ł.; Lipczyńska-Ilczuk, K.; Przybyłowicz, K.E.; Babuchowski, A.; Gajęcki, M.T. Correlations between Low Doses of Zearalenone, Its Carryover Factor and Estrogen Receptor Expression in Different Segments of the Intestines in Pre-Pubertal Gilts—A Study Protocol. *Toxins* **2021**, *13*, 379. [CrossRef] [PubMed]
33. Shigeyuki, U.; Dalton, T.P.; Derkenne, S.; Curran, C.P.; Miller, M.L.; Shertzer, H.G.; Nebert, D.W. Oral Exposure to Benzo[a]pyrene in the Mouse: Detoxication by Inducible Cytochrome P450 Is More Important Than Metabolic Activation. *Mol. Pharmacol.* **2004**, *65*, 1225–1237.

34. Basharat, Z.; Yasmin, A. Energy landscape of a GSTP1 polymorph linked with cytological function decay in response to chemical stressors. *Gene* **2017**, *609*, 19–27. [CrossRef]
35. Huszno, J.; Nowara, E.; Suwiński, R. The importance of genetic polymorphisms in cancer chemotherapy. *J. Oncol.* **2011**, *61*, 141–149.
36. Gajęcka, M.; Brzuzan, P.; Otrocka-Domagała, I.; Zielonka, Ł.; Lisieska-Żołnierczyk, S.; Gajęcki, M.T. The Effect of 42-Day Exposure to a Low Deoxynivalenol Dose on the Immunohistochemical Expression of Intestinal ERs and the Activation of CYP1A1 and GSTP1 Genes in the Large Intestine of Pre-pubertal Gilts. *Front. Vet. Sci.* **2021**, *8*, 644549. [CrossRef]
37. Zielonka, Ł.; Gajęcka, M.; Lisieska-Żołnierczyk, S.; Dąbrowski, M.; Gajęcki, M.T. The Effect of Different Doses of Zearalenone in Feed on the Bioavailability of Zearalenone and Alpha-zearalenol, and the Concentrations of Estradiol and Testosterone in the Peripheral Blood of Pre-pubertal Gilts. *Toxins* **2020**, *12*, 144. [CrossRef]
38. Bakhru, S.H.; Furtado, S.; Morello, A.P.; Mathiowitz, E. Oral delivery of proteins by biodegradable nanoparticles. *Adv. Drug. Deliv. Rev.* **2013**, *65*, 811–821. [CrossRef]
39. Lawrenz, B.; Melado, L.; Fatemi, H. Premature progesterone rise in ART-cycles. *Reprod. Biol.* **2018**, *18*, 1–4. [CrossRef]
40. Jakimiuk, E.; Kuciel-Lisieska, G.; Zwierzchowski, W.; Gajęcka, M.; Obremski, K.; Zielonka, Ł.; Skorska-Wyszyńska, E.; Gajęcki, M. Morphometric changes of the reproductive system in gilts during zearalenone mycotoxicosis. *Med. Weter.* **2006**, *62*, 99–102.
41. Rivera, H.M.; Stincic, T.L. Estradiol and the control of feeding behavior. *Steroids* **2018**, *133*, 44–52. [CrossRef]
42. Benagiano, M.; Bianchi, P.; D'Elios, M.M.; Brosens, I.; Benagiano, G. Autoimmune diseases: Role of steroid hormones. *Best Pract. Res. Cl. Ob.* **2019**, *60*, 24–34. [CrossRef] [PubMed]
43. Uvnäs-Moberg, K. The gastrointestinal tract in growth and reproduction. *Sci. Am.* **1989**, *261*, 78–83. Available online: https://www.jstor.org/stable/24987325 (accessed on 19 April 2022). [CrossRef] [PubMed]
44. Bulgaru, C.V.; Marin, D.E.; Pistol, G.C.; Taranu, I. Zearalenone and the Immune Response. *Toxins* **2021**, *13*, 248. [CrossRef]
45. Zhang, J.; Zheng, Y.; Tao, H.; Liu, J.; Zhao, P.; Yang, F.; Lv, Z.; Wang, J. Effects of Bacillus subtilis ZJ-2019-1 on Zearalenone Toxicosis in Female Gilts. *Toxins* **2021**, *13*, 788. [CrossRef]
46. Mahmoodzadeh, S.; Dworatzek, E. The Role of 17β-Estradiol and Estrogen Receptors in Regulation of Ca2+ Channels and Mitochondrial Function in Cardiomyocytes. *Front. Endocrinol.* **2019**, *10*, 310. [CrossRef]
47. Widodo, O.S.; Etoh, M.; Kokushi, E.; Uno, S.; Yamato, O.; Pambudi, D.; Okawa, H.; Taniguchi, M.; Lamid, M.; Takagi, M. Practical Application of Urinary Zearalenone Monitoring System for Feed Hygiene Management of a Japanese Black Cattle Breeding Herd—The Relationship between Monthly Anti-Müllerian Hormone and Serum Amyloid A Concentrations. *Toxins* **2022**, *14*, 143. [CrossRef]
48. Yan, Z.; Wang, L.; Wang, J.; Tan, Y.; Yu, D.; Chang, X.; Fan, Y.; Zhao, D.; Wang, C.; De Boevre, M.; et al. A QuEChERS-Based Liquid Chromatography Tandem Mass Spectrometry Method for the Simultaneous Determination of Nine Zearalenone-Like Mycotoxins in Pigs. *Toxins* **2018**, *10*, 129. [CrossRef]
49. Chodorowski, Z.; Sein Anand, J.; Robakowska, I.; Klimek, J.; Kaletha, K. The role of intestine in detoxification. *Przeg. Lek.* **2007**, *64*, 363–364.
50. Sergent, T.; Ribonnet, L.; Kolosova, A.; Garsou, S.; Schaut, A.; De Saeger, S.; Van Peteghem, C.; Larondelle, Y.; Pussemier, L.; Schneider, Y.J. Molecular and cellular effects of food contaminants and secondary plant components and their plausible interactions at the intestinal level. *Food Chem. Toxicol.* **2008**, *46*, 813–841. [CrossRef]
51. Martın, J.F.; Casqueiro, J.; Liras, P. Secretion systems for secondary metabolites: How producer cells send out messages of intercellular communication. *Curr. Opin. Microbiol.* **2005**, *8*, 282–293. [CrossRef]
52. Balaguer, P.; Delfosse, V.; Bourguet, W. Mechanisms of endocrine disruption through nuclear receptors and related pathways. *Curr. Opin. Endocrin. Metab. Res.* **2019**, *7*, 1–8. [CrossRef]
53. Vandenberg, L.N.; Colborn, T.; Hayes, T.B.; Heindel, J.J.; Jacobs, D.R.; Lee, D.-H.; Shioda, T.; Soto, A.M.; vom Saal, F.S.; Welshons, W.V.; et al. Hormones and endocrine-disrupting chemicals: Low-dose effects and nonmonotonic dose responses. *Endoc. Rev.* **2012**, *33*, 378–455. [CrossRef] [PubMed]
54. Bhasin, S.; Jasuja, R. Reproductive and Nonreproductive Actions of Testosterone. *Enc. Endocr. Dis.* **2019**, *2*, 721–734. [CrossRef]
55. Li, P.; Su, R.; Yin, R.; Lai, D.; Wang, M.; Liu, Y.; Zhou, L. Detoxification of Mycotoxins through Biotransformation. *Toxins* **2020**, *12*, 121. [CrossRef] [PubMed]
56. Zheng, W.; Feng, N.; Wang, Y.; Noll, L.; Xu, S.; Liu, X.; Lu, N.; Zou, H.; Gu, J.; Yuan, Y.; et al. Effects of zearalenone and its derivatives on the synthesis and secretion of mammalian sex steroid hormones: A review. *Food Chem. Toxicol.* **2019**, *126*, 262–276. [CrossRef]
57. Rogowska, A.; Pomastowski, P.; Sagandykova, G.; Buszewski, B. Zearalenone and its metabolites: Effect on human health, metabolism and neutralisation methods. *Toxicon* **2019**, *162*, 46–56. [CrossRef]
58. Tyagi, V.; Scordo, M.; Yoon, R.S.; Liporace, F.A.; Greene, L.W. Revisiting the role of testosterone: Are we missing something? *Rev. Urol.* **2017**, *19*, 16–24. [CrossRef]
59. Alvarez-Ortega, N.; Caballero-Gallardo, K.; Taboada-Alquerque, M.; Franco, J.; Stashenko, E.E.; Juan, C.; Juan-García, A.; Olivero-Verbel, J. Protective Effects of the Hydroethanolic Extract of *Fridericia chica* on Undifferentiated Human Neuroblastoma Cells Exposed to α-Zearalenol (α-ZEL) and β-Zearalenol (β-ZEL). *Toxins* **2021**, *13*, 748. [CrossRef]
60. Kalemba-Drożdż, M.; Kapiszewska, M. Genetic polymorphism in biosynthesis of estrogens. The risk of hormone-dependent neoplasms. In *Środowisko a Gospodarka Hormonalna u Kobiet. Tom I. Zaburzenia w Metabolizmie Estrogenów i ich Konsekwencje*; Oficyna

Wydawnicza AFM: Kraków, Poland, 2011; pp. 149–161. ISBN 978-83-7571-195-0. Available online: http://hdl.handle.net/11315/744 (accessed on 15 November 2011).
61. Singh, R.R.; Reindl, K.M. Glutathione S-Transferases in Cancer. *Antioxidants* **2021**, *10*, 701. [CrossRef]
62. Howie, A.F.; Forrester, L.M.; Glancey, M.J.; Schlager, J.J.; Powis, G.; Beckett, G.J.; Hayes, J.D.; Wolf, C.R. Glutathione S-transferase and glutathione peroxidase expression in normal and tumour human tissues. *Carcinogenesis* **1990**, *11*, 451–458. [CrossRef]
63. Bocedi, A.; Noce, A.; Marrone, G.; Noce, G.; Cattani, G.; Gambardella, G.; Di Lauro, M.; Di Daniele, N.; Ricci, G. Glutathione Transferase P1-1 an Enzyme Useful in Biomedicine and as Biomarker in Clinical Practice and in Environmental Pollution. *Nutrients* **2019**, *11*, 1741. [CrossRef] [PubMed]
64. Chatterjee, A.; Gupta, S. The multifaceted role of glutathione S-transferases in cancer. *Cancer Lett.* **2018**, *433*, 33–42. [CrossRef] [PubMed]
65. Ludvigsen, M.; Thorlacius-Ussing, L.; Vorum, H.; Stender, M.T.; Thorlacius-Ussing, O.; Honoré, B. Proteomic Characterization of Colorectal Cancer Tissue from Patients Identifies Novel Putative Protein Biomarkers. *Curr. Issues Mol. Biol.* **2021**, *43*, 1043–1056. [CrossRef] [PubMed]
66. Hokaiwado, N.; Takeshita, F.; Naiki-Ito, A.; Asamoto, M.; Ochiya, T.; Shirai, T. Glutathione S transferase pi mediates proliferation of androgen- independent prostate cancer cells. *Carcinogenesis* **2008**, *29*, 1134–1138. [CrossRef] [PubMed]
67. Knutsen, H.K.; Alexander, J.; Barregård, L.; Bignami, M.; Brüschweiler, B.; Ceccatelli, S.; Cottrill, B.; Dinovi, M.; Edler, L.; Grasl-Kraupp, B.; et al. Risks for animal health related to the presence of zearalenone and its modified forms in feed. *EFSA J.* **2017**, *15*, 4851. [CrossRef]
68. Gajęcki, M. Development Project NR12-0080-10 entitled. In *The Effect of Experimentally Induced Fusarium Mycotoxicosis on Selected Diagnostic and Morphological Parameters of the Porcine Digestive Tract*; The National Centre for Research and Development: Warsaw, Poland, 2013; pp. 1–180.
69. Heberer, T.; Lahrssen-Wiederholt, M.; Schat, H.; Abraham, K.; Pzyrembel, H.; Henning, K.J.; Schauzu, M.; Braeunig, J.; Goetz, M.; Niemann, L.; et al. Zero tolerances in food and animal feed—Are there any scientificalternatives? A European point of view on aninternational controversy. *Toxicol. Lett.* **2007**, *175*, 118–135. [CrossRef]
70. Smith, D.; Combes, R.; Depelchin, O.; Jacobsen, S.D.; Hack, R.; Luft, J.; Lammens, L.; von Landenberg, F.; Phillips, B.; Pfister, R.; et al. Optimising the design of preliminarytoxicity studies for pharmaceutical safetytesting in the dog. *Regul. Toxicol. Pharmacol.* **2005**, *41*, 95–101. [CrossRef]
71. Barański, W.; Gajęcka, M.; Zielonka, Ł.; Mróz, M.; Onyszek, E.; Przybyłowicz, K.E.; Nowicki, A.; Babuchowski, A.; Gajęcki, M.T. Occurrence of Zearalenone and Its Metabolites in the Blood of High-Yielding Dairy Cows at Selected Collection Sites in Various Disease States. *Toxins* **2021**, *13*, 446. [CrossRef]
72. Meerpoel, C.; Vidal, A.; Tangni, E.K.; Huybrechts, B.; Couck, L.; De Rycke, R.; De Bels, L.; De Saeger, S.; Van den Broeck, W.; Devreese, M.; et al. A Study of Carry-Over and Histopathological Effects after Chronic Dietary Intake of Citrinin in Pigs, Broiler Chickens and Laying Hens. *Toxins* **2020**, *12*, 719. [CrossRef]
73. Tohno, M.; Shimasato, T.; Moue, M.; Aso, H.; Watanabe, K.; Kawai, Y.; Yamaguchi, T.; Saito, T.; Kitazawa, H. Toll-like receptor 2 and 9 are expressed and functional in gut associated lymphoid tissues of presuckling newborn swine. *Vet. Res.* **2006**, *37*, 791–812. [CrossRef]
74. Arukwe, A. Toxicological housekeeping genes: Do they really keep the house? *Environ. Sci. Technol.* **2006**, *40*, 7944–7949. [CrossRef] [PubMed]
75. Spachmo, B.; Arukwe, A. Endocrine and developmental effects in Atlantic salmon (Salmo salar) exposed to perfluorooctane sulfonic or perfluorooctane carboxylic acids. *Aquat. Toxicol.* **2012**, *108*, 112–124. [CrossRef] [PubMed]

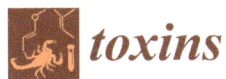

Article

Practical Application of Urinary Zearalenone Monitoring System for Feed Hygiene Management of a Japanese Black Cattle Breeding Herd—The Relationship between Monthly Anti-Müllerian Hormone and Serum Amyloid A Concentrations

Oky Setyo Widodo [1,2], Makoto Etoh [3], Emiko Kokushi [4], Seiichi Uno [4], Osamu Yamato [5], Dhidhi Pambudi [6], Hiroaki Okawa [7], Masayasu Taniguchi [1,8], Mirni Lamid [2] and Mitsuhiro Takagi [1,2,8,*]

1. Joint Graduate School of Veterinary Sciences, Yamaguchi University, Yamaguchi 753-8515, Japan; oky.widodo@fkh.unair.ac.id (O.S.W.); masa0810@yamaguchi-u.ac.jp (M.T.)
2. Department of Animal Husbandry, Faculty of Veterinary Medicine, Airlangga University, Surabaya 60115, Indonesia; mirnylamid@fkh.unair.ac.id
3. Ohita Agricultural Mutual Aid Association, Takeda 878-0024, Japan; mako_eto@nosai-oita.jp
4. Faculty of Fisheries, Kagoshima University, Kagoshima 890-0056, Japan; kokushi@fish.kagoshima-u.ac.jp (E.K.); uno@fish.kagoshima-u.ac.jp (S.U.)
5. Joint Faculty of Veterinary Medicine, Kagoshima University, Kagoshima 890-0065, Japan; osamu@vet.kagoshima-u.ac.jp
6. Department of Mathematics Education, Faculty of Teacher Training and Education, Sebelas Maret University, Surakarta 57126, Indonesia; dhidhipambudi@staff.uns.ac.id
7. Guardian Co., Ltd., Kagoshima 890-0033, Japan; okawa0117@guardian-vet.com
8. Laboratory of Theriogenology, Joint Faculty of Veterinary Medicine, Yamaguchi University, Yamaguchi 753-8515, Japan
* Correspondence: mtakagi@yamaguchi-u.ac.jp

Citation: Widodo, O.S.; Etoh, M.; Kokushi, E.; Uno, S.; Yamato, O.; Pambudi, D.; Okawa, H.; Taniguchi, M.; Lamid, M.; Takagi, M. Practical Application of Urinary Zearalenone Monitoring System for Feed Hygiene Management of a Japanese Black Cattle Breeding Herd—The Relationship between Monthly Anti-Müllerian Hormone and Serum Amyloid A Concentrations. *Toxins* **2022**, *14*, 143. https://doi.org/10.3390/toxins14020143

Received: 19 January 2022
Accepted: 11 February 2022
Published: 16 February 2022

Publisher's Note: MDPI stays neutral with regard to jurisdictional claims in published maps and institutional affiliations.

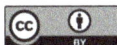

Copyright: © 2022 by the authors. Licensee MDPI, Basel, Switzerland. This article is an open access article distributed under the terms and conditions of the Creative Commons Attribution (CC BY) license (https:// creativecommons.org/licenses/by/ 4.0/).

Abstract: This study addresses an advantageous application of a urinary zearalenone (ZEN) monitoring system not only for surveillance of ZEN exposure at the production site of breeding cows but also for follow-up monitoring after improvement of feeds provided to the herd. As biomarkers of effect, serum levels of the anti-Müllerian hormone (AMH) and serum amyloid A (SAA) concentrations were used. Based on the results of urinary ZEN measurement, two cows from one herd had urinary ZEN concentrations which were two orders of magnitude higher (ZEN: 1.34 mg/kg, sterigmatocystin (STC): 0.08 mg/kg in roughages) than the levels of all cows from three other herds (ZEN: not detected, STC: not detected in roughages). For the follow-up monitoring of the herd with positive ZEN and STC exposure, urine, blood, and roughage samples were collected from five cows monthly for one year. A monitoring series in the breeding cattle herd indicated that feed concentrations were not necessarily reflected in urinary concentrations; urinary monitoring assay by ELISA may be a simple and accurate method that reflects the exposure/absorption of ZEN. Additionally, although the ZEN exposure level appeared not to be critical compared with the Japanese ZEN limitation in dietary feeds, a negative regression trend between the ZEN and AMH concentrations was observed, indicating that only at extremely universal mycotoxin exposure levels, ZEN exposure may affect the number of antral follicles in cattle. A negative regression trend between the ZEN and SAA concentrations could also be demonstrated, possibly indicating the innate immune suppression caused by low-level chronic ZEN exposure. Finally, significant differences ($p = 0.0487$) in calving intervals between pre-ZEN monitoring (mean ± SEM: 439.0 ± 41.2) and post-ZEN monitoring (349.9 ± 6.9) periods were observed in the monitored five cows. These preliminary results indicate that the urinary ZEN monitoring system may be a useful practical tool not only for detecting contaminated herds under field conditions but also provides an initial look at the effects of long-term chronic ZEN/STC (or other co-existing mycotoxins) exposure on herd productivity and fertility.

Keywords: AMH; cattle; long-term monitoring; sub-clinical contamination; SAA; urine; zearalenone

Key Contribution: The urinary ZEN monitoring system is an important practical tool for revealing the effects of long-term chronic ZEN/STC (or other co-existing mycotoxins) exposure on cows productivity and fertility. The long-term use of the ZEN-contaminated feed affected the calving interval.

1. Introduction

Recently, increasing attention has been paid to the impact of *Fusarium*-derived mycotoxins, as their prevalence seems to increase worldwide, despite efforts to minimize their concentration in animal feeds. Global warming and/or climate change are discussed as possible causes for higher exposure rates which may enhance the risk of harmful effects on both human and animal health [1–4]. Indeed, a large-scale global survey of mycotoxin contamination in more than 70,000 sample feeds collected from more than one hundred countries suggested that mycotoxins are almost ubiquitously detected contaminants [5]. The authors concluded that co-occurrence of *Fusarium*-derived mycotoxins (such as zearalenone (ZEN) and deoxynivalenol (DON) as the most important combinations) should be monitored more closely [5]. Based on a recent review, ZEN, one of the *Fusarium*-derived estrogenic-mycotoxins, is mainly formed at the pre-harvest stage, although continued fungal growth and ZEN synthesis may continue during poor storage conditions [6]. As controlling animals' exposure to mycotoxins is often difficult under farm conditions, where feed supplies may change rapidly, monitoring of urinary concentration of ZEN of farm animals such as cattle is presumed to be a suitable biomarker for ZEN exposure [7–9]. Previously, we have established a urinary ZEN-monitoring system with ELISA for initial screening purposes, followed by LC-MS/MS validation to detect ZEN and its related metabolites; α-zearalenol (α-ZEL) and β-zearalenol (β-ZEL) as well as sterigmatocystin (STC), as both toxins might occur together in diets for Japanese cattle [10–12]. Additionally, we have reported that monitoring ZEN or STC levels in urine is not only a practical and useful way of evaluating and detecting the naturally contamination status of cattle herds, but also assessing the efficiency of mycotoxin adsorbents (MAs) supplemented in dietary feed to reduce intestinal absorption of mycotoxins [10,11,13,14].

Multiple factors influence fungal growth and mycotoxin formation, including season, geographical location, drought, harvest time, processing, storage, and distribution, etc., [6], thus, the important first step in combating mycotoxins, especially in herds fed home-grown forage begins with measuring the level/status of mycotoxins contamination in the feed of individual herds during the stage of sub-clinical health condition. We have continued to monitor cattle herds in the field to detect subclinical ZEN-contaminated herds by using urinary ZEN monitoring. During this monitoring, we identified one herd which was speculated to have been fed rather high ZEN-contaminated roughage exceeding the standard value in Japan (>1 mg/kg) with urine samples by ELISA, following validated by LC-MS/MS assay of the dietary roughage. Given ethical and animal welfare concerns, and the high costs involved, it is hardly possible to conduct feeding trials with cattle exposed to ZEN contaminated feed to investigate the effects of chronic low levels of ZEN contamination. Therefore, we evaluated whether the identified cattle herd may serve as a useful tool for observing the effect of long-term exposure on urinary excretion of toxins as well as an indicator of the reproductive performance of female cattle.

The objectives of this field study were to (1) re-evaluate the urinary ZEN monitoring system for its practical usefulness in cattle farm conditions and (2) evaluate the follow-up monitoring results for 1 year, concomitant with the relationship between changes in both naturally occurring urinary ZEN and serum anti-Müllerian hormone (AMH) concentration, and STC concentrations. AMH is secreted by ovarian granulosa cells primarily from pre-antral and early antral follicles of females and is an endocrine marker closely associated with both gonadotrophin-responsive ovarian reserves and with the size of the pool of growing preantral and small antral follicles [15,16]. Additionally, serum amyloid A (SAA), which is one of the most reliable acute phase proteins (APPs) primarily produced by the liver induced by the inflammatory cytokines, such as interleukin (IL)-1, IL-6, and tumor necrosis factor (TNF)-α [17,18], was measured to monitor inflammation in each cow at the monthly sampling time, given our previous report that not only calving itself but also severe inflammation during the postpartum period indicated by high SAA concentration can affect the AMH concentration in cows [19].

2. Results

2.1. First Urinary ZEN Screening on Four JB Breeding Cattle Herds in the Neighborhood

Table 1 shows a summary of all results of the first screening of the four herds. The urinary ZEN concentrations of two samples from Herd C measured by ELISA exceeded the upper limit value that guarantees quantification within the range of the calibration curve used in the ELISA measurement (4050 ppt = 4050 pg/mL); thus, they were assumed to be >20,250 pg/mL without repeating ELISA measurements by using more diluted samples, whose concentration levels differed by two orders of magnitude compared to cows from the other three herds. Therefore, based on the results of the first urinary ZEN screening, it was assumed that the ZEN concentration in the roughage fed to herd C was much higher than that in the other herds. Thus, as the next step in our screening, both ZEN and STC concentrations in the dietary roughage from all herds were measured. The ZEN concentration of the roughage sample from Herd C was 1.34 mg/kg, which was higher than the Japanese national limit of ZEN, concomitant with STC exposure (0.08 mg/kg) (Table 1). Additionally, the results of LC/MS measurements performed later, i.e., the simultaneous detection of ZEN, its metabolites, and STC in the urine sample only from Herd C, clarified the ELISA results of urine samples and LC-MS/MS results of both ZEN and STC in roughage.

Table 1. Urinary ZEN concentrations at the first screening on four JB breeding cattle herds.

	ELISA			LC-MS/MS				LC-MS/MS	
Cow	Urinary ZEN Concentrations (pg/mL)	ZEN/Cre	ZEN/Cre	α-ZEL/Cre	β-ZEL/Cre	ΣZEN/Cre	STC/Cre	ZEN in Roughage (mg/kg)	STC in Roughage (mg/kg)
A1	2132.6	3280.9	ND	ND	ND	ND	ND	ND	ND
A2	1637.6	930.5	ND	ND	ND	ND	ND		
B1	1937.9	983.7	ND	ND	ND	ND	ND	ND	<0.04 **
B2	1528.5	979.8	ND	ND	ND	ND	ND		
C1	>20,250	>23,011.4 *	14,363.6	10,772.7	16,454.5	41,590.9	659.1	1.34	0.08
C2	>20,250	>21,315.8 *	11,915.8	8526.3	4736.8	25,178.9	442.1		
D1	1931.2	3862.4	ND	ND	ND	ND	ND	ND	ND
D2	985.2	1669.8	ND	ND	ND	ND	ND		

* The urinary ZEN concentrations of the two samples from Herd C ranged over the maximal standard concentration of the ELISA kit. Thus, ZEN/Cre were expressed based on the maximal standard concentrations. Cre: Creatinine. ** Sterigmatocystin was detected below the lower limit, but it was not reached the quantitative value. ND: Not detected.

2.2. Follow-up Monthly Monitoring in ZEN Detected JB Breeding Cattle Herd

Sampling could not be performed for Cow 4 in August 2020 because she was about to calve at the time of sampling. The monthly changes in both urinary ZEN concentrations measured by ELISA and serum AMH concentration are shown in Figure 1. During the 1-year follow-up period, two peaks of urinary ZEN concentrations were observed in August 2020 and between April and May 2021 with different concentrations in each cow, which were later confirmed by urinary ZEN and metabolite detection by LC-MS/MS measurement (Figure 1g). Additionally, STC was also detected in urine samples from four cows in July 2020 (Cow 1: 184.8), February (Cow 4: 508.5), March (Cow 1: 429.4, and Cow 2: 495.7), and one in June 2021 (Cow 1: 342.5) (Figure 1g). Alternatively, ZEN was only detected in May 2021 (0.03 mg/kg), and STC was detected in July 2020 (0.01 mg/kg), February (0.02 mg/kg), April (0.03 mg/kg), and May 2021 (0.05 mg/kg), suggesting that feed ZEN exposure does not correspond with urinary ZEN concentrations, and feed STC exposure does not seem to correspond with urinary STC concentrations (Figure 1h), which must be due to largely reflected by the influence of the sampling parts collected as roughage samples.

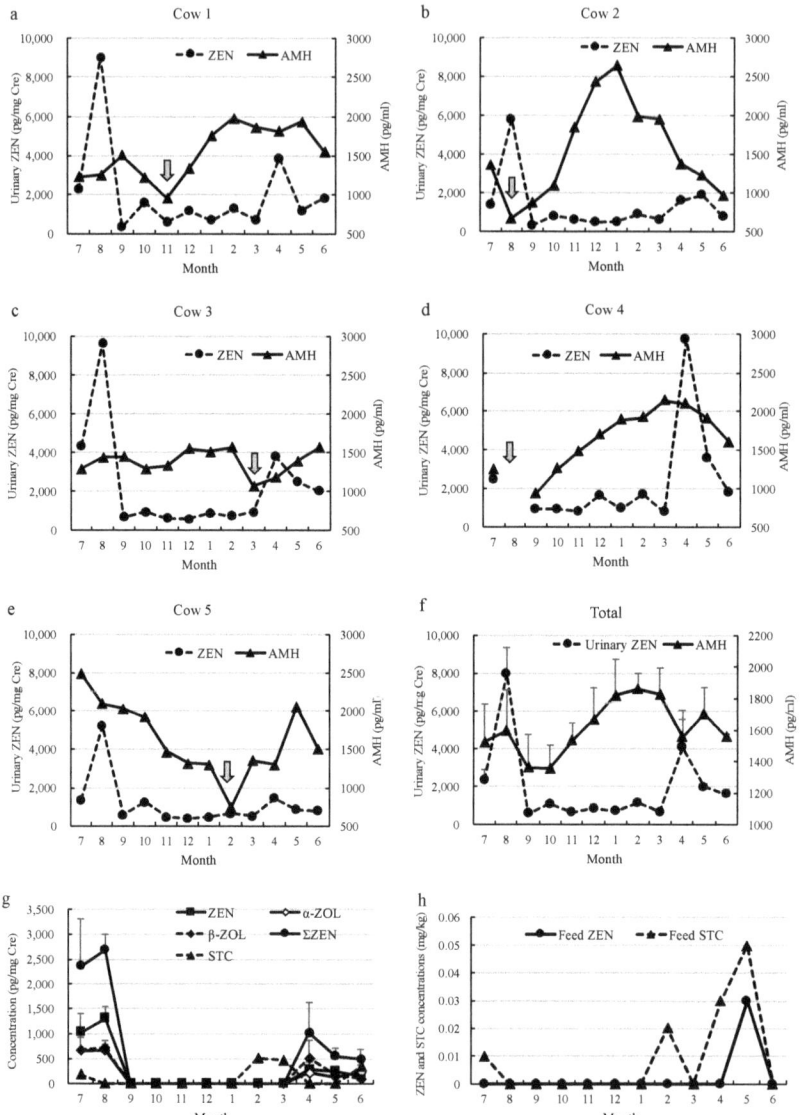

Figure 1. Monthly changes of both urinary ZEN concentration measured by ELISA and serum AMH concentration of each cow; (**a**) Cow 1, (**b**) Cow 2, (**c**) Cow 3, (**d**) Cow 4, and (**e**) Cow 5, ⇩: calving, (**f**) total; mean urinary ZEN concentration and AMH from five cows, (**g**) monthly changes of urinary ZEN, its metabolites, and STC concentrations measured by LC-MS/MS, (**h**) monthly changes of ZEN and STC concentrations in the dietary roughage measured by LC-MS/MS.

The estimated values of ZEN, AMH, and SAA for each month estimated by linear mixed model analysis are shown in Table 2 and Figure 1f. The ZEN value peaked in August, then decreased from September to March, and trended upward from April. Conversely, the AMH value dropped once in September, trended upward in March, then trended downward again in April. The SAA also showed a trend of increasing until March of the following year, although there have been increases and decreases since August.

Table 2. Estimated means and confidence intervals of ZEN, AMH, and SAA at each time point by mixture model.

	ZEN		AMH		SAA	
Date	Geometric Mean	95% CI	Arithmetic Mean	95% CI	Geometric Mean	95% CI
2020/7	2142.2	1373.8–3340.4	1521.6	1165.7–1877.5	2.8	1.5–4.9
2020/8	8056.5	4853.3–13373.8	1594.5	1135.0–2053.9	2.5	1.2–5.2
2020/9	521.1	334.2–812.6	1358.0	1002.1–1713.9	2.9	1.6–5.1
2020/10	1065.7	683.4–1661.7	1356.6	1000.7–1712.5	4.0	2.2–7.1
2020/11	627.1	392.9–1000.9	1532.9	1134.9–1930.8	3.4	1.8–6.4
2020/12	720.8	462.2–1123.9	1665.8	1309.9–2021.7	3.1	1.7–5.4
2021/1	676.9	434.1–1055.4	1820.8	1464.9–2176.7	4.9	2.8–8.7
2021/2	995.8	623.9–1589.5	1860.0	1462.1–2257.9	3.1	1.6–5.8
2021/3	669.9	419.7–1069.2	1828.1	1430.1–2226.0	5.2	2.8–9.8
2021/4	3194.8	2048.8–4981.8	1553.8	1197.9–1909.7	3.3	1.9–5.9
2021/5	1763.7	1131.0–2750.2	1704.4	1348.5–2060.3	3.0	1.7–5.3
2021/6	1414.2	885.9–2257.7	1554.7	1156.8–1952.6	2.2	1.2–4.2

95% CI: 95% confidence interval.

The results of the time-series regression between the ZEN and AMH values are shown in Table 3. Although neither correlation was significant, the effect of the ZEN value one month earlier on AMH displayed a negative regression trend ($\beta = -0.449$ [$-1.112, 0.214$], $p = 0.160$ in lag 1 month model). In other words, a low ZEN value one month prior tended to result in a high AMH value in the current month. The results of the examination of the time-series regression between the ZEN and AMH change values are shown in Table 4. Although no correlations were significant, a negative correlation trend was observed for the effect of the ZEN value from one month before AMH change ($\beta = -0.377$, lag 1 month). In other words, a low ZEN value in the current month suggested a tendency for AMH values to be higher in the next month.

Table 3. Regression between ZEN and AMH values.

	AMH				
	β		95% CI		p-Value
Simple correlation					
ZEN	−0.085	−0.787	–	0.617	0.793
Time-lagged correlation					
ZEN (lag 1 month)	−0.449	−1.112	–	0.214	0.160

The effects of ZEN on AMH values were evaluated by calculating the simple regression of ZEN values to AMH and the time-lagged regression, which examines the effect of ZEN values, one month earlier (lag 1 month), using a linear mixed model. β: Standardized regression coefficient. 95% CI: 95% confidence interval.

Table 4. Regression between ZEN and AMH changes.

	AMH Change over one Month				
	β		95% CI		p-Value
Time-lagged correlation					
ZEN (lag 0)	−0.024	−0.744	–	0.695	0.941
ZEN (lag 1 month)	−0.377	−1.039	–	0.285	0.230

The analysis was similarly for Table 3 evaluated by calculating the simple regression of ZEN value to AMH change over one month (lag 0 model) and time-lag regression to examine the effect of ZEN value one month earlier using a linear mixed model.

The results of the time series regression between SAA and ZEN values are shown in Table 5. Although both regressions were non-significant, the effect of the current month's ZEN value on SAA showed a negative regression trend ($\beta = -0.400$ $[-1.046, 0.246]$, $p = 0.198$ in lag 0 model). In other words, a high ZEN value may tend to result in a low SAA value in the current month. The results of the examination of the time series regression between SAA change and ZEN value are shown in Table 6. All regressions were non-significant, and the regression coefficients were small.

Table 5. Regression between ZEN and SAA values.

	SAA			
	β	95% CI		p-Value
Simple regression				
ZEN	−0.400	−1.046	– 0.246	0.198
Time-lagged regression				
ZEN (lag 1 month)	−0.333	−1.029	– 0.364	0.308

The effects of ZEN on SAA values were evaluated by calculating the simple regression of ZEN values to SAA and the time-lagged regression, which examines the effect of ZEN values one month earlier (lag 1 month), using a linear mixed model. β: standardized regression coefficient. 95%CI: 95% confidence interval.

Table 6. Regression between ZEN and SAA changes.

	SAA Change over one Month			
	β	95% CI		p-Value
Time-lagged regress				
ZEN (lag 0)	−0.245	−0.941	– 0.450	0.446
ZEN (lag 1 month)	0.065	−0.654	– 0.784	0.843

The analysis was similar for Table 5 evaluated by calculating the simple regression of ZEN value to SAA change over one month (lag 0 model) and the time-lag regression to examine the effect of ZEN value one month earlier using a linear mixed model.

The calving interval of the herd were 389.8 ± 35.3 ($n = 10$) in 2018, 471.7 ± 33.1 ($n = 18$) in 2019, 387.8 ± 15.0 ($n = 19$) in 2020, and 408.5 ± 24.6 ($n = 20$) in 2021, and tendency toward decreased calving intervals ($p = 0.099$) was observed between 2019 (pre-ZEN monitoring period) and 2020 (post-ZEN monitoring period). Table 7 shows the results of the calving intervals of the five cows examined during the pre- and post-ZEN monitoring periods. The number of calving intervals during the post-ZEN monitoring period (349.9 ± 6.9) was significantly lower ($p = 0.0487$) than the pre-ZEN monitoring period (439.0 ± 41.2).

Table 7. Mean calving intervals of the examined 5 cows during pre- and post-ZEN monitoring periods.

	Birthday	2017 (Pre)	2018 (Pre)	2019 (Pre) *	2020 (Post) **	2021 (Post)
Cow 1	9 January 2016	-	351	335	349	333
Cow 2	8 November 2014	690	-	380	321	349
Cow 3	7 April 2014	346	392	437	334	346
Cow 4	15 July 2015	-	600	-	377	355
Cow 5	27 December 2016	-	-	420	-	385
Mean of 5 cows		518.0 ± 172.0	447.7 ± 77.1	393.0 ± 22.7	345.3 ± 12.0	353.6 ± 8.6
Mean of the pre- and post-monitorin			439.0 ± 41.2 [a] ($n = 9$)		349.9 ± 6.9 [b] ($n = 9$)	

* Pre: Pre-ZEN monitoring period, ** Post: Post-ZEN monitoring period. [a,b]: $p < 0.05$.

3. Discussion

Currently, many reports have aimed to clarify and prevent the harmful effects of mycotoxins at each stage focused on three major factors. First, the characters, toxicity, and metabolites against the organs and/or systemic function of each mycotoxin (including emerging mycotoxins such as enniatin, beauvericine, and emodin) with both in vitro and in vivo approaches [20,21]. Second, the detection methods for these mycotoxins (including the case of multiple mycotoxins coexistence with different spp. of fungi) within dietary feeds and biological fluids, such as serum, urine, and milk, from animals [2,22–24]. Third, not only feed management and control strategies for fungal infection but also the degradation approaches by physical, chemical enzymatic, and biological methods to prevent the harmful effects of mycotoxins for the animals [1,3]. In cattle practice, acute exposure to high doses of mycotoxins is usually responsible for well-characterized clinical symptoms, such as reduced feed intake or diarrhea. Sub-chronic and chronic exposure to low doses has been less well characterized but is considered to be responsible for reduced performance, for reduced pathogen resistance, and more generally, for many of the causes of damaged health, and potentially the reproductive efficacy, of the herd [25]. Therefore, it is essential to first monitor the contamination status of mycotoxins in dietary feeds at each farm level to limit the exposure risks of mycotoxins. As previously suggested, one practical approach is to evaluate the feed contamination on each farm with an ELISA test kit for mycotoxin screening, followed by further validation of the suspected feed samples with LC-MS/MS [6]. Following these approaches, one objective of the present field trial/test was to 1) evaluate and apply the urinary ZEN monitoring system for its practical usefulness in cattle farm conditions. As expected, the results of our first screening indicated that (1) urinary ZEN measurements may be useful for monitoring or evaluating the level of intestinal absorption of ZEN from dietary feeds with follow-up by even small urinary samples (0.5 mL) from the same herd, (2) it was possible to detect ZEN naturally contaminated cattle herds by relatively high ZEN levels in feeds by ELISA as a rather simple method within the laboratory, concomitant with the coexistence of STC contamination of the dietary rice straw or WCS by following LC-MS/MS measurement, and (3) in a cattle herd (C) with confirmed ZEN exposure, monthly monitoring in the following year made it possible to monitor and control the exposure levels of dietary roughages derived from rice straw from within the same paddy field. To the best of our knowledge, this is the first practical verification test conducted in some cattle in which data are available encompassing the period from detection to follow-up using the urinary ZEN monitoring system.

The greatest advantage of using the urinary ZEN concentration monitoring system is that the ZEN concentration that is actually ingested and absorbed from the intestinal tract can be monitored and compared with other herds. As previously reported [12,26], the problem is that the concentration of mycotoxins produced in dietary feeds may vary greatly depending on the collection site of the feed sample to be collected. Indeed, in the present study, different results between the urinary ZEN concentration and the ZEN concentration in the roughages in August 2019 seem to clearly show this problem. Using the urinary ZEN monitoring system, it is possible to monitor the concentration of mycotoxins absorbed from the intestinal tract, and the absorbed concentration of mycotoxins may reflect the degree of contamination of the mycotoxins in the feed for each herd and its feed intake by animals. Since urinary ZEN concentration may be affected by the intake volumes of contaminated feeds, it seems to be a suitable method for monitoring and comparing mycotoxin exposure in cattle whose daily feed amount is fixed between each herd. In fact, in this study, although the urinary ZEN concentrations of the two heifers in Herd D (3862.4 and 1669.8) were like those of Herd A (3280.9 and 930.5), the urinary concentration was approximately 2 to 4 times higher than that of Herd B (983.7 and 979.8). Presumably, when comparing the daily feed volume, especially roughage, amounts for cows in Herd D were approximately half that of cows in Herd B. Naturally, the ZEN contamination level was lower than that of cows in Herd C, in which ZEN exposure was detected that time. However, in terms of the level of natural contamination of ZEN in roughage, that for cows in Herd D was higher than for cows in Herds A and B because the daily roughage feed for herd D was half that of Herds A and B. This demonstrates again that it can be inferred by performing ZEN monitoring to compare contamination levels within the rice straw in the present study. To investigate the effects of chronic mycotoxin exposure on the health status and productivity of livestock herds, a urinary mycotoxin monitoring system for monitoring mycotoxin intake from dietary feeds is indispensable. As we have demonstrated in this study, the simultaneous screening of cattle herds in the same area with similar breeding environments will be an important future strategy to understand the status of mycotoxin contamination of cattle herds. Additionally, the measurement results of ELISA and LC-MS/MS, the two measurement methods used for ZEN concentration measurement in this study, indicate that the urinary ZEN measurement using the ELISA method is an accurate, simple, and useful measurement method for evaluating the dynamics of mycotoxin infiltration at rather low concentrations and long-term chronic exposure.

The second purpose of the present study was to evaluate both ZEN (Fusarium mycotoxin called pre-harvest mycotoxin) and STC (Aspergillus mycotoxin called post-harvest mycotoxin) dynamics in the dietary roughage (rice straw and WCS) using the naturally ZEN (also STC)- contaminated herd (Herd C) detected in August 2019 as a model/examined herd, mainly by urinary ZEN monitoring during the year from July 2020 to June 2021. In addition, ZEN and its metabolites have been suggested to cause apoptosis of granulosa cell/atresia of follicles in several animals [27–30], the relationship between urinary ZEN and AMH concentration during the monitoring period was studied to clarify the effects of ZEN exposure on AMH secretion from antral follicles. In this regard, similar to our recently reported decrease in AMH concentration during the peripartum period [19], all five examined JB cows displayed a clear decline in AMH concentrations in the month of their calving with a large range of SAA concentrations (Cow 1: 3.1 mg/L, Cow 2: 23.4 mg/L, Cow 3: 4.9 mg/L, and Cow 5: 2.9 mg/L; data not shown). Thus, we deleted all AMH and SAA concentration data for the calving month of each cow from our data set in the present study. As a result, although it became clear that there was a large variation in AMH concentration in each month among each individual cow during 1 year period in the blood samplings (Figure 1a–e), our results regarding the relationship between ZEN and AMH suggest that natural exposure level of ZEN may affect AMH concentrations, and thus, the AFC in cattle ovaries (Figure 1f, Tables 3 and 4). Our results indicated that a low ZEN value one month prior may tend to result in a high AMH value in the current month, and a low ZEN value in the current month suggested a tendency for higher AMH values in the next month. Therefore, it was suggested that when AMH rises, it may be affected by the ZEN value of the previous month, and when AMH decreases, it may be affected by the ZEN value of the current month. Thus, the effects of ZEN on AMH secretion appeared early but recovery of AMH secretion after ZEN exposure may take some time. As an interesting result obtained from the present study, a negative regression trend between the concentrations of ZEN and SAA; a high ZEN value may tend to result in a low SAA value in the sampling month, were observed (Tables 6 and 7). ZEN has been reported to have immunotoxicity in addition to its endocrine disrupting effects [31,32]. Previous reports indicated that ZEN exposure altered the hepatic cellular immune response, and suppressed the secretion of proinflammatory cytokines, such as IL-1, IL-6, and TNF-α [31–33]. Therefore, the negative regression trend between urinary ZEN and SAA concentrations obtained in the present study is possibly due to innate immune suppression of cows by low-level chronic ZEN exposure. In the future, it will be necessary to increase the number of cow herds monitored, expand the scope of monitoring, and clarify that improving the feed while detecting the naturally exposed herd will lead to an improvement in productivity. At the same time, field tests in the process of improving the mycotoxins level in naturally contaminated feed will be important indicators of animal health risks.

Several incidences of STC contamination in food and feed (e.g., grains, grain-based products, maize, and rice) have also been reported in Japan [34–37]. Rice straw is considered one of the most important roughages used in the production of beef cattle in Japan, and

STC is a major mycotoxin produced in rice. However, the harmful or chronic effects of STC on cattle are not well understood, and there are no regulations or control measures for this toxin in Japan. Previous measures of large-scale in-feed mycotoxins confirm a large difference in the types of mycotoxins when multiple mycotoxins were detected in feed coexist in each country and region of the country [5]. In the present study, ZEN and STC co-exposure in rice straw (WCS) was also confirmed in the area screened, another prefecture in the Kyushu area where we previously detected co-exposure to ZEN and STC. Our results elucidate the characteristics of mycotoxin co-contamination of rice straw produced in Japan and future research should further expand the scope of the survey to understand the characteristics and relationships between the two mycotoxins.

ZEN and its metabolites exhibit distinct estrogenic properties that affect the reproductive system of several animal species, especially pigs [9,38,39]. In contrast, clinical signs of hyperestrogenism are not frequently observed in ruminating cows, and then only following the ingestion of highly contaminated silage or long-term exposure to contaminated feed materials [40–42]. In the present study, we simply compared the calving intervals of the monitored herd before and after introducing the urinary ZEN monitoring system and observed significantly reduced calving intervals of the herd. We previously reported the in vitro effects of acute ZEN exposure on bovine oocytes by using in vitro maturation, in vitro fertilization (IVF), and in vitro culture systems in cattle, and found that a high ZEN concentration (>1 mg/kg in the culture medium) might have a detrimental effect on the meiotic competence of bovine oocytes but does not affect fertilization and development after IVF [43]. Additionally, we reported that natural-feed ZEN contamination levels below the threshold value (i.e., below the maximum permissible ZEN concentration in Japan) did not affect embryo production in Japanese Black and Holstein cows undergoing superovulation [44]. Therefore, it was suggested that ZEN-contaminated feed affects the fertility of cattle by influencing the development of embryos in the uterus after implantation. In this study, the roughages harvested in 2019, which were fed prior to our first ZEN screening, were ZEN-contaminated, and the long-term use of the contaminated feed affected the calving interval. It is speculated that the introduction of the urinary ZEN monitoring system controlled ZEN contamination in the feeds, which shortened the calving interval of the herd. Obviously, further studies with an increased number of monitor herds in the field are needed.

In conclusion, our results demonstrate that the urinary ZEN monitoring system is an important practical tool, not only for detecting contaminated herds under field conditions but also for revealing the effects of long-term chronic ZEN/STC (or other co-existing mycotoxins) exposure on herd productivity and fertility. To date, several approaches have been developed to reduce mycotoxin contamination and exposure, including strategies involving agronomy, plant breeding and transgenics, biotechnology, toxin binding, and deactivating feed additives, and feed supplier/animal producer education [26]. As shown in the present field trial, herd management with a urinary ZEN monitoring system may be a possible novel concept for creating awareness among herd managers thereby preventing mycotoxin exposure in cattle herds.

4. Materials and Methods

All experiments were conducted according to the guidelines and regulations for the protection of experimental animals and guidelines stipulated by Yamaguchi University, Japan (no. 40, 1995; approved on 27 March 2017) and informed consent was obtained from the farmers.

4.1. Chemicals and Solvents

ZEN was purchased from MP Biomedicals (Heidelberg, Germany). The metabolites α-ZEL and β-ZEL were purchased from Sigma (St. Louis, MO, USA). Stock solutions of ZEN, α-ZEL, and β-ZEL, each at a concentration of 1 µg/mL in methanol, were stored under light protection at 4 °C. STC was purchased from MP Biomedicals (Heidelberg,

Germany). Stock solutions of 1 μg/mL STC in acetonitrile were stored in the dark at 4 °C, and high-performance liquid chromatography (HPLC)-grade methanol was purchased from FUJIFILM Wako Pure Chemical Co. (Osaka, Japan). β-Glucuronidase/arylsulfatase solution was purchased from Merck (Darmstadt, Germany). Sodium acetate was purchased from Kanto Chemical Co., Ltd. (Tokyo, Japan), and Tris was purchased from Nacalai Tesque Inc. (Kyoto, Japan).

4.2. Screening by Urinary ZEN Monitoring to Detect Cattle Herds Fed with Dietary Roughage with Elevated ZEN Contamination

Before the rice harvest period in September 2019, this screening was conducted at the Japanese Black (JB) breeding cattle production site to monitor the extent of ZEN contamination of rice straw and/or whole crop silage (WCS) stored by cattle farmers in the summer season when the mean temperature of daytime is higher than 30 °C. At the request of the managing veterinarian, urinary ZEN monitoring was performed in four herds (A, B, C, and D) of JB cows kept for breeding in the neighborhood in the Kyushu area, Japan, for which the veterinarian routinely provides veterinary treatments and consults with four farmers. All animals were housed indoors, and roughage and concentrates were fed separately. Feeding and management systems were similar in each herd and the dates of sampling and contents of the feeds in each herd are detailed in Table 8. As feed intake may reflect the ZEN exposure, urine samples were collected from two cows with similar body weight within each herd during natural urination after softly massaging the perineum. Regarding the number of cows to be sampled for urine in each herd, referring to our previous report [10], we considered samples from two cows to be sufficient to evaluate and estimate the contamination status of feed fed the same amount and same lot of feed. In addition, samples of all roughages, such as rice straw and WCS, were obtained from each herd to measure both ZEN and STC concentrations in the roughage. All concentrates fed to cattle in each herd were purchased from feed companies and are generally tested for mycotoxin contamination during the manufacturing stage. The urine and roughage samples were immediately placed into a cooler, protected from light, transported to the clinic office, and frozen. The frozen samples were sent to our laboratory and stored at -30 °C until our analysis of ZEN and creatinine (Crea) concentrations in the urine, and ZEN and STC concentrations in the roughage.

Table 8. Composition of feeds provided to the monitored herds kept for breeding purposes.

Herd	Date of Sample Collection	Forage Feeds/Day	Formula Feeds/Day
A ($n = 2$) (Both 12 y) *	10 July 2019	Home-grown rice straw 2 kg, Home-grown WCS (rice) 6 kg, Home-grown Italian ryegrass 4 kg Total: 12 kg	Commercially available concentrates 4 kg
B ($n = 2$) (3 y and 5 y)	24 June 2019	Home-grown rice straw 10 kg, Mixed of Italian ryegrass and Orchard grass 10 kg Total: 20 kg	Commercially available concentrates 1 kg, Wheat bran 1 kg, Maize 1 kg
C ($n = 2$) (8 y and 10 y)	19 August 2019	Home-grown rice straw 12~14 kg, Orchard grass 10 kg (once a week) Total: 12~14 kg	Commercially available concentrates 3 kg Wheat 0.5–1 kg
D ($n = 2$) (9 m and 10 m)	11 July 2019	Imported Oats-hey 2.25 kg, Bermuda-grass 2.25 kg Total: 4.5 kg	Commercially available concentrates 4.5 kg

* Age of the breeding cattle at sampling, y; years old, m; month old. WCS: whole crop silage.

4.3. Follow-up Monthly Monitoring on the Breeding Cattle Herd with Known Feed Contamination

Since contamination of rice straw/WCS from herd C collected in August 2019 exceeded the standard value of ZEN $\geq$ 1 mg/kg concomitant with STC was detected, this herd was selected for further monitoring. Therefore, monthly regular urinary ZEN monitoring of herd C was performed from July 2020 to help determine whether similar ZEN and STC exposure from the rice straw/WCS occurred year to year. For monitoring, five cows (Cows 1 to 5: mean 5.0 y: 3.6–6.3 y) in Herd C with similar body weight (approximately 500 kg) fed with the same roughage and concentrated feed were selected and monthly urine, blood, and roughage were sampled. We collected both urine and blood samples from the five cows at the beginning of each month, approximately 2 h after the morning feed, as per our previous methodology [10], and we also collected roughage samples fed to these cows. Both urine and blood samples were immediately stored on ice, protected from light, and transported to the laboratory, and were stored at −30 °C after centrifugation as dispensed urine and serum in microtubes until analysis. The collected roughages were also stored at −30 °C until measurement of both ZEN and STC concentrations.

Zearalenone concentrations in the collected urine samples were measured by ELISA every two months, as described below, and urine samples were measured monthly when deemed necessary by the herd manager monitoring the condition of the roughage being fed or by contamination status of the roughage by fungi at the monthly sampling. During the follow-up period, daily feeding was performed while sharing the urinary ZEN concentration measurement results with the herd manager and the managing veterinarian. When a high urinary ZEN concentration was confirmed, the roughage lot fed at the time of sampling was changed, and the urinary ZEN concentration was measured again in the following month for follow-up purposes, concomitant with measurement of both ZEN and STC concentrations of roughage samples by LC-MS/MS as mentioned below. Concentrations of urinary ZEN, its metabolites, α-ZEL, β-ZEL, and STC of all collected urine samples during the follow-up period were measured by LC-MS/MS within one assay for reconfirmation of results by the ELISA assay and urinary STC measurement. A schematic representation of the experimental design is shown in Figure 2.

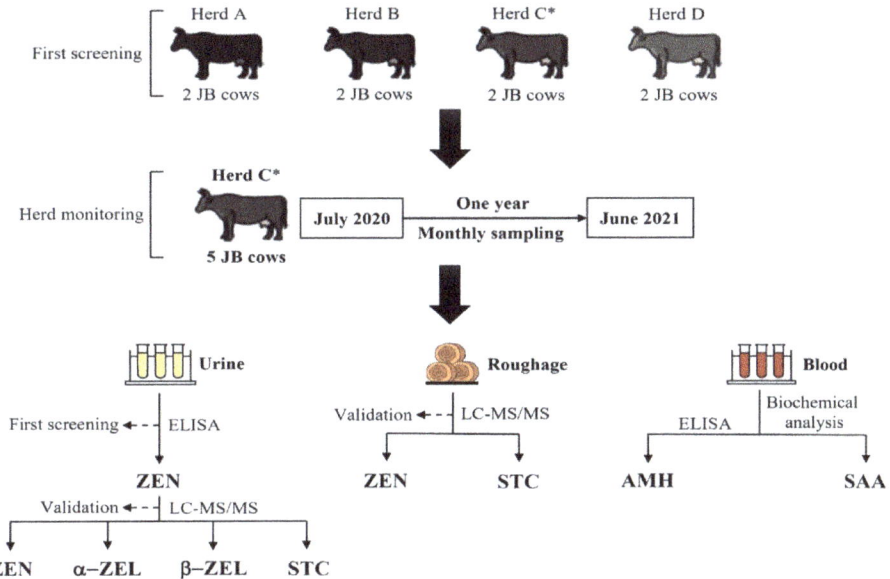

Figure 2. Schematic representation of the experimental design. C*, herd with high contamination: urinary ZEN concentrations exceeding the standard concentration of the ELISA kit, and ZEN-contaminated roughage exceeding the standard value in Japan (>1 mg/kg). α-ZEL: α-zearalenol; β-ZEL: β-zearalenol; AMH: anti-Müllerian hormone; SAA: serum amyloid A; STC: sterigmatocystin; ZEN: zearalenone.

4.4. Reproductive Records

As a reproductive record, the calving intervals of the herd were compared for each year from 2017 to 2021. Additionally, the reproductive records from the five cows examined between pre-ZEN monitoring (2017 to 2019) and post-ZEN monitoring periods (2020 and 2021) were evaluated to confirm the impact of introducing the ZEN monitoring system on herd fertility.

4.5. Analytical Methods of ZEN in Urine and Feed Samples

Zearalenone concentration in urine was determined using a commercially available kit (RIDASCREEN Zearalenon; R-Biopharm AG, Garmstadt, Germany) according to the manufacturer's instructions, with minor modifications. Briefly, a urine sample (0.1 mL: 5-fold dilution of the kit) was added into 3 mL of 50 mM sodium acetate buffer (pH 4.8) and the solution was incubated for 15 h at 37 °C in the presence of 10 µL of β-glucuronidase/arylsulfatase solution. Thereafter, the samples were loaded onto a C18 solid-phase extraction (SPE) column (Strata; Phenomenex, Torrance, CA, USA), which had been preconditioned with 3 mL of methanol, followed by 2 mL of 20 mM Tris buffer (pH 8.5)/methanol (80:20). After washing the SPE column with 2 mL of 20 mM Tris buffer (pH 8.5)/methanol (80:20) and 3 mL of methanol (40%), the column was centrifuged for 10 min at $500 \times g$ to dry the column. The analytes were then eluted slowly (flow rate: 15 drops/min) with 1 mL of methanol (80%). The eluate was evaporated to dryness at 60 °C using a centrifugation evaporator. The dried residue was redissolved in 50 µL of methanol, 450 µL of sample dilution buffer was added, the solution was mixed thoroughly, and an aliquot of 50 µL was used for the ELISA assay. To determine the ZEN concentration in the urine sample, RIDA SOFT Win (R-Biopharm) was used to calculate the absorbance at 450 nm using a microplate spectrophotometer. The cross-reactivity rates using this particular ELISA kit for α-ZEL, β-ZEL, and Zeranol were 41.6, 13.8%, and 27.7%, respectively, based on the manufacturer's instruction, and the mean recovery rate of the ELISA assay based on the three trials was 84% ± 14%.

Urine creatinine concentrations were determined using a commercial kit (Sikarikit-S CRE, Kanto Chemical, Tokyo, Japan), according to the manufacturer's instructions, and were measured using a 7700 Clinical Analyzer (Hitachi High-Tech, Tokyo, Japan). All urine concentrations were expressed as a ratio of creatinine (pg/mg creatinine), as described previously [10].

Based on the results of the first screening and measurement of urinary ZEN concentrations by ELISA, both the urine and roughage samples in herds expected to have high ZEN infiltration in the feed were retested using a liquid chromatography-tandem mass spectrometry (LC-MS/MS) measurement system not only for the confirmation of the ELISA results but also for measuring the ZEN metabolites, α-ZEL and β-ZEL. Additionally, as per our previous reports, urinary STC levels were concomitantly higher in cattle fed ZEN-contaminated rice straw in Japan; thus, it was speculated that co-contamination of both ZEN and STC was observed. Therefore, in the retest, the STC concentration in urine and roughage was also measured according to our previous reports [10,12].

The LC-MS/MS method and validation have been described in our previous report [10]. Briefly, each urine sample (0.5 mL) was mixed with 3.0 mL of 50 mM ammonium acetate buffer (pH 4.8) and 8 µL of glucuronidase/arylsulfatase solution and incubated for 12 h at 37 °C. The solution was loaded onto a C18 SPE column, which was preconditioned with 3 mL 100% methanol and 2 mL Tris buffer, followed by the addition of 2 mL Tris buffer and 3 mL of 40% methanol. After washing the SPE column with approximately 1 mL of 80% methanol, the volume of the eluted solution was adjusted to 1 mL. Then, 20 µL of the reconstituted solution was injected into the LC-MS/MS system. The LC-MS/MS analyses were performed on an API 2000 MS/MS system (Applied Biosystems, Foster City, CA, USA) equipped with an electrospray ionization (ESI) interface and a 1200 Infinity Series HPLC system (Agilent Technologies, Santa Clara, CA, USA). The detection limits for ZEN, α-ZEL, and β-ZEL were 0.04 ng/mL, 0.05 ng/mL, and 0.05 ng/mL, respectively, while the mean recovery rates for ZEN, α-ZEL, and β-ZEL were 90%, 109%, and 90%, respectively. STC concentrations of the same eluted solution described above were also determined by LC-MS/MS using an API 2000 system equipped with an ESI as previously described [12]. Briefly, after elution with approximately 1 mL of 80% methanol, the volume was adjusted to exactly 1 mL, and 20 µL of the solution was injected into the LC-MS/MS system. Chromatographic separation was performed on an Inertsil ODS-3 column (4.6 i.d. × 100 mm, 5 µm; GL Sciences, Tokyo, Japan) at 40 °C. A mobile phase consisting of methanol/water/acetic acid (97:3:0.01, v:v:v) was used (200 µL/min) to separate the analyte in isocratic mode. Measurements were performed for 15 min. The limit of detection (LoD) was 0.2 ng/mL. ZEN, α-ZEL, β-ZEL, and STC concentrations in the urine are expressed as a ratio to creatinine (pg/mg creatinine).

Both STC and ZEN concentrations in the roughage samples were measured using an API 3200 LC-MS/MS system (AB Sciex, Tokyo, Japan) equipped with an electrospray ionization (ESI) interface and a Prominence HPLC system (Shimadzu Corp., Kyoto, Japan), according to the Food and Agricultural Materials Inspection Center [45] at Shokukanken Inc., Gunma, Japan. In brief, representative samples of stored straw (2 g) and concentrate (10 g) were homogenized and chopped into small pieces. Each sample was placed in a sample tube, to which 20 mL of 84% acetonitrile was added. The tubes were shaken for 1 h and centrifuged for 10 min at 500× g at room temperature. The supernatant (10 mL) was loaded onto a MultiSep 226 Aflazon + multifunctional column (Romer Labs, Union, MO, USA). Subsequently, 1 mL of the eluent was mixed with 1 mL acetic acid (1 + 100) and centrifuged for 5 min at 500× g. Next, 10 µL of supernatant was injected into the LC-MS/MS system under the following conditions: column, Synergi 4 µm Polar-RP 80 A (2 mm × 150 mm, 4 µm); oven temperature, 40 °C; eluent flow, 200 µL/min; and solvent, methanol (A) + 1 mM Ammonium acetate in 0.1% aqueous acetic acid (B). An ESI probe was used in the positive mode for the STC analysis and the negative mode for the ZEN analysis. The detection limit for each analyte was 0.01 mg/kg. The mean STC and ZEN recovery rates were 90.5%–93.5% and 95.3%–98.5%.

4.6. Analytical Methods of AMH and SAA in Serum Samples

Serum AMH concentration was measured using a bovine AMH ELISA kit (AnshLabs, Webster, TX, USA), according to a previous report [46] to monitor the ovarian AFC of the examined cows during the follow-up period. Briefly, undiluted plasma (50 µL) was used for the assay, which had a limited detection of 11 pg/mL and a coefficient of variation of 2.9%, according to the manufacturer's instructions. Based on our previous studies [19], it is clear that the blood AMH concentration in cattle is lower than usual during the peripartum period; thus, in this study, the AMH concentration in each cow's calving month during the monitoring period was evaluated with particular care. Additionally, SAA concentrations were measured using an automated biochemical analyzer (Pentra C200; HORIBA ABX SAS, Montpellier, France) with a special SAA reagent for animal serum or plasma (VET-SAA 'Eiken' reagent; Eiken Chemical Co. Ltd., Tokyo, Japan) to monitor the inflammation status of each cow during sampling. The SAA concentration was calculated using a standard curve generated using a calibrator (VET-SAA calibrator set; Eiken Chemical Co. Ltd., Tokyo, Japan).

4.7. Data Management and Statistical Analysis

Monthly estimates for ZEN, AMH, and SAA were calculated using mixed model analysis with subject as a variable factor, because they contain missing data due to calving of the examined cows. Because the ZEN and SAA values approximate a lognormal distribution, the geometric mean estimate was calculated. The AMH value approximates a normal distribution; therefore, the arithmetic mean estimate was calculated. The effects of ZEN and AMH values were evaluated by calculating the simple regression of ZEN values with AMH and the time-lagged regression, which examines the effect of ZEN values one month earlier (lag 1 month), using a linear mixed model. Furthermore, the effects of ZEN on AMH change were evaluated by defining the change in AMH value over one month as the change from the previous month. The analysis was similarly evaluated by calculating the simple regression of ZEN value to AMH change (lag 0 model) and the time-lag regression to examine the effect of ZEN value one month earlier using a linear mixed model. In other words, the lag 1-month model evaluates the effect of the ZEN value of the current month on the AMH change until the next month. In addition, the effect of ZEN on SAA was also evaluated using the same linear mixed model as described above. A two-sided p-value ≤ 0.05 was considered statistically significant. All statistical analyses were performed using SPSS for Windows (version 24.0; IBM Japan, Tokyo, Japan).

All results of the reproductive records of the herds obtained are expressed as the mean ± SEM. Statistical analyses were performed using BellCurve for Excel software (Social Survey Research Information Co., Ltd., Tokyo, Japan). Calving intervals of the herd from 2017 to 2021 were compared using a one-way analysis of variance, followed by a post-hoc test (Tukey-Kramer). Additionally, calving intervals during the pre- (2017 and 2019) and post-ZEN monitoring (2020 and 2021) periods of the examined five cows were compared between the groups using Student's t-test to determine the effects of introducing the monthly urinary ZEN monitoring system on the reproductive efficacies of the breeding herd. Statistical significance was set at $p \leq 0.05$, whereas p-values ranging between 0.05 and 0.1 were considered to indicate a trend toward significance.

Author Contributions: Conceptualization, O.S.W., M.E., M.L. and M.T. (Mitsuhiro Takagi); formal analysis, O.S.W., E.K., S.U., O.Y., D.P., H.O., and M.T. (Mitsuhiro Takagi); investigation, O.S.W., M.E., and M.T. (Mitsuhiro Takagi); methodology, E.K., S.U., O.Y., M.T. (Masayasu Taniguchi) and M.T.(Mitsuhiro Takagi); project administration, M.T. (Mitsuhiro Takagi); resources, M.T.(Masayasu Taniguchi) and M.T. (Mitsuhiro Takagi); supervision, M.T. (Masayasu Taniguchi), M.L. and M.T. (Mitsuhiro Takagi); visualization, O.S.W.; writing—original draft, O.S.W., D.P. and M.T.(Mitsuhiro Takagi); writing—review and editing, O.S.W., M.E., E.K., S.U., O.Y., D.P., H.O., M.T. (Masayasu Taniguchi), M.L. and M.T. (Mitsuhiro Takagi) All authors have read and agreed to the published version of the manuscript.

Funding: This work was supported by JSPS KAKENHI Grant Number JP21K05920.

Institutional Review Board Statement: All experiments were conducted according to the guidelines and regulations for the protection of experimental animals and guidelines stipulated by Yamaguchi University, Japan (no. 40, 1995; approved on 27 March 2017).

Informed Consent Statement: Informed consent was obtained from all farmers involved in this study.

Data Availability Statement: The original contributions presented in the study are included in the article/supplementary material; further inquiries can be directed to the corresponding author.

Acknowledgments: The authors would like to express our sincerely gratitude to J. Fink-Gremmels, Utrecht University, The Netherlands, for her critical reading of this manuscript and encouragement to promote our research activity.

Conflicts of Interest: The authors declare that the research was conducted in the absence of any commercial or financial relationships that could be construed as a potential conflict of interest.

References

1. Liew, W.P.P.; Mohd-Redzwan, S. Mycotoxin: Its impact on gut health and microbiota. *Front. Cell Infect. Microbiol.* **2018**, *8*, 60. [CrossRef]
2. Vandicke, J.; De Visschere, K.; Croubels, S.; De Saeger, S.; Audenaert, K.; Haesaert, G. Mycotoxins in Flanders fields: Occurrence and correlations with *Fusarium* species in whole-plant harvested maize. *Microorganism* **2019**, *7*, 571. [CrossRef]
3. Li, P.; Su, R.; Yin, R.; Lai, D.; Wang, M.; Liu, Y.; Zhou, L. Detoxification of mycotoxins through biotransformation. *Toxins* **2020**, *12*, 121. [CrossRef] [PubMed]
4. Raduly, Z.; Szabo, L.; Madar, A.; Pocsi, I.; Csernoch, L. Toxicological and medical aspects of aspergillus-derived mycotoxins entering the feed and food chain. *Fronit. Microbiol.* **2020**, *10*, 2908. [CrossRef] [PubMed]
5. Gruber-Dorninger, C.; Jenkins, T.; Schatzmayr, G. Global mycotoxin occurrence in feed: A ten-year survey. *Toxins* **2019**, *11*, 375. [CrossRef]

6. Liu, J.; Applegate, T. Zearalenone (ZEN) in livestock and poultry: Does, toxicokinetics, toxicity and estrogenicity. *Toxins* **2020**, *12*, 377. [CrossRef] [PubMed]
7. Prelusky, D.B.; Warner, R.M.; Trenholm, H.L. Sensitive analysis of the mycotoxin zearalenone and its metabolites in biological fluids by high-performance liquid chromatography. *J. Chromatogr.* **1989**, *494*, 267–277. [CrossRef]
8. Usleber, A.; Renz, V.; Martlbauer, E.; Terplan, G. Studies on the application of enzyme immunoassays for the *Fusarium* mycotoxins deoxynivalenol, 3-acetyldeoxynivalenol, and zearalenone. *J. Vet. Med. B.* **1992**, *39*, 617–627. [CrossRef]
9. Kleinova, M.; ZELlner, P.; Kahlbacher, H.; Hochsteiner, W.; Lindner, W. Metabolic profiles of the mycotoxin zearalenone and of the growth promoter zeranol in urine, liver, and muscle of heifers. *J. Agric. Food. Chem.* **2002**, *50*, 4769–4776. [CrossRef]
10. Takagi, M.; Uno, S.; Kokushi, E.; Shiga, S.; Mukai, S.; Kuriyagawa, T.; Takagaki, K.; Hasunuma, H.; Matsumoto, D.; Okamoto, K.; et al. Measurement of urinary zearalenone concentrations for monitoring natural feed contamination in cattle herds-on farm trials. *J. Anim. Sci.* **2011**, *89*, 287–296. [CrossRef]
11. Hasunuma, H.; Takagi, M.; Kawamura, O.; Taniguchi, C.; Nakamura, M.; Chuma, T.; Uno, S.; Kokushi, E.; Matsumoto, D.; Tshering, C.; et al. Natural contamination of dietary rice straw with zearalenone and urinary zearalenone concentrations in a cattle herd. *J. Anim. Sci.* **2012**, *90*, 1610–1616. [CrossRef] [PubMed]
12. Fushimi, Y.; Takagi, M.; Uno, S.; Kokushi, E.; Nakamura, M.; Hasunuma, H.; Shinya, U.; Duguchi, E.; Fink-Gremmels, J. Measurement of sterigmatocystin concentrations in urine for monitoring the contamination of cattle feed. *Toxins* **2014**, *6*, 3117–3128. [CrossRef] [PubMed]
13. Toda, K.; Uno, S.; Kokushi, E.; Shiiba, A.; Hasunuma, H.; Matsumoto, D.; Ohtani, M.; Yamato, O.; Shinya, U.; Wijayagunawardane, M.; et al. Fructo-oligosaccharide (DFA III) feed supplementation for mitigation of mycotoxin exposure in cattle—clinical evaluation by a urinary zearalenone monitoring system. *Toxins* **2018**, *10*, 223. [CrossRef]
14. Sasazaki, N.; Uno, S.; Kokushi, E.; Toda, K.; Hasunuma, H.; Matsumoto, D.; Miyashita, A.; Yamato, O.; Okawa, H.; Ohtani, M.; et al. Mitigation of sterigmatocystin exposure in cattle by difructose anhydride III feed supplementation and detection of urinary sterigmatocystin and serum amyloid A concentrations. *Arch. Anim. Breed.* **2021**, *64*, 257–264. [CrossRef]
15. Monniaux, D.; di Clemente, N.; Touzé, J.L.; Belville, C.; Rico, C.; Bontoux, M.; Picard, J.Y.; Fabre, S. Intrafollicular steroids and anti-mullerian hormone during normal and cystic ovarian follicular development in the cow. *Biol. Reprod.* **2008**, *79*, 387–396. [CrossRef]
16. Monniaux, D.; Drouilhet, L.; Rico, C.; Estienne, A.; Jarrier, P.; Touze, J.L.; Sapa, J.; Phocas, F.; Dupont, J.; Dalbies-Tran, R.; et al. Regulation of anti-Mullerian hormone production in domestic animals. *Reprod. Fertil. Dev.* **2013**, *25*, 1–16. [CrossRef]
17. Berg, L.C.; Thomsen, P.D.; Andersen, P.H.; Jensen, H.E.; Jacobsen, S. Serum amyloid A is expressed in histologically normal tissues from horses and cattle. *Vet. Immunol. Immunopathol.* **2011**, *144*, 155–159. [CrossRef]
18. Zhang, S.; Yang, F.; Oguejiofor, C.F.; Wang, D.; Dong, S.; Yan, Z. Endometrial expression of the acute phase molecule SAA is more significant than HP in reflecting the severity of endometritis. *Res. Vet. Sci.* **2018**, *121*, 130–133. [CrossRef]
19. Okawa, H.; Monniaux, D.; Mizokami, C.; Fujikura, A.; Takano, T.; Sato, S.; Shinya, U.; Kawashima, C.; Yamato, O.; Fushimi, Y.; et al. Association between anti-Müllerian hormone concentration and inflammation markers in serum during the peripartum period in dairy cows. *Animals* **2021**, *11*, 1241. [CrossRef]
20. Reisinger, N.; Schurer-Waldheim, S.; Mayer, E.; Debevere, S.; Antonissen, G.; Sulyok, M.; Nagl, V. Mycotoxin occurrence in maize silage-A neglected risk for bovine gut health? *Toxins* **2019**, *11*, 577. [CrossRef]
21. Kinkade, C.W.; Rivera-Nunez, Z.; Gorcyzca, L.; Aleksunes, L.M. Impact of Fusarium-derived mycoestrogens on female reproduction: A systematic review. *Toxins* **2021**, *13*, 373. [CrossRef] [PubMed]
22. Lee, M.J.; Kim, H.J. Development of an immunoaffinity chromatography and LC-MS/MS method for the determination of 6 zearalenones in animal feed. *PLoS ONE* **2018**, *5*, e0193584. [CrossRef] [PubMed]
23. Panasiuk, L.; Jedziniak, P.; Pietruazka, K.; Piatkowska, M.; Bocian, L. Frequency and levels of regulated and emerging mycotoxins in silage in Poland. *Mycotoxin Res.* **2019**, *35*, 17–25. [CrossRef] [PubMed]
24. Nualkaw, K.; Poapolathep, S.; Zhang, Z.; Zhang, Q.; Giorgi, M.; Li, P.; Logrieco, F.; Poapolathep, A. Simultaneous determination of multiple mycotoxins in swine, poultry and dairy feeds using ultra high-performance liquid chromatography-tandem mass spectrometry. *Toxins* **2020**, *12*, 253. [CrossRef] [PubMed]
25. Guerre, P. Mycotoxin and gut microbiota interactions. *Toxins* **2020**, *12*, 769. [CrossRef]
26. Bryden, W.L. Mycotoxin contamination of the feed supply chain: Implications for animal productivity and feed security. *Anim. Feed Sci.* **2012**, *173*, 134–158. [CrossRef]
27. Minervini, F.; Giannoccaro, A.; Fornelli, F.; Dell' Aquila, M.E.; Minoia, P.; Visconti, A. Influence of mycotoxin zearalenone and its derivatives (alpha and beta zearalenol) on apoptosis and proliferation of cultured granulosa cells from equine ovaries. *Reprod. Biol. Endocrinol.* **2006**, *4*, 62. [CrossRef]
28. Zhu, L.; Yuan, H.; Guo, C.; Lu, Y.; Deng, S.; Yang, Y.; Wei, Q.; Wen, L.; He, Z. Zearalenone induces apoptosis and necrosis in porcine granulosa cells via a caspase-3- and caspase-9-dependent mitochondrial signaling pathway. *J. Cell Physiol.* **2012**, *227*, 1814–1820. [CrossRef]
29. Zhang, G.L.; Feng, Y.L.; Song, J.L.; Zhou, X.S. Zearalenone: A mycotoxin with different toxic effect in domestic and laboratory animals' granulosa cells. *Front. Genet.* **2018**, *9*, 667. [CrossRef]
30. Li, L.; Yang, M.; Li, C.; Yang, F.; Wang, G. Understanding the toxin effects of β-zearalenol and HT-2 on bovine granulosa cells using iTRAQ-based proteomics. *Animals* **2020**, *10*, 130. [CrossRef]

31. Pistol, G.C.; Gras, M.A.; Marin, D.E.; Israel-Roming, F.; Stancu, M.; Taranu, I. Natural feed contaminant zearalenone decreases the expressions of important pro- and anti-inflammatory mediators and mitogen-activated protein kinase/NF-$_k$B signaling molecules in pigs. *Br. J. Nutr.* **2014**, *111*, 452–464. [CrossRef]
32. Bulgaru, C.V.; Marin, D.E.; Pistol, G.C.; Taranu, I. Zearalenone and the immune response. *Toxins* **2021**, *13*, 248. [CrossRef]
33. Lee, P.-Y.; Liu, C.-C.; Wang, S.-C.; Chen, K.-Y.; Lin, T.-C.; Liu, P.-L.; Chiu, C.-C.; Chen, I.-C.; Lai, Y.-H.; Cheng, W.-C. Mycotoxin zearalenone attenuates innate immune responses and suppresses NLRP3 inflammasome activation in LPS-activated macrophages. *Toxins* **2021**, *13*, 593. [CrossRef] [PubMed]
34. Kobayashi, N.; Kubosaki, A.; Takahashi, Y.; Yanai, M.; Konuma, R.; Uehara, S.; Chiba, T.; Watanabe, M.; Terajima, J.; Sugita-Konishi, Y. Distribution of sterigmatocystin-producing aspergilli in Japan. *Food Safety* **2018**, *6*, 67–73. [CrossRef] [PubMed]
35. Nomura, M.; Aoyama, K.; Ishibashi, T. Sterigmatocystin and aflatoxin B1 contamination of corn, soybean meal, and formula feed in Japan. *Mycotoxin Res.* **2018**, *34*, 21–27. [CrossRef]
36. Kobayashi, N.; Sakurai, K.; Nakarai, R.; Shigaki, K.; Horikawa, K.; Honda, M.; Sugiura, Y.; Watanabe, M.; Takino, M.; Sugita-Konishi, Y. Microflora of mycotoxigenic fungi in rice grains in Kyushu region of Japan and their changes during storage under non-controlled conditions. *Biocont. Sci.* **2019**, *24*, 161–166. [CrossRef]
37. Yoshinari, T.; Takeuchi, H.; Kosugi, M.; Taniguchi, M.; Waki, M.; Hashiguchi, S.; Fujiyoshi, T.; Shichinohe, Y.; Nakajima, M.; Ohnishi, T.; et al. Determination of sterigmatocystin in foods in Japan: Method validation and occurrence data. *Food Addit. Contam. Part A* **2019**, *36*, 1404–1410. [CrossRef]
38. Fink-Gremmels, J.; Malekinejad, H. Clinical effects and biochemical mechanisms associated with exposure to the mycoestrogen zearalenone. *Anim. Feed Sci. Technol.* **2007**, *37*, 326–341. [CrossRef]
39. Minervini, F.; Dell'Aquila, M.E. Zearalenone and reproductive function in farm animals. *Int. J. Mol. Sci.* **2008**, *9*, 2570–2584. [CrossRef]
40. Weaver, H.A.; Kurtz, H.T.; Behrens, J.C.; Robinson, T.S.; Seguin, B.E.; Bates, F.Y.; Mirocha, J.C. Effect of zearalenone of dairy cows. *Am. J. Vet. Res.* **1986**, *47*, 659–662.
41. Weaver, H.A.; Kurtz, H.T.; Behrens, J.C.; Robinson, T.S.; Seguin, B.E.; Bates, F.Y.; Mirocha, J.C. Effects of zearalenone on the fertility of virgin dairy heifers. *Am. J. Vet. Res.* **1986**, *47*, 1395–1397. [PubMed]
42. Fink-Gremmels, J. The role of mycotoxins in the health and performance of dairy cows. *Vet. J.* **2008**, *176*, 84–92. [CrossRef] [PubMed]
43. Takagi, M.; Mukai, S.; Kuriyagawa, T.; Takagaki, K.; Uno, S.; Kokushi, E.; Otoi, T.; Budiyanto, A.; Shirasuna, K.; Miyamoto, A.; et al. Detection of zearalenone and its metabolites in naturally contaminated follicular fluids by using LC/MS/MS and in vitro effects of zearalenone on oocyte maturation in cattle. *Reprod. Toxicol.* **2008**, *26*, 164–169. [CrossRef]
44. Takagi, M.; Hirai, T.; Shiga, S.; Uno, S.; Kokushi, E.; Otoi, T.; Deguchi, E.; Tshering, C.; Fink-Gremmels, J. Relationship between urinary zearalenone concentration and embryo production in superovulated cattle. *Arch. Anim. Breed.* **2013**, *36*, 360–366. [CrossRef]
45. FAMIC (Food and Agricultural Materials Inspection Center, Japan). Shiryobunsekikijun. FAMIC, Saitama. Available online: http://www.famic.go.jp/ffis/feed/bunseki/bunsekikijun.html (accessed on 20 April 2012). (In Japanese).
46. Fushimi, Y.; Monniaux, D.; Takagi, M. Efficacy of a single measurement of plasma anti-Muüllerian hormone concentration for ovum pick-up donor selection of Japanese Black heifers in herd breeding programs. *J. Reprod. Dev.* **2019**, *65*, 369–374. [CrossRef]

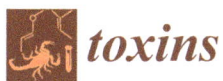

Article

The Effect of Low Doses of Zearalenone (ZEN) on the Bone Marrow Microenvironment and Haematological Parameters of Blood Plasma in Pre-Pubertal Gilts

Magdalena Mróz [1], Magdalena Gajęcka [1,*], Katarzyna E. Przybyłowicz [2], Tomasz Sawicki [2], Sylwia Lisieska-Żołnierczyk [3], Łukasz Zielonka [1] and Maciej Tadeusz Gajęcki [1]

[1] Department of Veterinary Prevention and Feed Hygiene, Faculty of Veterinary Medicine, University of Warmia and Mazury in Olsztyn, Oczapowskiego 13/29, 10-718 Olsztyn, Poland; magdzia.mroz@gmail.com or magdalena.mroz@uwm.edu.pl (M.M.); lukaszz@uwm.edu.pl (Ł.Z.); gajecki@uwm.edu.pl (M.T.G.)

[2] Department of Human Nutrition, Faculty of Food Sciences, University of Warmia and Mazury in Olsztyn, Słoneczna 45F, 10-719 Olsztyn, Poland; katarzyna.przybylowicz@uwm.edu.pl (K.E.P.); tomasz.sawicki@uwm.edu.pl (T.S.)

[3] Independent Public Health Care Centre of the Ministry of the Interior and Administration, and the Warmia and Mazury Oncology Centre in Olsztyn, Wojska Polskiego 37, 10-228 Olsztyn, Poland; lisieska@wp.pl

* Correspondence: mgaja@uwm.edu.pl; Tel.: +48-89-523-37-73; Fax: +48-89-523-36-18

Abstract: The aim of this study was to determine whether low doses of zearalenone (ZEN) influence the carry-over of ZEN and its metabolites to the bone marrow microenvironment and, consequently, haematological parameters. Pre-pubertal gilts (with a body weight of up to 14.5 kg) were exposed to daily ZEN doses of 5 μg/kg BW (group ZEN5, n = 15), 10 μg/kg BW (group ZEN10, n = 15), 15 μg/kg BW (group ZEN15, n = 15), or were administered a placebo (group C, n = 15) throughout the entire experiment. Bone marrow was sampled on three dates (exposure dates 7, 21, and 42—after slaughter) and blood for haematological analyses was sampled on 10 dates. Significant differences in the analysed haematological parameters (WBC White Blood Cells, MONO—Monocytes, NEUT—Neutrophils, LYMPH—Lymphocytes, LUC—Large Unstained Cells, RBC—Red Blood Cells, HGB—Haemoglobin, HCT—Haematocrit, MCH—Mean Corpuscular Volume, MCHC—Mean Corpuscular Haemoglobin Concentrations, PLT—Platelet Count and MPV—Mean Platelet Volume) were observed between groups. The results of the experiment suggest that exposure to low ZEN doses triggered compensatory and adaptive mechanisms, stimulated the local immune system, promoted eryptosis, intensified mycotoxin biotransformation processes in the liver, and produced negative correlations between mycotoxin concentrations and selected haematological parameters.

Keywords: zearalenone; low dose; bone marrow microenvironment; haematology; pre-pubertal gilts

Key Contribution: The administered ZEN doses and the duration of ZEN exposure were negatively correlated with three haematological parameters in pre-pubertal gilts.

1. Introduction

Zearalenone (ZEN) and its metabolites (ZELs), α-zearalenol (α-ZEL) and β-zearalenol (β-ZEL), are the most ubiquitous mycotoxins in plant materials. They are frequently referred to as xenobiotics. These mycotoxins disrupt reproductive functions because they are structurally similar to oestradiol [1,2]. Alpha-ZEL is the main ZEN metabolite that affects pigs. Other animal species, including broilers, cows, and sheep, are more susceptible to β-ZEL, which is characterized by lower levels of metabolic activity [3]. Zearalenone's activity is determined by biotransformation processes in plants and animals as well as the immune status of the reproductive system (due to variations in steroid hormone levels during maturation, reproduction, and pregnancy) and the gastrointestinal system of the exposed individuals [4–7].

Different doses of mycotoxins induce various effects [7]. The symptoms and toxic effects of high mycotoxin doses have been extensively researched [8]. Low monotonic doses of mycotoxins are well tolerated by animals during prolonged exposure, and these compounds can meet the animals' life needs or exert therapeutic effects [9–11]. The adverse effects of low mycotoxin doses have also been well documented [12]. These effects can be attributed to hormesis, namely exposure to the highest doses below the No Observed Adverse Effect Level (NOAEL) that induce subclinical (asymptomatic) states or interact positively with the host organism in various stages of life [13–16]. In turn, doses corresponding to the Lowest Observed Adverse Effect Level (LOAEL) induce clear clinical symptoms of mycotoxicosis. The lowest measurable dose that interacts positively with the host body in different stages of life is known as the Minimal Anticipated Biological Effect Level (MABEL) [16].

The dose-response relationship has been also undermined by the low dose hypothesis. The above applies particularly to hormonally active chemical compounds, including mycoestrogens such as ZEN and ZELs, which disrupt the functioning of the endocrine system (ED), even when ingested in small quantities [5,17]. This ambiguous dose-response relationship does not justify direct analyses or meta-analyses of the risk (clinical symptoms or the results of laboratory analyses) associated with the transition from high to low doses [18]. The concept of the lowest identifiable dose that produces counter-intuitive effects is becoming increasingly popular in biomedical sciences. For this reason, the relevant mechanisms should be investigated to support rational decision-making in selected processes [7,19]. Substances that both disrupt and contribute to homeostasis have undermined the traditional concepts in toxicology, in particular "the dose makes the poison" adage. Zearalenone and ZELs induce different responses in mammals when administered in low doses [13]. Similar observations have been made by Knutsen et al. [12]. According to the Scientific Panel on Contaminants in the Food Chain (CONTAM), the influence of ZEN on animal health should be re-evaluated based on the animals' responses to the lowest detectable doses of ZEN (MABEL; the highest values of NOAEL and LOAEL), including the parent compound and its metabolites, in feed [7,12,20,21].

Hematopoietic stem cells (controlled primarily by the local bone marrow microenvironment as well as by long-range signals from, for example, the endocrine system [22], such as oestrogens or xenobiotics) cannot cross the bone marrow microenvironment barrier. Only mature blood cells containing specific membrane proteins are able to bind to the vascular endothelium and reach peripheral blood. Blood vessels act as a barrier that prevents immature blood cells from leaving the bone marrow microenvironment. Different types of haematopoietic cells have specific roles: red blood cells (RBC) contain haemoglobin, a specific protein that transports oxygen within the body [23], white blood cells (WBC) participate in immune functions and help fight infections, and platelets (PLT) participate in blood clotting at the sites of vascular injury [24].

The bone marrow microenvironment is an interesting object of scientific inquiry [25]. Red marrow is highly vascular, soft, gelatinous-spongy tissue, which fills the cavities of long bones and the spaces between trabeculae in cancellous bones, such as the wing of ilium. Red marrow is the primary producer of blood cells in the body, and it actively participates in haematopoiesis. Each day, red marrow produces 200 billion new morphotic elements in the blood. It is composed of delicate, highly vascular, fibrous tissue, and it contains hematopoietic stem cells, which give rise to various types of blood cells that are transported to the bloodstream upon maturation [26]. Yu and Scadden [27] described bone marrow as a carrier with sub-compartments that support different haematopoietic activities.

The aim of the present study was to determine whether exposure to low ZEN doses (MABEL [5 µg/kg body weight—BW], the highest values of NOAEL [10 µg/kg BW], and LOAEL [15 µg/kg BW]) administered *per os* to pre-pubertal gilts over a period of 6 weeks influences the concentrations of ZEN and ZELs in the bone marrow microenvironment and induces changes in selected haematological parameters.

2. Results

The presented results provide the basis for continuing research on the assessment of the impact of very low doses of ZEN on the macroorganism. There is a specific interaction between the mycotoxin level in the bone marrow microenvironment and the hematological values of the test animals. Preliminary data analysis documents that it is a set of highly individualized results for the parent substance and the absence of essential ZEN metabolites. The presented experimental design confirmed the correctness of the use of the method (chromatography), classified as precision medicine: medicine that allows the assessment of a single organism as well as the entire population. The existing values of the concentration of the undesirable substance in the bone marrow microenvironment contributed to the negative values of the Pearson's r coefficient for white and red blood cells and platelets.

2.1. Experimental Feed

The analysed feed did not contain mycotoxins, or its mycotoxin content was below the sensitivity of the method (VBS). The concentrations of masked mycotoxins were not analysed.

2.2. Clinical Observations

The results presented in this paper were acquired during a large-scale experiment where clinical signs of ZEN mycotoxicosis were not observed. However, changes in specific tissues or cells were frequently noted in analyses of selected serum biochemical parameters, heart muscle, coronary artery, genotoxicity of caecal water, selected steroid concentrations, gut microbiota parameters, and the animals' body weight gains. Samples for laboratory analyses were collected from the same pre-pubertal gilts. The results of these analyses were presented in our previous studies [7,16,28,29].

2.3. Concentrations of Zearalenone and Its Metabolites in the Bone Marrow Microenvironment

Zearalenone concentrations in the bone marrow microenvironment did not differ significantly between the experimental groups, but the lowest values were noted on the first two exposure dates (5.64 ng/g on D1; 4.69 ng/g on D2) in group ZEN5 (5 µg ZEN/kg BW) (see Table 1). In turn, significant differences at $p \leq 0.05$ were observed between group ZEN5 and group ZEN10 (7.74 ng/g and 7.35 ng/g, respectively) on D3. Significant differences at $p \leq 0.01$ were noted between group ZEN5 and group ZEN15 (7.74 ng/g and 7.03 ng/g, respectively) on D3, and in group ZEN15 between D2 and D3 vs. D1 (6.84 ng/g and 7.03 ng/g vs. 8.17 ng/g, respectively). Similar values had been reported in other tissues, such as the heart muscle [19]. Zearalenone metabolites, α-ZEL and β-ZEL, were not detected (values below the sensitivity of the method).

2.4. Carry-OVER Factor (CF)

The carry-over of ZEN from the intestinal lumen to the bone marrow microenvironment collected from the wing of ilium (posterior superior iliac spine), was influenced by the administered dose and time of exposure in each group (see Table 1). The lowest values of the CF were noted in group ZEN5 (in particular on D1 and D3 at 7×10^{-5} and 6×10^{-5}, respectively), and the highest CF values were observed in group ZEN15 (in particular on D3 at 98×10^{-7}). The values of the CF determined in this study were proportionally higher relative to the values noted in the blood serum [28] and the heart muscle [19] of the same animals.

Table 1. The carry-over factor (CF) and mean ($\bar{x}$) concentrations of ZEN and ZELs (ng/g) in the bone marrow microenvironment of pre-pubertal gilts.

Exposure Date	Feed Intake [kg/Day]	Total ZEN Doses in Groups Respectively [µg/kg BW]	Group ZEN5 [ng/g]	CF Group ZEN5	Group ZEN10 [ng/g]	CF Group ZEN10	Group ZEN15 [ng/g]	CF Group ZEN15
			Zearalenone					
D1	0.8	80.5/161.9/242.7	5.64 ± 3.24	7×10^{-5}	6.35 ± 3.56	39×10^{-6}	8.17 ± 0.45	33×10^{-6}
D2	1.1	101.01/196.9/298.2	4.69 ± 4.28	46×10^{-6}	7.08 ± 0.10	35×10^{-6}	6.84 ± 0.18 ••	22×10^{-6}
D3	1.6	128.3/481.4/716.7	7.74 ± 0.26	6×10^{-5}	7.35 ± 0.25 *	15×10^{-6}	7.03 ± 0.14 **,••	98×10^{-7}
			α-ZEL and β-ZEL					
D1–D3		not applicable			0			

Abbreviation: D1, exposure day 7; D2, exposure day 21; D3, exposure day 42. Experimental groups: Group ZEN5, 5 µg ZEN/kg BW; Group ZEN10, 10 µg ZEN/kg BW; Group ZEN15, 15 µg ZEN/kg BW. LOD > values below the limit of detection were expressed as 0. Statistically significant differences were determined at * $p \leq 0.05$ and **,•• $p \leq 0.01$; *, ** statistical difference between group ZEN5 vs. group ZEN10 and group ZEN15 on exposure date D3; •• statistical difference in group 3 between exposure date D1 and exposure dates D2 and D3.

2.5. Results of Haematological Analyses

Only statistically significant differences in all animal groups are presented in the figure drawings. The results of this study and the findings of other authors indicate that even very low concentrations of mycotoxins in feed materials can lead to changes in blood homeostasis in pre-pubertal gilts [10,30–32]. The significant differences in the haematological parameters of pre-pubertal gilts exposed to various doses of ZEN (MABEL, highest NOAEL values, and LOAEL) for 6 weeks did not exceed the reference range [32,33]. In view of the above, the results noted in group C were unambiguous (see Supplementary Materials—Table S1), and they could be used as a reference in a risk assessment analysis, where each result is considered within a range of positive control (increase) or negative control (decrease) values during subchronic exposure to the mycotoxin.

2.6. Haematological Analyses

2.6.1. General Analysis

Significant differences were rarely noted, mostly in erythrocyte parameters in the middle (see Figure 1) and at the end of the experiment (see Figure 2), and in the percentages of white blood cells on the first and last date of exposure (see Figure 2). At the beginning of the experiment, the analysed parameters were generally lower in group C, whereas the reverse was noted towards the end of the study. Significant differences were not observed on date 9.

2.6.2. Accompanying Factors

The results of this study could have been influenced by several accompanying factors, including (i) the manner of ZEN transmission to the body, (ii) ZEN dose, (iii) and/or the kinetic effects of mycotoxin bioassimilation [13]. The latter can be subdivided into several sub-processes, beginning from mycotoxin extraction from the feed matrix to its absorption, distribution, and deposition in tissues, and mycotoxin modification [15]. This is a very important consideration, but it was not studied in the described experiment.

The above can have two effects: (i) higher demand for energy needed for biotransformation and constitutive growth of pre-pubertal gilts [7,34], and (ii) a milder response to the applied mycotoxin doses in the peripheral vascular system (*vena cava cranialis*) from which samples for metabolic analyses were collected. As a result, the exposure to low doses of ZEN with low values of the CF to intestinal tissues (towards the end of the experiment) and the liver probably induced minor but significant changes in the values of selected haematological parameters. Changes in WBC (White Blood Cells), EOS (Eosinophils), BASO (Basophils), MONO (Monocytes), RBC—Red Blood Cells; HGB—Haemoglobin, and

HCT—Haematocrit, values were observed mainly in the first three weeks of exposure (between sampling dates 1 and 6; see Tables 2–4).

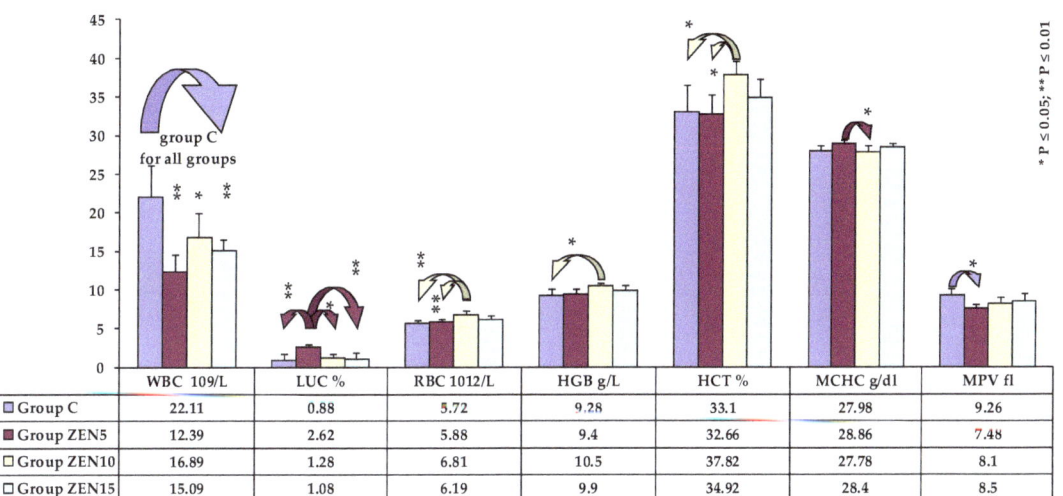

Figure 1. Selected haematological parameters on the fourth analytical date ($\bar{x}$, SD) Key: C, control group; Group ZEN5, 5 µg ZEN/kg BW; Group ZEN10, 10 µg ZEN/kg BW; Group ZEN15, 15 µg ZEN/kg BW. Statistically significant differences: * at $p \leq 0.05$; ** at $p \leq 0.01$.

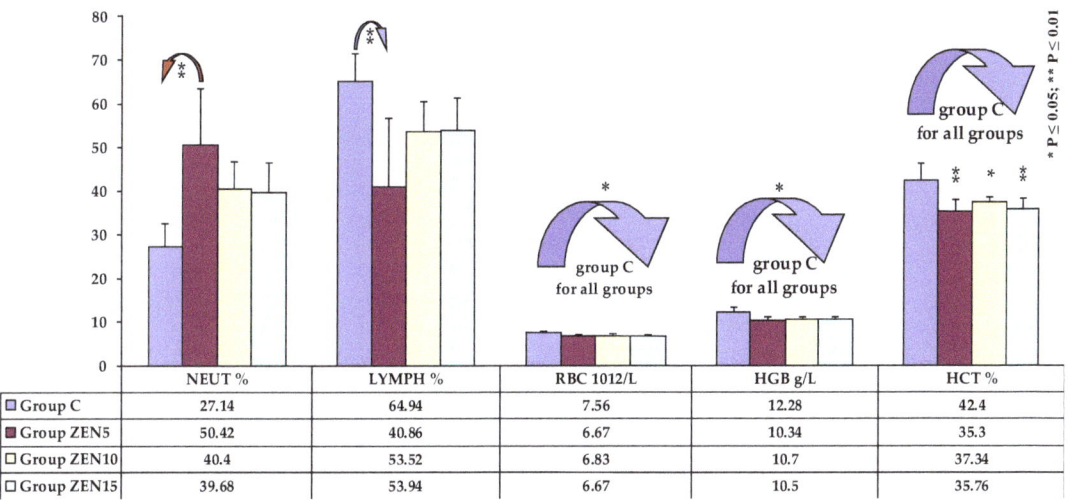

Figure 2. Selected haematological parameters on the tenth analytical date ($\bar{x}$, SD). Key: C, control group; Group ZEN5, 5 µg ZEN/kg BW; Group ZEN10, 10 µg ZEN/kg BW; Group ZEN15, 15 µg ZEN/kg BW. Statistically significant differences: * at $p \leq 0.05$; ** at $p \leq 0.01$.

Table 2. Selected haematological parameters in group ZEN5 on different analytical dates ($\bar{x}$, SD).

Blood Collection Dates	WBC 10^9/L	MONO %	LUC %	MPV fl
1	15.52 ± 7.58	5.32 ± 1.06	0.88 ± 0.63 [bb]	7.36 ± 1.61 [cc,ff]
2	18.8 ± 4.84	4.94 ± 1.07	1.72 ± 0.99	8.94 ± 0.99 [a]
3	18.8 ± 2.71	6.04 ± 3.69	1.42 ± 0.94	7.68 ± 0.55 [c,f]
4	12.39 ± 2.1 [ee]	4.3 ± 1.02	2.62 ± 0.31	7.48 ± 0.54 [c,ff]
5	17.23 ± 0.57	3.56 ± 0.55	1.26 ± 0.38	9.44 ± 1.44
6	15.45 ± 1.41	6.78 ± 0.91	0.84 ± 0.76 [bb]	8.14 ± 0.59
7	12.46 ± 1.37 [ee]	3.84 ± 0.89	1.44 ± 0.73	8.44 ± 0.87
8	15.04 ± 10.37	6.4 ± 2.59	0.8 ± 0.53 [b]	8.82 ± 1.42
9	24.55 ± 5.39	5.78 ± 1.18	0.6 ± 0.35 [bb]	8.82 ± 1.35
10	10.44 ± 3 [ee]	2.82 ± 0.84 [d]	0.72 ± 0.37 [bb]	9.66 ± 1.88

Key: Group ZEN5, 5 µg ZEN/kg BW; WBC, White Blood Cells; MONO, Monocytes; LUC, Large Unstained Cells; MPV, Mean Platelet Volume. Statistical symbols: [a], relative to date 1; [b], relative to date 4; [c], relative to date 5; [d], relative to date 6; [e], relative to date 9; [f], relative to date 10. Statistically significant differences: [a,b,c,d] and [f] at $p \leq 0.05$; [bb,cc,ee] and [ff] at $p \leq 0.01$.

Significant differences in PLT (Platelet Count) and PLT clump values were also noted on the same dates (see Table 5). These changes were probably induced by compensatory mechanisms [35].

2.7. Correlation Coefficients

Linear correlation coefficients (Pearson's r) were calculated to assess the relationships between ZEN concentrations in the bone marrow microenvironment and the values of blood morphotic components (RBC, WBC, and PLT) on different exposure dates and in different experimental groups (see Table 6). These blood components were selected because erythropoiesis, leukopoiesis, and thrombopoiesis take place during the last processes of hemopoiesis in the bone marrow environment. The strength of the examined correlations can be evaluated based on the values presented in Table 6 [36]. A correlation is negative when $r < 0$. The strength of correlations is evaluated on the following scale: $r < 0$ to -0.2, no negative linear correlation; $r = -0.21$ to -0.39, weak negative correlation; $r = -0.4$ to -0.69, moderate negative correlation; $r = -0.7$ to -0.9, relatively strong negative correlation; $r > -0.9$, very strong negative correlation. The correlation coefficient denotes a statistical relationship, and it does not imply a cause-effect relationship.

In a negative correlation, an increase in the value of one variable is accompanied by a decrease in the value of another variable, which was observed in this study. A negative correlation coefficient must be lower than -0.710 (relatively strong negative correlation) to explain more than 50% of the variance in the examined values. A relatively strong negative correlation was noted in PLT values on D1 in group ZEN5 and on D3 in groups ZEN5 and ZEN10 (see Table 6), in WBC values on D2 in groups ZEN5 and ZEN15, and in RBC values on D1 in group ZEN15, on D2 in group ZEN10, and on D3 in groups ZEN5 and ZEN15. A moderate positive correlation was observed in PLT values on D1 in group ZEN10, which could be attributed to the lowest ZEN concentration at a relatively low value of CF. These findings indicate that ZEN dose and time of exposure exert a negative effect on the haematopoietic activity of the evaluated blood morphotic components in the bone marrow microenvironment.

Table 3. Selected white blood cell markers in group ZEN10 on different analytical dates ($\bar{x}$, SD).

Blood Collection Dates	WBC 10⁹/L	NEUT %	LYMPH %	LUC %	RBC 10¹²/L	HGB g/L	HCT %	MCV fl	MCHC g/dL	HDW g/dL
1	21.86 ± 2.67 ᵈ	37.68 ± 3.89	55.7 ± 3.89	0.8 ± 0.64	6.68 ± 0.54	10.79 ± 0.65	37.08 ± 2.19	55.6 ± 1.81	29.1 ± 1.23	1.58 ± 0.13 ᵃᵃ,ᵇᵇ
2	22.74 ± 3.6 ᵃ,ᵈ	43.7 ± 12.26 ᵃ	50.02 ± 12.12 ᵃ	0.86 ± 0.69	6.57 ± 0.38 ᶜ	10.22 ± 0.36 ᵇ,ᶜᶜ	34.98 ± 1.27 ᵇᵇ,ᶜᶜ	53.3 ± 2.52	29.12 ± 0.57 ᵃ	1.57 ± 0.04 ᵃ,ᵇ
3	19.55 ± 3.03	45.14 ± 5.14 ᵃ	46.94 ± 3.13 ᵃᵃ	0.98 ± 0.62	6.56 ± 0.17 ᶜ	10.18 ± 0.34 ᵇ,ᶜᶜ	35.48 ± 0.74 ᵇᵇ,ᶜᶜ	54.14 ± 2.49	28.7 ± 0.51	1.6 ± 0.08 ᵃ,ᵇᵇ
4	16.89 ± 2.94	29.58 ± 7.88	63.9 ± 7.68	1.28 ± 0.37	6.81 ± 0.39	10.5 ± 0.36	37.82 ± 1.63	55.6 ± 1.75	27.78 ± 0.8	1.54 ± 0.09 ᵃ
5	22.6 ± 6.49 ᵃ,ᵈ	43.34 ± 11.1	48.62 ± 10.43 ᵃ	1.86 ± 0.34 ᶜ	6.83 ± 0.46	10.28 ± 0.76 ᵇ,ᶜ	35.7 ± 2.87 ᵇᵇ,ᶜᶜ	52.22 ± 1.6 ᵃ	28.72 ± 0.38	1.54 ± 0.05 ᵃ
6	15.36 ± 3.68	33.7 ± 6.15	57.92 ± 6.89	1.22 ± 0.61	6.71 ± 0.33	10.62 ± 0.97	38.06 ± 2.54	56.68 ± 1.98	27.86 ± 0.86	1.55 ± 0.07 ᵃ,ᵇ
7	13.59 ± 2.68	27.28 ± 8.23	66.96 ± 8.07	0.66 ± 0.45	6.51 ± 0.42 ᵇ,ᶜ	10.34 ± 0.28 ᶜ	37.56 ± 1.11	57.86 ± 2.94	27.48 ± 0.54	1.43 ± 0.06
8	15.43 ± 5.68	34.08 ± 5.43	58.78 ± 5.47	1.64 ± 0.01	7.35 ± 0.33	11.54 ± 0.6	40.54 ± 2.56	55.18 ± 3.32	28.44 ± 0.6	1.44 ± 0.05
9	19.81 ± 3.64	39.6 ± 5.69	53.58 ± 6.26	0.52 ± 0.15	7.47 ± 0.41	11.7 ± 0.43	40.92 ± 0.86	54.84 ± 2.3	28.54 ± 0.94	1.53 ± 0.06 ᵃ
10	12.85 ± 3.75	40.4 ± 6.31	53.52 ± 6.83	0.88 ± 0.21	6.83 ± 0.4	10.7 ± 0.55	37.34 ± 1.23	54.74 ± 2.65	28.62 ± 0.79	1.54 ± 0.08 ᵃ

Key: Group ZEN10, 10 μg ZEN/kg BW; WBC, White Blood Cells; NEUT, Neutrophils; LYMPH, Lymphocytes; LUC, Large Unstained Cells; RBC, Red Blood Cells; HGB, Haemoglobin; HCT, Haematocrit; MCV, Mean Corpuscular Volume; MCHC, Mean Corpuscular Haemoglobin Concentrations; HDW, Haemoglobin Distribution Width. Statistical symbols: ᵃ, relative to date 7; ᵇ, relative to date 8; ᶜ, relative to date 9; ᵈ, relative to date 10. Statistically significant differences: ᵃ,ᵇ,ᶜ and ᵈ at $p \leq 0.05$, ᵃᵃ,ᵇᵇ and ᶜᶜ at $p \leq 0.01$.

Table 4. Selected haematological parameters in group ZEN15 on different analytical dates ($\bar{x}$, SD).

Blood Collection Dates	WBC 10^9/L	NEUT %	LYMPH %	EOS %	MPV fl
1	22.01 ± 3.85 [ee,ff]	52.92 ± 7.91	39.96 ± 8.22 [e]	2.4 ± 1.47	8.22 ± 1.65
2	19.83 ± 1.35 [e,f]	43.7 ± 6.64	48.62 ± 5.62	1.32 ± 0.52	7.68 ± 1.55 [a]
3	20.73 ± 2.21 [e,f]	44.92 ± 7.66	46.42 ± 6.85	1.96 ± 0.65	7.50 ± 0.45
4	15.09 ± 14.43	38.54 ± 7.92	55.38 ± 7.23	0.64 ± 0.27 [a]	8.51 ± 1.12
5	22.33 ± 5.96 [ee,ff]	48.16 ± 12.12	45.62 ± 10.12	1.22 ± 0.43	7.58 ± 1.05 [aa,b,c]
6	16.66 ± 3.96	37 ± 5.58	54.14 ± 5.95	1.6 ± 0.41	7.84 ± 1.09
7	10.79 ± 2.53	26.44 ± 6.28 [a,d]	66.12 ± 4.45	0.74 ± 0.23 [a]	7.44 ± 1.32
8	19.04 ± 2.47	41.32 ± 11.48	49.64 ± 11.23	1.9 ± 0.76	8.38 ± 2.72
9	14.8 ± 10.25	29.02 ± 20.07 [a]	40.37 ± 27.41 [e]	1.15 ± 0.82	8.85 ± 2.46
10	10.73 ± 1.78	39.68 ± 6.79	53.94 ± 7.3	1.44 ± 1.05	8.28 ± 1.05 [aa,b,cc]

Key: Group ZEN15, 15 µg ZEN/kg BW; WBC, White Blood Cells; NEUT, Neutrophils; LYMPH, Lymphocytes; EOS, Eosinophils; MPV, Mean Platelet Volume. Statistical symbols: [a], relative to date 1; [b], relative to date 3; [c], relative to date 4; [d], relative to date 5; [e], relative to date 7; [f], relative to date 10. Statistically significant differences: [a,b,c,d,e] and [f] at $p \leq 0.05$; [aa,cc,ee] and [ff] at $p \leq 0.01$.

Table 5. Platelet count in the experimental groups on different analytical dates ($\bar{x}$, SD).

Blood Collection Dates	PLT 10^9/L Group ZEN5	PLT 10^9/L Group ZEN10	PLT Clumps % Group ZEN10	PLT 10^9/L Group ZEN15	PLT Clumps % Group ZEN15
1	405.4 ± 295.39	690.2 ± 121.87 [e]	26.4 ± 14.75	479.8 ± 214.68	19.8 ± 18.07
2	522.6 ± 112.81	763 ± 107.01 [d,ee]	19.8 ± 18.07	668 ± 144.82 [d,e]	19.8 ± 18.07
3	745 ± 54.41 [e]	813.2 ± 149.05 [c,dd,ee]	0 ± 0	753.8 ± 167.69 [a,dd,ee]	0 ± 0
4	741.4 ± 89.6 [e]	734.6 ± 131.75 [d,e]	26.4 ± 14.75	501.6 ± 62.13 [b]	33 ± 0 [b]
5	517.2 ± 162.41	800.2 ± 212.97 [c,dd,ee]	33 ± 0 [bb]	718.2 ± 129.56 [a,d,ee]	26.4 ± 14.75
6	645.2 ± 140.47	650.6 ± 238.35	19.8 ± 18.07	635.4 ± 38.01 [e]	19.8 ± 18.07
7	463.6 ± 83.09	569.4 ± 132.14	26.4 ± 14.75	607.8 ± 203.15	13.2 ± 18.07
8	454 ± 317.27	617.2 ± 180.88	13.2 ± 18.07	626.6 ± 263.92 [e]	19.8 ± 18.07
9	595.6 ± 172.33	497.2 ± 101.9	33 ± 0 [bb]	394 ± 294.02	24.75 ± 16.5
10	369.4 ± 118.85	478.2 ± 151.9	33 ± 0 [bb]	386.6 ± 158.7	33 ± 0 [b]

Key: PLT count in groups 1, 2, and 3; PLT clumps in groups 2 and 3. Statistical symbols: [a], relative to date 1; [b], relative to date 3; [c], relative to date 7; [d], relative to date 9; [e], relative to date 10. Statistically significant differences: [a,b,c,d] and [e] at $p \leq 0.05$; [bb,dd] and [ee] at $p \leq 0.01$.

Table 6. Correlation coefficients (Pearson's r).

Exposure Date	Experimental Groups	PLT	WBC	RBC
D1	Group ZEN5	−0.739	−0.362	−0.456
D1	Group ZEN10	0.685	−0.502	−0.189
D1	Group ZEN15	−0.590	−0.336	−0.869
D2	Group ZEN5	−0.251	−0.851	−0.424
D2	Group ZEN10	−0.559	−0.325	−0.832
D2	Group ZEN15	−0.682	−0.797	−0.565
D3	Group ZEN5	−0.772	−0.230	−0.752
D3	Group ZEN10	−0.731	−0.451	−0.300
D3	Group ZEN15	−0.436	−0.128	−0.738

Key: Ratio of ZEN concentrations in the bone marrow microenvironment and blood morphotic components (RBC, WBC, and PLT) on different exposure dates (D1, D2, and D3: exposure days 7, 21, and 42, respectively). The mycotoxin was administered once daily before morning feeding (group ZEN5, 5 µg ZEN/kg BW; group ZEN10, 10 µg ZEN/kg BW; group ZEN15, 15 µg ZEN/kg BW). Samples were collected from pre-pubertal gilts immediately before slaughter.

3. Discussion

In this study and in our previous research, attempts were made to fill the gap in knowledge about the in vivo effects of low and very low doses of ZEN and its metabolites on mammals [7,16,28,29]. The present study was undertaken to address the general scarcity of published data on the influence of feed contamination with ZEN and its metabolites on haematopoietic activity and the bone marrow microenvironment in pre-pubertal gilts. In this study, selective ZEN doses, in each range of their values, influenced ZEN concentrations in the bone marrow microenvironment on different dates of exposure.

3.1. Zearalenone and Its Metabolites in the Bone Marrow Microenvironment

The first exposure date (D1) marks the end of stimulatory processes after seven days of exposure to an undesirable substance, such as ZEN. The final effects of adaptive processes [37], accompanied by decreased haematopoiesis in the bone marrow microenvironment, are manifested on D2 [28]. These processes can be accompanied by increased Ca^{2+} levels, in particular in the mitochondria [38], and changes in the activity of selected enzymes, such as hydroxysteroid dehydrogenases [39], thus disrupting steroidogenesis [13]. Excess ZEN (which was not biotransformed or was recovered after enterohepatic recirculation) probably led to hyperestrogenism on D3. The resulting "free ZEN" can affect steroidogenesis [28].

The present findings demonstrate that the process of ZEN absorption in the bone marrow microenvironment was highly individualised, due to considerable differences in standard deviation values and specifically due to the absence of ZEN metabolites in the analysed tissue in pre-pubertal gilts. Low ZEN concentrations and the absence of ZEN metabolites in the bone marrow microenvironment on all exposure dates confirm the previous suggestion that the physiological demand for exogenous oestrogen-like compounds [28] in pre-pubertal gilts is high due to supraphysiological hormone levels [40]. However, the values noted in this study were higher than those reported in the blood serum [28] or the heart muscle [19] of the same pre-pubertal gilts. This observation could be attributed to a much higher number of oestrogen receptors in the bone marrow microenvironment than in other tissues or organs [41,42]. In menopausal females, the reproductive system, followed by the bone marrow microenvironment, are most sensitive to the presence of gonadal hormones (long-range signals) [43]. This order is reversed in maturing females (the signals are initiated by oestradiol–oestrogen receptors [44]), which could explain higher ZEN concentrations in the bone marrow environment of pre-pubertal gilts. Exposure to higher ZEN doses leads to the production of "free ZEN", which plays different and not always positive roles. Oestradiol and "free ZEN" levels increase proportionally to the ZEN dose. These compounds decrease the concentrations of progesterone and testosterone [28], but they also play important protective roles in skeletal homeostasis [42], which is an important consideration in pre-pubertal gilts.

The above observations are confirmed by ZEN concentrations on D1 in all experimental groups. According to most researchers, metabolites are produced during the biotransformation of ZEN in pigs [45]. Therefore, the absence of metabolites in the bone marrow microenvironment could be regarded as a consequence of biotransformation processes in pre-pubertal gilts, where ZEN does not induce hyperestrogenism, but compensates for the physiological deficiency of endogenous oestrogens [40]. The above situation could result from a higher demand of the host organism for compounds with high estrogenic activity, such as ZEN and its metabolites (whose concentrations were below the sensitivity of the method) [46], or perhaps these were the physiological values that are required for the body to function [5]. This implies that it was a satisfactory effect of exposure to very low doses of ZEN during the ongoing detoxification processes. Other explanations are also possible: (i) the seventh day of exposure to an undesirable substance such as ZEN marks the end of adaptive processes [37], or (ii) ZEN is utilized as a substrate that regulates the expression of genes encoding HSDs, which act as molecular switches for the modulation of steroid hormone pre-receptors [28], or (iii) undesirable substances undergo enterohepatic circulation before they are completely eliminated from the body [47], and/or (iv) the gut microbiome exhibits specific behaviour during exposure to ZEN [29]. The above factors, alone or in combination, could affect the concentrations of ZEN in the bone marrow microenvironment, because ZEN is a promiscuous compound that can decrease the values of hematopoietic parameters [48].

On the other two exposure dates, similar correlations were noted in the average concentrations of ZEN in the bone marrow microenvironment. On these dates, ZEN concentrations were higher, but still low or very low, and ZEN metabolites were not detected. These observations could be attributed to the accumulation of ZEN (due to the saturation of active oestrogen receptors [48] and other factors that determine the concentrations of steroid hormones [45]) during prolonged exposure. However, due to the general scarcity of studies investigating the influence of low ZEN doses on the bone marrow environment and haematopoiesis, our results cannot be compared with the findings of other authors. According to the hormesis principle, exposure to very low ZEN doses affects the synthesis and secretion of sex steroid hormones. Therefore, very low ZEN doses were biotransformed in an identical manner, but the parent compound (ZEN) and, possibly, its metabolites were utilized more efficiently or completely by the macroorganism and, in particular, the bone marrow microenvironment. The interactions between endogenous and environmental (exogenous) steroids could also be influenced by other endogenous factors [49].

3.2. White Blood Cells

Haematological parameters somewhat exceeded the upper reference limit, in particular the percentage of lymphocytes, which increased in groups ZEN5 and ZEN10 on D1-relative lymphocytosis [50]. The increase in the percentage of lymphocytes was accompanied by a decrease in the percentage of neutrocytes. Contrary results were reported by [51], where very high ZEN concentrations exerted apoptotic effects on lymphocytes in vitro. In the present study, apoptotic effects were observed only on blood sampling date 10.

Based on the observations made by Etim et al. [52], the fact that haematological parameters were within the reference ranges indicates that feed composition had no negative effect on their values throughout the experiment. However, in view of the results of another study by Etim et al. [31], the fact that the values of WBC, NEUT, and LYMPH were within the reference ranges, but were lower than in group C, suggests that feed components did not stimulate the immune system. The neutrophil-to-lymphocyte ratio must be analysed (see Figure 3) to validate the hypothesis that the immune system was more stimulated by nutritional factors (including ZEN) and dietary stress than by functional stress [32,53]. The sizeable increase in the percentage of EOS in total WBC counts in group ZEN5, relative to group C during the entire experiment, should also be considered. In the remaining experimental groups, the percentage of EOS was lower than in group C. This observation suggests that ZEN can exert allergizing effects, which was confirmed in our previous study [54].

The observed decrease in WBC counts in all groups during the experiment points to probable immune suppression (as a consequence of gilt maturation), but this trend was least pronounced in group ZEN5. It should also be noted that during ZEN exposure, lymphocytes migrate to tissues with a physiologically higher number of oestrogen receptors, which intensifies proliferation processes and stimulates vascular filling [55]. Similar observations were made by Przybylska-Gornowicz et al. [56].

The decrease in WBC counts in the experimental groups suggests that ZEN affects adaptive processes by inducing reversible changes in the morphological and functional organization of the local immune system [50,55].

3.3. Red Blood Cells

Red blood cell counts remained stable throughout the experiment. Considerable differences were noted on blood sampling dates 4 and 10, with a rising trend in group C. In the experimental groups, a decrease in Fe levels [7] had no effect on RBC counts. Haemoglobin distribution width values were stable, but very low, and they were accompanied by a drop in glucose levels [7]. The above values are characteristic of pre-pubertal animals [57].

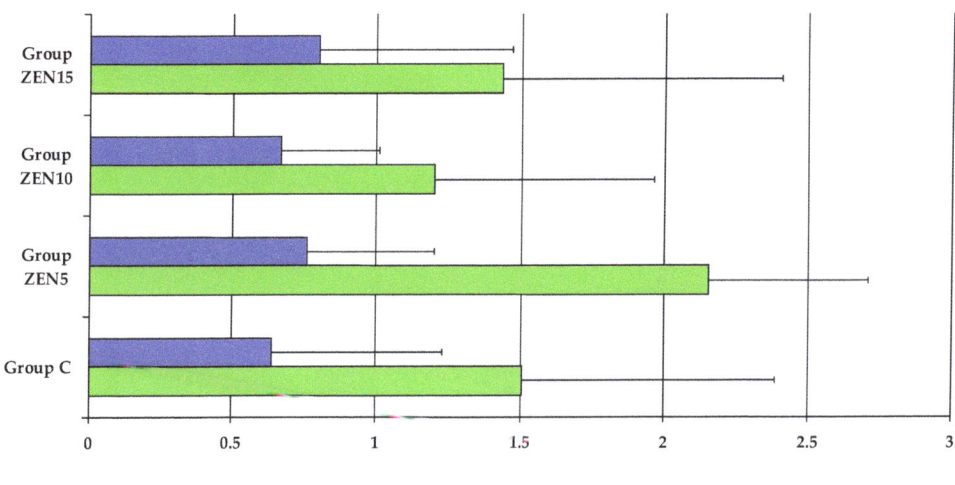

Figure 3. Selected haematological parameters in groups ($\bar{x}$). Key: C, control group; Group ZEN5, 5 µg ZEN/kg BW; Group ZEN10, 10 µg ZEN/kg BW; Group ZEN15, 15 µg ZEN/kg BW.

Erythrocytes, the main morphotic components of the blood, are highly sensitive to endogenous factors such as oxidation. Red blood cells have effective antioxidant mechanisms that remove reactive oxygen species that are produced outside or inside erythrocytes [58]. According to Tatay et al. [59], ZEN is a powerful antioxidant, and one of the side effects of ZEN exposure is a decrease in RBC counts, which could be attributed to "antioxidant competition". Similar suggestions were made by other authors who reported that ZEN induced eryptosis in mature human erythrocytes [60]. According to the cited authors, eryptosis can take place even at low concentrations of ZEN.

Eryptosis can also be induced by a mechanistic increase in intracellular Ca^{2+} levels [61,62], oxidative stress, energy depletion [63], and exposure to undesirable substances such as ZEN [56]. However, the loss of extracellular Ca^{2+} can also inhibit the eryptotic effect [64] due to anaemia and microcirculatory disorders. Microcirculatory disorders are observed in various tissues during exposure to ZEN, and they lead to numerous extravasations and vasodilation [65,66] in pre-pubertal female mammals, due to the relaxation of smooth muscle cells in vessel walls, in particular in large veins, large arteries, and smaller arterioles. An analysis of RBC values clearly indicates that all of the tested ZEN doses decreased erythrocyte counts and induced eryptosis [41].

3.4. Platelets

Platelet counts were above the norm in all groups, which is indicative of thrombocytosis [67]. The percentage of PLT Clumps was also elevated (pseudothrombocytopenia). These results could be explained by inadequate analytical standards or blood artefacts [68]. It should also be noted that platelets participate in the early stages of liver regeneration, but the underlying mechanisms of action have not yet been fully elucidated [69]. The liver is the main organ responsible for the biotransformation (detoxification) of undesirable substances such as ZEN [13]. The observed differences in values can be attributed to: (i) intensified proliferation in group ZEN5, and (ii) the influence of substances that stimulate proliferation in maturing animals [7,67,70].

In an analysis of PLT values, a positive correlation coefficient was noted only once. On the remaining exposure dates, the correlation coefficient assumed negative values, and it revealed the presence of a relatively strong negative correlation on three occasions. The strongest negative correlations were noted on D1 (during the highest exposure to ZEN) and D3 (during prolonged hyperestrogenism resulting from the accumulation of ZEN).

3.5. Summary and Conclusions

The exposure to very low doses of ZEN, administered *per os* to pre-pubertal gilts over a period of 42 days, induced a specific response in the bone marrow microenvironment. Zearalenone metabolites were not detected, and the concentration of the parent compound was higher in the bone marrow microenvironment than in other tissues. Low doses of ZEN affected haematopoiesis and induced completely different responses in selected haematological parameters than high doses (LOAEL). Zearalenone's multidirectional effects on blood morphotic components at the beginning and end of the experiment were probably modified by compensatory and adaptive mechanisms. Zearalenone also induced reversible changes in the morphological and functional organization of the local immune system. The values of the analysed haematological parameters pointed to eryptosis and the stimulation of detoxifying organs such as the liver, where the intensity of biotransformation processes decreases under exposure to low doses of the studied mycotoxin. Further research is needed to elucidate the mechanisms responsible for changes in the haematological parameters of pre-pubertal gilts exposed to low doses of ZEN.

The results of these observations should play an important role in clinical veterinary practice, where ZEN could become a biomarker of the subclinical state of pre-pubertal gilts.

4. Materials and Methods

4.1. General Information

All experimental procedures involving animals were carried out in compliance with Polish regulations setting forth the terms and conditions of animal experimentation (Opinions No. 12/2016 and 45/2016/DLZ of the Local Ethics Committee for Animal Experimentation of 27 April 2016 and 30 November 2016).

4.2. Experimental Feed

Analytical samples of ZEN were dissolved in 96 μL of 96% ethanol (SWW 2442-90, Polskie Odczynniki SA, Katowice, Poland) in doses appropriate for different BW. Feed was placed in gel capsules saturated with the solution and kept at room temperature to evaporate the alcohol. All groups of gilts received the same feed throughout the experiment. The animals were weighed at weekly intervals, and the results were used to adjust individual mycotoxin doses [12,16,29].

The feed administered to all experimental animals was supplied by the same producer. Friable feed was provided *ad libitum* twice daily, at 8:00 a.m. and 5:00 p.m., throughout the experiment. The composition of the complete diet, as declared by the manufacturer, is presented in Table 7 [12,16,29].

Table 7. Declared composition of the complete diet.

Parameters	Composition Declared by the Manufacturer (%)
Soybean meal	16
Wheat	55
Barley	22
Wheat bran	4.0
Chalk	0.3
Zitrosan	0.2
Vitamin-mineral premix [1]	2.5

[1] Composition of the vitamin-mineral premix per kg: vitamin A, 500.000 IU; iron, 5000 mg; vitamin D3, 100.000 IU; zinc, 5000 mg; vitamin E (alpha-tocopherol), 2000 mg; manganese, 3000 mg; vitamin K, 150 mg; copper ($CuSO_4 \cdot 5H_2O$), 500 mg; vitamin B_1, 100 mg; cobalt, 20 mg; vitamin B_2, 300 mg; iodine, 40 mg; vitamin B_6, 150 mg; selenium, 15 mg; vitamin B_{12}, 1500 μg; L-lysine, 9.4 g; niacin, 1200 mg; DL-methionine+cystine, 3.7 g; pantothenic acid, 600 mg; L-threonine, 2.3 g; folic acid, 50 mg; tryptophan, 1.1 g; biotin, 7500 μg; phytase+choline, 10 g; ToyoCerin probiotic+calcium, 250 g; antioxidant+mineral phosphorus and released phosphorus, 60 g; magnesium, 5 g; sodium and calcium, 51 g.

The proximate chemical composition of the diets fed to pigs in groups C, ZEN5, ZEN10, and ZEN15 was determined using the NIRS™ DS2500 F feed analyser (FOSS, Hillerød, Denmark), a monochromator-based NIR reflectance and transflectance analyser with a scanning range of 850–2500 nm [12,16,29].

Toxicological Analysis in Feed

Feed was analysed for the presence of mycotoxins and their metabolites: ZEN, α-ZEL, and deoxynivalenol (DON). Mycotoxin concentrations in feed were determined by separation in immunoaffinity columns (Zearala-Test™ Zearalenone Testing System, G1012, VICAM, Watertown, MA, USA; DON-Test™ DON Testing System, VICAM, Watertown, MA, USA). The feed samples were ground in a laboratory mill. 25 g of the ground sample was taken up in 150 mL of acetonitrile (90%) to extract the mycotoxins. 10 mL of the resulting solution was withdrawn and diluted with 40 mL of water. Again, 10 mL of the next solution was taken and passed through the immunoaffinity column (VICAM). The immunoaffinity bed in the column was subsequently washed with demineralized water (Millipore Water Purification System, Millipore S.A., Molsheim, France). The column was eluted with 99.8% methanol (LIChrosolvTM, No. 1.06 007, Merck-Hitachi, München, Germany) to wash away the bound mycotoxin. The obtained solutions were analyzed by high-performance liquid chromatography (HPLC system, Hewlett Packard type 1050 and 1100, Beeston Court, United Kingdom) coupled with a diode array detector (DAD) and a fluorescence detector (FLD) and chromatography columns (Atlantis T3, 3 µm 3.0 150 mm Column No. 186003723, Waters, AN Etten-Leur, Ireland). Mycotoxins were separated using a mobile phase of acetonitrile:water:methanol (46:46:8, $v/v/v$). The flow rate was 0.4 mL/min. The limit of detection was set at 5 µg/kg of feed for DON and 2 µg/kg of feed for ZEN, based on validation of chromatographic methods for the determination of ZEN and DON levels in feed materials and feeds. Chromatographic methods were validated at the Department of Veterinary Prevention and Feed Hygiene, Faculty of Veterinary Medicine, University of Warmia and Mazury in Olsztyn, Poland [11].

4.3. Experimental Animals

The experiment was performed at the Department of Veterinary Prevention and Feed Hygiene of the Faculty of Veterinary Medicine at the University of Warmia and Mazury in Olsztyn Poland on 60 clinically healthy pre-pubertal gilts with initial BW of 14.5 ± 2 kg. The animals were housed in the same building, in adjoining pens with latticework walls, and had free access to water. They were randomly assigned to three experimental groups (group ZEN5, group ZEN10, and group ZEN15; $n = 15$) and a control group (group C; $n = 15$) [71,72]. Group ZEN5 gilts were orally administered ZEN at 5 µg/kg BW, Group ZEN10, 10 µg/kg BW, and Group ZEN15, 15 µg/kg BW. Group C animals were orally administered a placebo. Zearalenone was administered daily in gel capsules before morning feeding. Feed was the carrier, and group C pigs were administered the same gel capsules, but without mycotoxins [12,16,29].

4.3.1. Toxicological Analysis of Bone Marrow Microenvironment
Tissues Samples

Five prepubertal gilts from every group were euthanized on analytical date 1 (D1, exposure day 7), date 2 (D2, exposure day 21), and date 3 (D3, exposure day 42) by intravenous administration of pentobarbital sodium (Fatro, Ozzano Emilia, Bologna, Italy) and bleeding. Samples were taken from the iliac wing (posterior superior iliac spine) immediately after cardiac arrest and were rinsed with phosphate buffer. The collected samples were stored at a temperature of −20 °C.

Extraction Procedure

The presence of ZEN, α-ZEL, and β-ZEL in the bone marrow microenvironment was determined with the use of immunoaffinity columns. The samples of bone marrow environment (3 mL) were transferred to centrifuge tubes homogenized with 7 mL of methanol (99.8%) for 4 min. The tubes were vortexed 4 times at 5 min intervals, after which they were centrifugated at 5000 rpm for 15 min. 5 mL was taken from the suspension obtained and taken up in 20 mL of deionized water, and only from this solution, 12.5 mL was taken for zearalenone extraction. The supernatant was carefully collected and passed through immunoaffinity columns (Zearala-TestTM Zearalenone Testing System, G1012, VICAM, Watertown, MA, USA) at the rate of 1–2 drops per second. The immunoaffinity bed in the column was subsequently washed with demineralized water (Millipore Water Purification System, Millipore S.A., Molsheim, France). The column was eluted isocratic with 99.8% methanol (LIChrosolvTM, No. 1.06 007, Merck-Hitachi, Germany) to wash away the bound mycotoxin. After extraction, the eluents were placed in a water bath at a temperature of 50 °C and were evaporated in a stream of nitrogen. Dry residues were stored at −20 °C until chromatographic analysis. Next, 0.5 mL of 99.8% acetonitrile (ACN) was added to dry residues to dissolve the mycotoxin. The process was monitored with the use of internal standards (Cayman Chemical 1180 East Ellsworth Road Ann Arbor, MI 48108, USA, ZEN-catalog number 11353; Batch 0593470-1; α-ZEN-catalog number 16549; Batch 0585633-2; β-ZEN-catalog number 19460; Batch 0604066-7), and the results were validated by mass spectrometry.

Chromatographic Quantification of ZEN and Its Metabolites

Zearalenone and its metabolites were quantified at the Institute of Dairy Industry Innovation in Mrągowo, Poland. The biological activity of ZEN, α-ZEL, and β-ZEL in the bone marrow microenvironment was determined by combined separation methods, involving immunoaffinity columns (Zearala-TestTM Zearalenone Testing System, G1012, VICAM, Watertown, MA, USA), Agilent 1260 liquid chromatography (LC) system, and a mass spectrometry (MS, Agilent 6470, Santa Clara, United States) system. Samples were analyzed on a chromatographic column (Atlantis T3, 3 μm 3.0 × 150 mm, column No. 186003723, Waters, AN Etten-Leur, Ireland). The mobile phase was composed of 70% acetonitrile (LiChrosolvTM, No. 984 730 109, Merck-Hitachi, Mannheim, Germany), 20% methanol (LiChrosolvTM, No. 1.06 007, Merck-Hitachi, Mannheim, Germany), and 10% deionized water (MiliporeWater Purification System, Millipore S.A. Molsheim, France) with the addition of 2 mL of acetic acid per 1 L of the mixture. The flow rate was 0.4 mL/min, and the temperature of the oven column was 40 °C. The chromatographic analysis was completed in 4 min. The column was flushed with 99.8% methanol (LIChrosolvTM, No. 1.06 007, Merck-Hitachi, Mannheim, Germany) to remove the bound mycotoxin. The flow rate was 0.4 mL/min, and the temperature of the oven column was 40 °C. The chromatographic analysis was completed in 4 min.

Mycotoxin concentrations were determined with an external standard and were expressed in ppb (ng/mL). Matrix-matched calibration standards were applied in the quantification process to eliminate matrix effects that can decrease sensitivity. Calibration standards were dissolved in matrix samples based on the procedure that was used to prepare the remaining samples. The material for calibration standards was free of mycotoxins. The limits of detection (LOD) for ZEN, α-ZEL, and β-ZEL were determined as the concentration at which the signal-to-noise ratio decreased to 3. The concentrations of ZEN, α-ZEL, and β-ZEL were determined in each group and on three analytical dates (see Table 1).

Carryover Factor

Carryover toxicity takes place when an organism is able to survive under exposure to low doses of mycotoxins. Mycotoxins can compromise tissue or organ functions [73] and modify their biological activity [7,28]. The CF was determined in the bone marrow microenvironment when the daily dose of ZEN (5 μg ZEN/kg BW, 10 μg ZEN/kg BW, or 15 μg ZEN/kg BW) administered to each animal was equivalent to 560–32251.5 μg ZEN/kg of the complete diet, depending on daily feed intake. Mycotoxin concentrations in tissues were expressed in terms of the dry matter content of the samples.

The CF was calculated as follows:

CF = toxin concentration in tissue [ng/g]/toxin concentration in diet [ng/g].

Statistical Analysis

Data were processed statistically at the Department of Discrete Mathematics and Theoretical Computer Science, Faculty of Mathematics and Computer Science of the University of Warmia and Mazury in Olsztyn, Poland. The bioavailability of ZEN and its metabolites in the bone marrow microenvironment was analysed in group C and three experimental groups on three analytical dates. The results were expressed as means ($\pm$) with standard deviation (SD). The following parameters were analysed: (i) differences in the mean values for three ZEN doses (experimental groups) and the control group on both analytical dates, and (ii) differences in the mean values for specific ZEN doses (groups) on both analytical dates. In both cases, the differences between mean values were determined by one-way ANOVA. If significant differences were noted between groups, the differences between paired means were determined by Tukey's multiple comparison test. If all values were below LOD (mean and variance equal zero) in any group, the values in the remaining groups were analysed by one-way ANOVA (if the number of the remaining groups was higher than two), and the means in these groups were compared against zero by Student's t-test. Differences between groups were determined by Student's t-test. The results were regarded as highly significant at $p < 0.01$ (**) and as significant at $0.01 < p < 0.05$ (*). Data were processed statistically using Statistica v.13 software (TIBCO Software Inc., Silicon Valley, CA, USA, 2017). Dose–response relationships were determined by Pearson's correlation analysis. Differences were regarded as significant at $p \leq 0.05$. The results were presented as means $\pm$ standard error of the mean (S.E.M.).

4.4. Blood Sampling for Metabolic Profile Analysis

Blood for haematology tests was sampled from the *vena cava cranialis* ten times: on the first day (first date) of the experiment and on nine successive dates. Blood was sampled within 20 s after the immobilization of pre-pubertal gilts [74]. Blood was sampled from 5 gilts from every group on each sampling date.

4.5. Haematology Tests

Blood samples of 2 mL were collected from pre-pubertal gilts into test tubes containing EDTAK$_2$ (Ethylenediaminetetraacetic acid dipotassium salt dihydrate) (Sigma Aldrich, Darmstadt, Germany) as anticoagulant. The samples were thoroughly mixed and analysed to determine: Red Blood Cell (RBC) counts, Mean Corpuscular Volume (MCV), Mean Corpuscular Haemoglobin Concentrations (MCHC), Mean Corpuscular Haemoglobin (MCH), Haematocrit (HCT), and White Blood Cell (WBC) counts in a Medonic (Siemens, Plantation, FL, USA) haematology analyser according to the procedure recommended by the manufacturer. Measurements were performed in K2-EDTA whole blood by laser flow cytometry in the Siemens Advia 2120I (Erlangen, Germany) haematology analyser equipped with: (i) optical peroxide biosensor which measures dispersed light and light absorbed by individual cells by hydrodynamic focusing on a cell stream in a flow-through cuvette, (ii) laser optics for measuring high-angular and low-angular light dispersion and absorption by individual cells, where the laser diode was the source of light; the measurement was performed to evaluate red blood cells, platelets, and lobulation of nuclei in white blood cells, (iii) HGB (Haemoglobin) colorimeter, for measuring lamp voltage corresponding to the amount of transmitted light, and (iv) PEROX and BASO leukocytes cytograms (ADVIA 2120i -Siemens Healthcare®, Bayer, Germany) reagents, for generating differential cytograms.

Randomly selected samples were analysed in two replications. Repeatable results were obtained.

4.6. Statistical Analysis

The results were grouped based on: (i) duration of the experiment in group C and the experimental groups on a given sampling date, and (ii) sampling dates for a given parameter. The results were processed in the Statistica application (Statistica 9.0, StatSoft Kraków, Poland). Differences between groups (parameter or sampling date) were determined by ANOVA. The use of ANOVA was justified by the Brown-Forsythe test for the equality of group variances. When differences between groups were statistically significant ($p < 0.01$, highly significant differences; $0.01 < p < 0.05$, significant differences; $p > 0.05$, no differences), Tukey's HSD test was used to identify the groups that were significantly different. Linear correlations between the concentrations of ZEN in bone marrow environment in fixed groups were determined based on the values of the Pearson's correlation coefficient [75]. Data were processed in Statistica v. 13 (TIBCO Software Inc., Silicon Valley, CA, USA, 2017).

Supplementary Materials: The following supporting information can be downloaded at: https://www.mdpi.com/article/10.3390/toxins14020105/s1, Table S1: Selected haematological parameters in group C on different analytical dates ($\bar{x}$, SD).

Author Contributions: The experiments were conceived and designed by M.M., M.G. and M.T.G. The experiments were performed by M.M., K.E.P., T.S., S.L.-Ż. and M.G. Data were analysed and interpreted by M.M. and M.G. The manuscript was drafted by M.M. and M.G., and critically edited by Ł.Z. and M.T.G. All authors have read and agreed to the published version of the manuscript.

Funding: The study was supported by the "Healthy Animal—Safe Food" Scientific Consortium of the Leading National Research Centre (KNOW) pursuant to a decision of the Ministry of Science and Higher Education No. 05-1/KNOW2/2015. Project financially supported by the Minister of Education and Science under the program entitled "Regional Initiative of Excellence" for the years 2019–2022, Project No. 010/RID/2018/19, amount of funding 12.000.000 PLN.

Institutional Review Board Statement: Not applicable.

Informed Consent Statement: Not applicable.

Data Availability Statement: Not applicable.

Conflicts of Interest: The authors declare no conflict of interest.

References

1. Wielogórska, E.; Elliott, C.T.; Danaher, M.; Connolly, L. Validation and application of a reporter gene assay for the determination of estrogenic endocrine disruptor activity in milk. *Food Chem. Toxicol.* **2014**, *69*, 260–266. [CrossRef] [PubMed]
2. Zhang, Q.; Ding, N.; Zhang, L.; Zhao, X.; Yang, Y.; Qu, H.; Fang, X. Biological Databases for Hematology Research. *Genomics* **2016**, *14*, 333–337. [CrossRef] [PubMed]
3. Flores-Flores, M.E.; Lizarraga, E.; de Cerain, A.L.; González-Peñas, E. Presence of mycotoxins in animal milk: A review. *Food Control* **2015**, *53*, 163–176. [CrossRef]
4. Broekaert, N.; Devreese, M.; De Baere, S.; De Backer, P.; Croubels, S. Modified *Fusarium* mycotoxins unmasked: From occurrence in cereals to animal and human excretion. *Food Chem. Toxicol.* **2015**, *80*, 17–31. [CrossRef]
5. Kowalska, K.; Habrowska-Górczyńska, D.E.; Piastowska-Ciesielska, A. Zearalenone as an endocrine disruptor in humans. *Environ. Toxicol. Pharmacol.* **2016**, *48*, 141–149. [CrossRef]
6. Dunbar, B.; Patel, M.; Fahey, J.; Wira, C. Endocrine control of mucosal immunity in the female reproductive tract: Impact of environmental disruptors. *Mol. Cell. Endocrinol.* **2012**, *354*, 85–93. [CrossRef]
7. Rykaczewska, A.; Gajęcka, M.; Dąbrowski, M.; Wiśniewska, A.; Szcześniewska, J.; Gajęcki, M.T.; Zielonka, Ł. Growth performance, selected blood biochemical parameters and body weights of pre-pubertal gilts fed diets supplemented with different doses of zearalenone (ZEN). *Toxicon* **2018**, *152*, 84–94. [CrossRef]
8. Zachariasova, M.; Dzumana, Z.; Veprikova, Z.; Hajkovaa, K.; Jiru, M.; Vaclavikova, M.; Zachariasova, A.; Pospichalova, M.; Florian, M.; Hajslova, J. Occurrence of multiple mycotoxins in European feeding stuffs, assessment of dietary intake by farm animals. *Anim. Feed Sci. Technol.* **2014**, *193*, 124–140. [CrossRef]
9. Frizzell, C.; Ndossi, D.; Verhaegen, S.; Dahl, E.; Eriksen, G.; Sørlie, M.; Ropstad, E.; Muller, M.; Elliott, C.T.; Connolly, L. Endocrine disrupting effects of zearalenone, alpha- and beta-zearalenol at the level of nuclear receptor binding and steroidogenesis. *Toxicol. Lett.* **2011**, *206*, 210–217. [CrossRef]

10. Gajęcka, M.; Tarasiuk, M.; Zielonka, Ł.; Dąbrowski, M.; Gajęcki, M. Risk assessment for changes in metabolic profile and body weight of pre-pubertal gilts during long-term monotonic exposure to low doses of zearalenone (ZEN). *Res. Vet. Sci.* **2016**, *109*, 169–180. [CrossRef]
11. Zielonka, Ł.; Waśkiewicz, A.; Beszterda, M.; Kostecki, M.; Dąbrowski, M.; Obremski, K.; Goliński, P.; Gajęcki, M. Zearalenone in the Intestinal Tissues of Immature Gilts Exposed *per os* to Mycotoxins. *Toxins* **2015**, *7*, 3210–3223. [CrossRef] [PubMed]
12. Knutsen, H.K.; Alexander, J.; Barregård, L.; Bignami, M.; Brüschweiler, B.; Ceccatelli, S.; Cottrill, B.; Dinovi, M.; Edler, L.; Grasl-Kraupp, B.; et al. Risks for animal health related to the presence of zearalenone and its modified forms in feed. *EFSA J.* **2017**, *15*, 4851. [CrossRef]
13. Gajęcka, M.; Zielonka, Ł.; Gajęcki, M. Activity of zearalenone in the porcine intestinal tract. *Molecules* **2017**, *22*, 18. [CrossRef] [PubMed]
14. Calabrese, E.J. Paradigm lost, paradigm found: The re-emergence of hormesis as a fundamental dose response model in the toxicological sciences. *Environ. Pollut.* **2005**, *138*, 378–411. [CrossRef] [PubMed]
15. Freire, L.; Sant'Ana, A.S. Modified mycotoxins: An updated review on their formation, detection, occurrence, and toxic effects. *Food Chem. Toxicol.* **2018**, *111*, 189–205. [CrossRef] [PubMed]
16. Cieplińska, K.; Gajęcka, M.; Nowak, A.; Dąbrowski, M.; Zielonka, Ł.; Gajęcki, M.T. The gentoxicity of caecal water in gilts exposed to low doses of zearalenone. *Toxins* **2018**, *10*, 350. [CrossRef] [PubMed]
17. Vandenberg, L.N.; Colborn, T.; Hayes, T.B.; Heindel, J.J.; Jacobs, D.R.; Lee, D.-H.; Shioda, T.; Soto, A.M.; vom Saal, F.S.; Welshons, W.V.; et al. Hormones and endocrine-disrupting chemicals: Low-dose effects and nonmonotonic dose responses. *Endoc. Rev.* **2012**, *33*, 378–455. [CrossRef] [PubMed]
18. Grenier, B.; Applegate, T.J. Modulation of intestinal functions following mycotoxin ingestion: Meta-analysis of published experiments in animals. *Toxins* **2013**, *5*, 396–430. [CrossRef] [PubMed]
19. Gajęcka, M.; Majewski, M.S.; Zielonka, Ł.; Grzegorzewski, W.; Onyszek, E.; Lisieska-Żołnierczyk, S.; Juśkiewicz, J.; Babuchowski, A.; Gajęcki, M.T. Concentration of Zearalenone, Alpha-Zearalenol and Beta-Zearalenol in the Myocardium and the Results of Isometric Analyses of the Coronary Artery in Prepubertal Gilts. *Toxins* **2021**, *13*, 396. [CrossRef]
20. EFSA. Scientific Opinion on the risks for public health related to the presence of zearalenone in food. *EFSA J.* **2011**, *9*, 2197. [CrossRef]
21. Pastoor, T.P.; Bachman, A.N.; Bell, D.R.; Cohen, S.M.; Dellarco, M.; Dewhurst, I.C.; Doe, J.E.; Doerrer, N.G.; Embry, M.R.; Hines, R.N.; et al. A 21st century roadmap for human health risk assessment. *Crit. Rev. Toxicol.* **2014**, *44*, 1–5. [CrossRef] [PubMed]
22. Kumar, R.S.; Goyal, N. Estrogens as regulator of hematopoietic stem cell, immune cells and bone biology. *Life Sci.* **2021**, *269*, 119091. [CrossRef] [PubMed]
23. Hamza, E.; Metzinger, L.; Metzinger-Le Meuth, V. Uremic Toxins Affect Erythropoiesis during the Course of Chronic Kidney Disease: A Review. *Cells* **2020**, *9*, 2039. [CrossRef]
24. Molica, F.; Stierlin, F.; Fontana, P.; Kwak, B.R. Pannexin- and Connexin-Mediated Intercellular Communication in Platelet Function. *Int. J. Mol. Sci.* **2017**, *18*, 850. [CrossRef] [PubMed]
25. Johnson, C.B.; Zhang, J.; Lucas, D. The Role of the Bone Marrow Microenvironment in the Response to Infection. *Front. Immunol.* **2020**, *11*, 585402. [CrossRef]
26. Tjon, J.M.-L.; Langemeijer, S.M.C.; Halkes, C.J.M. Anti Thymocyte Globulin-Based Treatment for Acquired Bone Marrow Failure in Adults. *Cells* **2021**, *10*, 2905. [CrossRef] [PubMed]
27. Yu, V.W.C.; Scadden, D.T. Heterogeneity of the bone marrow niche. *Curr. Opin. Hematol.* **2016**, *23*, 331–338. [CrossRef]
28. Rykaczewska, A.; Gajęcka, M.; Onyszek, E.; Cieplińska, K.; Dąbrowski, M.; Lisieska-Żołnierczyk, S.; Bulińska, M.; Babuchowski, A.; Gajęcki, M.T.; Zielonka, Ł. Imbalance in the Blood Concentrations of Selected Steroids in Prepubertal Gilts Depending on the Time of Exposure to Low Doses of Zearalenone. *Toxins* **2019**, *11*, 561. [CrossRef]
29. Cieplińska, K.; Gajęcka, M.; Dąbrowski, M.; Rykaczewska, A.; Zielonka, Ł.; Lisieska-Żołnierczyk, S.; Bulińska, M.; Gajęcki, M.T. Time-dependent changes in the intestinal microbiome of gilts exposed to low zearalenone doses. *Toxins* **2019**, *11*, 296. [CrossRef]
30. Gajęcka, M.; Tarasiuk, M.; Zielonka, Ł.; Dąbrowski, M.; Nicpoń, J.; Baranowski, M.; Gajęcki, M.T. Changes in the metabolic profile and body weight of pre-pubertal gilts during prolonged monotonic exposure to low doses of zearalenone and deoxynivalenol. *Toxicon* **2017**, *125*, 32–43. [CrossRef]
31. Etim, N.N.; Williams, M.E.; Akpabio, U.; Offiong, E.E. Haematological parameters and factors affecting their values. *Agric. Sci.* **2014**, *2*, 37–47. [CrossRef]
32. Goyarts, T.; Dänicke, S.; Brüssow, K.P.; Valenta, H.; Ueberschär, K.H.; Tiemann, U. On the transfer of the Fusarium toxins deoxynivalenol (DON) and zearalenone (ZON) from sows to their fetuses during days 35–70 of gestation. *Toxicol. Lett.* **2007**, *171*, 38–49. [CrossRef] [PubMed]
33. Winnicka, A. *Reference Values of Basic Laboratory Tests in Veterinary Medicine*; SGGW Publishers: Warszawa, Poland, 2008; ISBN 978-83-7244-974-0.
34. Li, Q.; Patience, J.F. Factors involved in the regulation of feed and energy intake of pigs. *Anim. Feed Sci. Technol.* **2016**, *233*, 22–33. [CrossRef]
35. Bryden, W.L. Mycotoxin contamination of the feed supply chain: Implications for animal productivity and feed security. *Anim. Food Sci Technol.* **2012**, *173*, 134–158. [CrossRef]

36. Lin, K.S.; Uemura, S.; Thwin, K.K.M.; Nakatani, N.; Ishida, T.; Yamamoto, N.; Tamura, A.; Saito, A.; Mori, T.; Hasegawa, D.; et al. Minimal residual disease in high-risk neuroblastoma shows a dynamic and disease burden-dependent correlation between bone marrow and peripheral blood. *Transl. Oncol.* **2021**, *14*, 101019. [CrossRef]
37. Benagiano, M.; Bianchi, P.; D'Elios, M.M.; Brosens, I.; Benagiano, G. Autoimmune diseases: Role of steroid hormones. *Best Pr. Res. Clin. Obstet. Gynaecol.* **2019**, *60*, 24–34. [CrossRef]
38. Wilkenfeld, S.R.; Linc, C.; Frigo, D.E. Communication between genomic and non-genomic signaling events coordinate steroid hormone actions. *Steroids* **2018**, *133*, 2–7. [CrossRef]
39. Gajęcka, M.; Otrocka-Domagała, I. Immunocytochemical expression of 3β- and 17β-hydroxysteroid dehydrogenase in bitch ovaries exposed to low doses of zearalenone. *Pol. J. Vet. Sci.* **2013**, *16*, 55–62. [CrossRef]
40. Lawrenz, B.; Melado, L.; Fatemi, H. Premature progesterone rise in ART-cycles. *Reprod. Biol.* **2018**, *18*, 1–4. [CrossRef]
41. Nakada, D.; Oguro, H.; Levi, B.P.; Ryan, N.; Kitano, A.; Saitoh, Y.; Takeichi, M.; Wendt, G.R.; Morrison, S.J. Estrogen increases haematopoietic stem cell self-renewal in females and during pregnancy. *Nature* **2014**, *505*, 555–558. [CrossRef]
42. Balla, B.; Sárvári, M.; Kósa, J.P.; Kocsis-Deák, B.; Tobiás, B.; Árvai, K.; Takács, I.; Podani, J.; Liposits, Z.; Lakatos, P. Long-term selective estrogen receptor-beta agonist treatment modulates gene expression in bone and bone marrow of ovariectomized rats. *J. Steroid Biochem.* **2019**, *188*, 185–194. [CrossRef]
43. Pinkas, J.; Gujski, M.; Wierzbińska-Stępniak, A.; Owoc, A.; Bojar, I. The polymorphism of oestrogen receptor alpha is important for metabolic consequences associated with menopause. *Endokrynol. Polska* **2016**, *67*, 608–619. [CrossRef] [PubMed]
44. Satirapod, C.; Wang, N.; MacDonald, J.A.; Sun, M.; Woods, D.C.; Tilly, J.L. Estrogen regulation of germline stem cell differentiation as a mechanism contributing to female reproductive aging. *Aging* **2020**, *12*, 7313–7333. [CrossRef] [PubMed]
45. Zheng, W.; Feng, N.; Wang, Y.; Noll, L.; Xu, S.; Liu, X.; Lu, N.; Zou, H.; Gu, J.; Yuan, Y.; et al. Effects of zearalenone and its derivatives on the synthesis and secretion of mammalian sex steroid hormones: A review. *Food Chem. Toxicol.* **2019**, *126*, 262–276. [CrossRef] [PubMed]
46. Yang, D.; Jiang, T.; Lin, P.; Chen, H.; Wang, L.; Wang, N.; Zhao, F.; Tang, K.; Zhou, D.; Wang, A.; et al. Apoptosis inducing factor gene depletion inhibits zearalenone-induced cell death in a goat Leydig cell line. *Reprod. Toxicol.* **2017**, *67*, 129–139. [CrossRef]
47. Hennig-Pauka, I.; Koch, F.J.; Schaumberger, S.; Woechtl, B.; Novak, J.; Sulyok, M.; Nagl, V. Current challenges in the diagnosis of zearalenone toxicosis as illustrated by a field case of hyperestrogenism in suckling piglets. *Porc. Health Manag.* **2018**, *4*, 18. [CrossRef]
48. Fañanas-Baquero, S.; Orman, I.; Aparicio, F.B.; de Miguel, S.B.; Merino, J.G.; Yañez, R.; Sainz, Y.F.; Sánchez, R.; Dessy-Rodríguez, M.; Alberquilla, O.; et al. Natural estrogens enhance the engraftment of human hematopoietic stem and progenitor cells in immunodeficient mice. *Haematologica* **2021**, *106*, 1659–1670. [CrossRef]
49. Luisetto, M.; Almukhtar, N.; Ahmadabadi, B.N.; Hamid, G.A.; Mashori, G.R.; Khan, K.R.; Khan, F.A.; Cabianca, L. Endogenus Toxicology: Modern Physio- Pathological Aspects and Relationship with New Therapeutic Strategies. An Integrative Discipline Incorporating Concepts from Different Research Discipline Like Biochemistry, Pharmacology and Toxicology. *Arch Cancer Sci Ther.* **2019**, *3*, 001–004. [CrossRef]
50. Elegido, A.; Graell, M.; Andrés, P.; Gheorghe, A.; Marcos, A.; Nova, E. Increased naive CD4+ and B lymphocyte subsets are associated with body mass loss and drive relative lymphocytosis in anorexia nervosa patients. *Nutr. Res.* **2017**, *39*, 43–50. [CrossRef]
51. Ren, Z.; Deng, H.; Deng, Y.; Liang, Z.; Deng, J.; Zuo, Z.; Hu, Y.; Shen, L.; Yu, S.; Cao, S. Combined effects of deoxynivalenol and zearalenone on oxidative injury and apoptosis in porcine splenic lymphocytes in vitro. *Exp. Toxicol. Pathol.* **2017**, *69*, 612–617. [CrossRef]
52. Etim, N.A.N.; Offiong, E.E.A.; Williams, M.E.; Asuquo, L.E. Influence of nutrition on blood parameters of pigs. *Am. J. Biol. Life Sci.* **2014**, *2*, 46–52. Available online: http://www.opensciencenline.com/journal/ajbls (accessed on 10 January 2022).
53. Sutherland, M.A.; Bryer, P.J.; Krebs, N.; McGlone, J.J. Tail docking in pigs: Acute physiological and behavioural responses. *Animal* **2008**, *2*, 292–297. [CrossRef]
54. Gajęcki, M.; Gajęcka, M.; Zielonka, Ł.; Jakimiuk, E.; Obremski, K. Zearalenone as a potential allergen in the alimentary tract—A review. *Pol. J. Food Nutr. Sci.* **2006**, *56*, 263–268.
55. Gajęcka, M.; Przybylska-Gornowicz, B. The low doses effect of experimental zearalenone (ZEN) intoxication on the presence of Ca^{2+} in selected ovarian cells from pre-pubertal bitches. *Pol. J. Vet. Sci.* **2012**, *15*, 711–720. [CrossRef] [PubMed]
56. Przybylska-Gornowicz, B.; Tarasiuk, M.; Lewczuk, B.; Prusik, M.; Ziółkowska, N.; Zielonka, Ł.; Gajęcki, M.; Gajęcka, M. The Effects of Low Doses of Two Fusarium Toxins, Zearalenone and Deoxynivalenol, on the Pig Jejunum. A Light and Electron Microscopic Study. *Toxins* **2015**, *7*, 4684–4705. [CrossRef]
57. Bao, X.; Wan, M.; Gu, Y.; Song, Y.; Zhang, Q.; Liu, L.; Meng, H.; Xia, Y.; Shi, H.B.; Su, Q.; et al. Red cell distribution width is associated with hemoglobin A1C elevation, but not glucose elevation. *J. Diabetes Complicat.* **2017**, *31*, 1544–1548. [CrossRef]
58. Paiva-Martins, F.; Barbosa, S.; Silva, M.; Monteiro, D.; Pinheiro, V.; Mourão, J.L.; Fernandes, J.; Rocha, S.; Belo, L.; Santos-Silva, A. The effect of olive leaf supplementation on the constituents of blood and oxidative stability of red blood cells. *J. Funct. Foods* **2014**, *9*, 271–279. [CrossRef]
59. Tatay, E.; Espín, S.; García-Fernández, A.J.; Ruiz, M.J. Oxidative damage and disturbance of antioxidant capacity by zearalenone and its metabolites in human cells. *Toxicol. Vitro* **2017**, *45*, 334–339. [CrossRef]

60. Jilani, K.; Lang, F. Ca(2+)-dependent suicidal erythrocyte death following zearalenone exposure. *Arch. Toxicol.* **2013**, *87*, 1821–1828. [CrossRef]
61. Pyrshev, K.A.; Klymchenko, A.S.; Csúcs, G.; Demchenko, A.P. Apoptosis and eryptosis: Striking differences on biomembrane level. *BBA-Biomembrane* **2018**, *1860*, 1362–1371. [CrossRef]
62. Qadri, S.M.; Bissinger, R.; Solh, Z.; Oldenborg, P.A. Eryptosis in health and disease: A paradigm shift towards understanding the (patho)physiological implications of programmed cell death of erythrocytes. *Blood Rev.* **2017**, *31*, 349–361. [CrossRef] [PubMed]
63. Lang, E.; Lang, F. Mechanisms and pathophysiological significance of eryptosis, the suicidal erythrocyte death. *Semin. Cell Dev. Biol.* **2015**, *39*, 35–42. [CrossRef] [PubMed]
64. Chan, W.Y.; Lau, P.M.; Yeung, K.W.; Kong, S.K. The second generation tyrosine kinase inhibitor dasatinib induced eryptosis in human erythrocytes-An in vitro study. *Toxicol. Lett.* **2018**, *295*, 10–21. [CrossRef] [PubMed]
65. Gajęcka, M.; Rybarczyk, L.; Jakimiuk, E.; Zielonka, Ł.; Obremski, K.; Zwierzchowski, W.; Gajęcki, M. The effect of experimental long-term exposure to low-dose zearalenone on uterine histology in sexually immature gilts. *Exp. Toxicol. Pathol.* **2012**, *64*, 537–542. [CrossRef] [PubMed]
66. Gajęcka, M.; Zielonka, Ł.; Dąbrowski, M.; Mróz, M.; Gajęcki, M. The effect of low doses of zearalenone and its metabolites on progesterone and 17β-estradiol concentrations in peripheral blood and body weights of pre-pubertal female Beagle dogs. *Toxicon* **2013**, *76*, 260–269. [CrossRef]
67. Yorbik, O.; Mutlu, C.; Tanju, I.A.; Celik, D.; Ozcan, O. Mean platelet volume in children with attention deficit hyperactivity disorder. *Med. Hypotheses* **2014**, *82*, 341–345. [CrossRef]
68. Dai, Q.; Zhang, G.; Lai, C.; Du, Z.; Chen, L.; Chen, Q.; Peng, L.; Wang, Y.; Yang, H.; Ye, L.; et al. Two cases of false platelet clumps flagged by the automated haematology analyser Sysmex XE-2100. *Clin. Chim. Acta.* **2014**, *429*, 152–156. [CrossRef]
69. Meyer, J.; Lejmi, E.; Fontana, P.; Morel, P.; Gonelle-Gispert, C.; Bühler, L. A focus on the role of platelets in liver regeneration: Do platelet-endothelial cell interactions initiate the regenerative process? *J. Hepatol.* **2015**, *63*, 1263–1271. [CrossRef]
70. Wysokiński, A.; Szczepocka, E. Platelet parameters (PLT, MPV, P-LCR) in patients with schizophrenia, unipolar depression and bipolar disorder. *Psychiatry Res.* **2016**, *237*, 238–245. [CrossRef]
71. Heberer, T.; Lahrssen-Wiederholt, M.; Schafft, H.; Abraham, K.; Pzyrembel, H.; Henning, K.J.; Schauzu, M.; Braeunig, J.; Goetz, M.; Niemann, L.; et al. Zero tolerances in food and animal feed-Are there any scientific alternatives? A European point of view on an international controversy. *Toxicol. Lett.* **2007**, *175*, 118–135. [CrossRef]
72. Smith, D.; Combes, R.; Depelchin, O.; Jacobsen, S.D.; Hack, R.; Luft, J.; Lammens, L.; von Landenberg, F.; Phillips, B.; Pfister, R.; et al. Optimising the design of preliminary toxicity studies for pharmaceutical safety testing in the dog. *Regul. Toxicol. Pharm.* **2005**, *41*, 95–101. [CrossRef]
73. Meerpoel, C.; Vidal, A.; Tangni, E.K.; Huybrechts, B.; Couck, L.; De Rycke, R.; De Bels, L.; De Saeger, S.; Van den Broeck, W.; Devreese, M.; et al. A Study of Carry-Over and Histopathological Effects after Chronic Dietary Intake of Citrinin in Pigs, Broiler Chickens and Laying Hens. *Toxins* **2020**, *12*, 719. [CrossRef]
74. Kowalski, A.; Kaleczyc, J.; Gajęcki, M.; Zieliński, H. Adrenaline, noradrenaline and cortisol levels in pigs during blood collection (In Polish). *Med. Weter.* **1996**, *52*, 716–718.
75. Williams, M.S.; Ebel, E.D. Estimating correlation of prevalence at two locations in the farm-to-table continuum using qualitative test data. *Int. J. Food Microbiol.* **2017**, *245*, 29–37. [CrossRef]

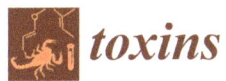

Review

Biosensors for Deoxynivalenol and Zearalenone Determination in Feed Quality Control

Krisztina Majer-Baranyi [1,*], Nóra Adányi [1] and András Székács [2]

[1] Food Science Research Group, Institute of Food Science and Technology, Hungarian University of Agriculture and Life Sciences, Herman Ottó út 15, H-1022 Budapest, Hungary; adanyine.kisbocskoi.nora@uni-mate.hu

[2] Agro-Environmental Research Centre, Institute of Environmental Sciences, Hungarian University of Agriculture and Life Sciences, Herman Ottó út 15, H-1022 Budapest, Hungary; szekacs.andras@uni-mate.hu

* Correspondence: majerne.baranyi.krisztina@uni-mate.hu

Abstract: Mycotoxin contamination of cereals used for feed can cause intoxication, especially in farm animals; therefore, efficient analytical tools for the qualitative and quantitative analysis of toxic fungal metabolites in feed are required. Current trends in food/feed analysis are focusing on the application of biosensor technologies that offer fast and highly selective and sensitive detection with minimal sample treatment and reagents required. The article presents an overview of the recent progress of the development of biosensors for deoxynivalenol and zearalenone determination in cereals and feed. Novel biosensitive materials and highly sensitive detection methods applied for the sensors and the application of these sensors to food/feed products, the limit, and the time of detection are discussed.

Keywords: biosensors; zearalenone; deoxynivalenol; immunosensors; feed; antibody; aptamer; molecularly imprinted polymer

Key Contribution: This paper exhaustively reviews the recent trends in biosensing of two *Fusarium* mycotoxins of prime toxicological importance, deoxynivalenol and zearalenone, in the last decade (2011–2021). Techniques are classified according to the biological recognition element (antibodies, aptamers, and molecularly imprinted polymers) and according to the detection method (optical and electrochemical biosensors) used in them. Analytical performance parameters are comparatively discussed, highlighting the great practical utility of biosensing these mycotoxins.

1. Introduction

Mycotoxin contamination is one of the most important problems in food and feed safety. According to previous studies, 25–50% of crops harvested worldwide are contaminated with different types of mycotoxins [1]. *Fusarium* species are the most widespread pathogens in cereals, and *Fusarium* toxins are the most reported mycotoxins in raw agricultural commodities [2]. Therefore, mycotoxins produced by *Fusarium* moulds significantly affect feed quality and safety and also represent a prominent issue in feed quality control after the most hazardous contaminants aflatoxins of *Aspergillus* origin. Accordingly, as most alerts in official food and feed monitoring mostly refer to aflatoxin contamination [3], most monitoring activities and analytical method development efforts are geared towards aflatoxins. Nonetheless, growing attention is paid to *Fusarium* mycotoxins as well, partly due to their spread caused by climate change and partly due to their well-known toxicological significance. Among *Fusarium* mycotoxins, deoxynivalenol (DON) and zearalenone (ZON), as well as their metabolites 3- and 15-acetyl-DON, α-, and β-zearalenol, are of special importance as they are formed under field conditions prior to harvest, being highly stable during storage and difficult to degrade by thermal processing [4–6]. Especially wheat, barley, oats, rye, corn, and triticale are vulnerable to *Fusarium* infection, and compared to other cereals, they are also frequently contaminated mostly with DON and ZON [7].

Low-level contamination of *Fusarium* toxins is very frequent. DON and ZON are typically found in more than 50% and about 80%, respectively, of food samples tested in studies conducted between 2010 and 2015 in the EU [8]. DON, also known as vomitoxin, is of primary concern due to its genotoxicity, but it can also cause slow growth, lowered milk production in cattle, feed refusal, reduced egg production in laying hens, intestinal haemorrhage, and suppression of immune responses. ZON is problematic due to its hormonal effects causing changes in the reproductive system and reduced fertility. The use of toxin-contaminated feeds in livestock farming can cause a variety of adverse health effects in farm animals and a corresponding high degree of economic loss. Furthermore, contaminated feed can pose a health risk to humans indirectly, while mycotoxin carry-over is possible to milk, meat, and eggs; therefore, systematic control of mycotoxin content in feeds is of great importance. Although ZON, DON, and their metabolites are not of major concern due to their occurrence in milk, their presence has been reported in several studies. In an Italian study, 185 cow's milk-based infant formula products were investigated for ZON and its metabolites. ZON, α-, and β-zearalenol were detected in 9%, 26%, and 28.6% of the samples, respectively, with a maximum level of the latter metabolite of 73.2 ng/mL [9]. A technical survey from New Zealand reported that 0.06–0.08% of ZON residues mainly in form of α- and β-zearalenol can be secreted into milk, while DON residues occur in milk mainly in form of its diepoxy derivative exerting lower toxicity than the parent mycotoxin [10]. The EU has established maximum permitted levels and guidance levels of certain mycotoxins in feed, which should be routinely monitored. The guidance levels for ZON is 100–500 µg/kg in complementary and complete feeding-stuffs and 2–3 mg/kg for feed material, and for DON, it is 900 µg/kg in complementary and complete feeding-stuffs, 8 mg/kg in cereals and cereal products, and 12 mg/kg in maize by-products [11]. Commonly used techniques, such as high-performance liquid chromatography (HPLC) hyphenated with different detectors [12–14], liquid chromatography coupled with mass spectrometry (LC-MS) [15], liquid chromatography-tandem mass spectrometry (LC-MS/MS) [16–18], and gas chromatography-tandem mass spectrometry (GC-MS/MS) [19,20], for mycotoxin determination in food and feed have been powerful tools, as they provide proper sensitivity and accuracy in quantitative determination, but they are time-consuming, laborious, expensive, and require advanced instrumentation and trained staff [21]. In contrast, technically simple thin-layer chromatography (TLC) is also an excellent tool for rapid routine testing [22,23]; however, its sensitivity is unsatisfactory because of the even stricter EU limits. It is therefore essential to develop analytical methods that can detect the target analytes with sufficient sensitivity and accuracy and at the same time are inexpensive, fast, rely on simple measurement techniques, and allow on-site applications. The development and use of biosensors in food and feed analysis may efficiently address this challenge. This paper aims to provide an overview of recent advances and current trends in biosensor development for ZON and DON determination.

2. The Use of Sensorics for Determination of DON and ZON

Biosensors can be defined as a device incorporating an active biological sensing element (an enzyme, a tissue, living cells, antibodies, molecularly imprinted polymers (MIP), aptamers, DNA/RNA) connected to a transducer that converts the observed physical or chemical changes into a measurable signal. Biosensors can be classified according to the applied recognition elements (enzyme sensors, immunosensors, aptasensors, etc.) and also according to the signal transduction method: optical, electrochemical, piezoelectric, and thermometric; however, the latter application is not common in food and feed analysis. For mycotoxin determination, immunosensors are the most commonly applied analytical tools among biosensors, but beside that, MIP-based sensors and aptasensors (as artificial recognition element-based sensors) are also emerging techniques. Immunosensors employ antibodies, antibody fragments, antigens, or antigen conjugates as biomolecular recognition elements, and the specific antigen-antibody binding event is detected and converted to a measurable signal by the transducer. The basic working principle of the immunosensor set-up is that the specific binding of the antibody or antigen immobilised on the transducer to the antigen or antibody in the sample produces an analytical signal that varies dynamically with the concentration of the analyte of interest. The formation of the immunocomplex can be determined either by label-free methods by directly measuring the physical changes induced by the binding event or by label-based modes using detection specific labels. For mycotoxin determination, both labelled and label-free immunosensors incorporated with various types of transducers are extensively researched and developed.

2.1. Optical Immunosensors

Nowadays, beside electrochemical immunosensors, the use of optical transducers has taken the lead in immunosensor development for mycotoxin determination because optical detection allows the construction of sensitive, simple, inexpensive, and portable analytical devices for on-site monitoring and also enables direct, real-time detection of various analytes. Optical biosensing can be divided into two general modes: label-free and label-based mode. Label-free biosensors do not require the use of any label to monitor the biorecognition event, while label-based protocols use specific labels like fluorescent dyes, enzymes, or nanoparticles, and the optical signal is generated by colorimetric, fluorescent, or luminescent methods [24,25]. Although these label-based methods are very sensitive and widely used, the performance of the sensor depends on the efficiency of the labelling step. Thus, the use of label-free biosensors may be preferable to the use of label-based ones, as they offer simple, rapid measuring procedures and enable real-time monitoring of the binding reaction. Of course, label-free optical biosensors also have disadvantages, especially in the determination of small molecules such as mycotoxins, as the sensor response often depends on the size of the analyte, and these analytes are mostly not chromogenic or fluorescent [26].

2.1.1. Label-Free Optical Immunosensors

Surface plasmon resonance (SPR) technique has gained great attention in biosensor development lately. The technique was introduced in the early 1990s and since then become a powerful analytical tool in the risk assessment of contaminants in food and feed [27]. The SPR phenomenon occurs at the gold surface of the sensor chip when an incident polarised laser light beam strikes the surface at a particular angle through a prism (Figure 1A). It generates electron charge density waves called plasmons, which cause intensity reduction of the reflected light at this angle [28]. In the SPR immunosensor, immunogens (antibody or antigen) are immobilised on the gold layer of the chip mounted on a glass support. The binding of the analyte to the sensor surface causes a local change in refractive index, and corresponding shifts of the coupling angle are monitored in real time. SPR-based biosensors have received considerable attention in the past decades as they allow fast, reliable, and label-free detection of analytes [29]. In addition, they are suitable for real-time monitoring of the interaction kinetics; moreover, the biosensor chips are reusable. Another advantage of the SPR technique is that several measurements can be performed in parallel on a single sensor using multi-channel measurement. As several mycotoxins may be present simultaneously in feed or food samples, multiplex analysis is particularly relevant. Despite the fact that the SPR technique in biosensor research is being studied very extensively [30–33], only a few sensor development efforts suitable for ZON or DON determination have been investigated in recent years.

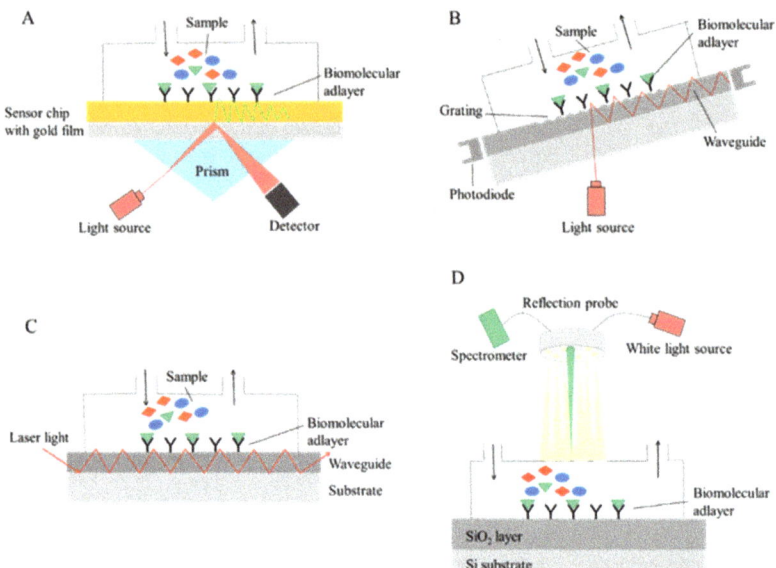

Figure 1. Operating principles of label-free optical immunosensors. (**A**) Surface plasmon resonance (SPR); (**B**) optical waveguide lightmode spectroscopy (OWLS); (**C**) planar waveguide; (**D**) white light reflectance spectroscopy.

Recently, Wei et al. [34] reported an SPR-based biosensor for the simultaneous determination of aflatoxin B1 (AFB1), ochratoxin A (OTA), ZON, and DON in corn and wheat. The limit of detection (LOD) for AFB1, OTA, ZON, and DON were identified as 0.59 ng/mL, 1.27 ng/mL, 7.07 ng/mL, and 3.26 ng/mL, respectively. Average recoveries were between 85% and 115%. Joshi et al. [35] developed two types of SPR-based biosensors for the detection of mycotoxins in barley. First, a double 3-plex assay was developed for the detection of DON, ZON, and T-2 toxin on the first chip and for OTA, fumonisin B1 (FB1), and AFB1 on the second chip using SPR. After determining the optimal conditions, the assay was transferred to a 6-plex format (six different mycotoxins determined on a single chip) in a portable nanostructured imaging surface plasmon resonance (iSPR) instrument, and the two assays were compared. The advances of iSPR technique over conventional SPR are the visualisation of the entire sensor surface in real time to monitor hundreds of molecular interactions simultaneously, and also multiplex detection is available. Results showed that DON, T-2, ZON, and FB1 could be detected at sufficient levels in barley samples according to the EC guidelines, but for OTA and AFB1, sensitivities should be improved when SPR was used for determination. The portable 6-plex iSPR was less sensitive but still allowed detection of DON, T-2, ZON, and FB1 at relevant levels. The sensitivities (IC_{50} values) obtained by iSPR biosensor in an assay buffer for T-2, FB1, and ZON were 10 ng/mL, 8 ng/mL, and 25 ng/mL, respectively.

A rapid and sensitive iSPR assay was developed for *Fusarium* toxins by Hossain and Maragos [36] using secondary antibody with gold nanoparticles (AuNPs) as an amplification tag to determine DON, ZON, and T-2 toxin in wheat. LODs were 15 µg/kg for DON, 24 µg/kg for ZON, and 12 µg/kg for T-2 toxin. Sensor chips could be reused for over 46 cycles without significant signal loss, and it took 17.5 min to measure a sample, including the regeneration steps. The same research group developed an iSPR-based immunosensor for T-2 and T-2 toxin 3-glucoside (T2-G), so-called "masked" mycotoxin, determination in wheat, which is a niche in the field of research [37]. In their experiment on a carboxyl functionalised sensor surface, T-2-protein conjugate was immobilised using 1-ethyl-3-(3-dimethylaminopropyl) carbodiimide with N-hydroxysuccinimide (EDC-NHS) method. A competitive immunoassay format was applied to detect the mycotoxins, and a secondary antibody labelled with AuNPs was used for signal amplification. The LOD was 48 µg/kg of T-2 and 36 µg/kg of T-2-G; the recoveries ranged between 86–90%. Hu et al. [38] could achieve LODs for AFB1, OTA, and ZON as low as 8, 30, and 15 pg/mL, respectively, with their iSPR immunosensor using AuNPs for signal amplification.

Another emerging technique in the field of optical immunosensor development is the optical waveguide lightmode spectroscopy (OWLS) technique that enables monitoring molecular interactions on the sensor surface in a label-free manner in real-time (Figure 1B). The basic principle of the OWLS method is that linearly polarised He-Ne laser light is coupled by a diffraction grating into the waveguide layer. The incoupling is a resonance phenomenon that occurs at a defined angle of incidence that depends on the refractive index of the medium covering the surface of the waveguide. In the waveguide layer, light is guided by total internal reflection to the edges, where it is detected by photodiodes. By varying the angle of incidence of the light, the mode spectrum can be obtained from which effective refractive indices are calculated for both the electric and magnetic modes. The sensor consists of a glass substrate with a lower refractive index and a thin (160–220 nm) waveguide layer with a higher refractive index mounted on the top in which a fine optical grating (2400–3600 line/mm) is formed for in- or outcoupling of the light [39].

For DON measurement, Majer-Baranyi et al. [40] presented a label-free OWLS-based immunosensor. In their research, the sensor was modified by 3-aminopropyltriethoxysilane (APTS), and a DON-ovalbumin conjugate was immobilised via glutaraldehyde (GA). With the optimised sensor, DON content of spiked wheat flour samples was investigated using a competitive assay method where DON was quantitatively detectable in the 0.005–50 mg/kg concentration range, and it took 10 min to measure a sample, offering fast and sensitive determination of DON. Székács et al. [41] developed a competitive OWLS-based immunosensor for ZON determination in maize samples. In the competitive assay method, a ZON-bovine serum albumin (BSA) conjugate was immobilised on the sensor surface using three different surface modification methods. According to their results, the epoxy-modified sensors provided lower binding efficacy and reproducibility; when using amino-silanised sensor chips for immobilisation either by GA (APTS/GA) or succinic anhydride (SA) and EDC-NHS (APTS/SA/EDC-NHS) the detection range of ZON were the same in both cases, but for further application, the APTS/SA/EDC-NHS sensor was chosen due to the better reproducibility and longer shelf-life. The LOD of ZON was 0.002 pg/mL, and the dynamic measuring range was between 0.01 and 1 pg/mL.

Recently, another waveguide-based immunosensor for ZON detection was published also using a planar waveguide (PW) for the sensor set-up [42] (Figure 1C). The working principle of the sensor is as follows: circularly polarised laser light is incoupled into the planar waveguide, which propagates through by multiple internal reflections, and the outcoming light is collected by a charge-coupled device (CCD) array photodetector. The sensing principle is based on the different behaviour of the s- and p-components of polarised light. Changes in the refractive index of the covering media cause phase shifts between p- and s-polarisations of light, which are converted to a multiperiodic signal by a polariser and detected by a CCD photodetector. For ZON determination, polyclonal ZON-specific antibodies were immobilised on the functionalised surface, and the binding of ZON was detected in a direct manner. The LOD of the method was 0.01 ng/mL, and the dynamic working range was between 0.01–1000 ng/mL.

Another emerging label-free optical sensor technique is white light reflectance spectroscopy (WLRS), where a broadband light from a light source is emitted and guided vertically to the surface by a reflection probe consisting of six fibres distributed on the periphery of the circle-shaped probe, while the reflected light from the sample is collected by the optical fibre positioned in the centre of the probe and directed to the spectrometer (Figure 1D). The sensor consists of two layers: a Si substrate and, on top of this, a thicker silicon dioxide layer where the biomolecules can be immobilised. The emitted white light is reflected from the sensor consisting of layers with different refractive indexes, resulting in an interference spectrum that is recorded by the spectrometer. Due to biomolecular interactions on the surface, the spectra shift to higher wavelengths [43]. A fast WLRS-based immunosensor for DON determination in wheat and maize samples was reported by Anastasiadis et al. [44], where DON-ovalbumin conjugate was immobilised on the aminosilanised sensor surface. A competitive immunoassay was performed where DON presented in the sample and DON immobilised on the sensor surface were competed for the anti-DON monoclonal antibody binding sites. The primary immunoreaction was followed by a signal enhancement step using an anti-mouse IgG secondary antibody. With the optimised sensor, wheat and maize samples were investigated. In the spiked grain samples, the LOD of DON was 62.5 µg/kg in both cases, while the linear response range was broadened up to 12.5 mg/kg. The measurement was completed within 17 min, including regeneration step, and a single chip could be reused 20 times.

The statistical parameters of the measurements, the cross reactivity, and the matrix analysed of optical immunosensors for DON and ZON detection are summarized in Table 1.

Table 1. Statistics of measuring parameters, cross reactivity, and the matrix analysed of optical immunosensors for DON and ZON detection.

Mycotoxin	Method	Detection Range	LOD	Matrix	Selectivity/cross Reactivity	Reference
AFB1 OTA ZON DON	SPR	0.99–21.92 ng/mL 1.98–28.22 ng/mL 10.37–103.31 ng/mL 5.31–99.37 ng/mL	0.59 ng/mL, 1.27 ng/mL, 7.07 ng/mL, 3.26 ng/mL	Spiked corn and wheat	AFB2 19.1% OTB 6.2% α-ZEL 15,3% 15-AcDON 16.2%	[34]
DON ZON T-2	iSPR	48–2827 µg/kg 54–790 µg/kg 42–1836 µg/kg	15 µg/kg 24 µg/kg 12 µg/kg	wheat	15-AcDON 150% α-ZEL 104% HT-2 n.s.	[36]
T-2 T2-G	iSPR		1.2 ng/mL 0.9 ng/mL	spiked wheat	15-AcDON < 1% HT-2Glc < 1% HT-2 < 1%	[37]
AFB1 OTA ZON	iSPR		8 pg/mL 30 pg/mL 15 pg/mL	spiked peanut	n.d.	[38]
DON	OWLS	0.01–100 ng/mL	0.005 ng/mL	spiked wheat flour	n.d.	[40]
ZON	OWLS	0.01–1 pg/mL	0.002 pg/mL	spiked maize	α-ZEL 25.2% Zeranol 12.8%	[41]
ZON	PW	0.01–1000 ng/mL	0.01 ng/mL	ZON standard	AFB1 n.s. OTA n.s.	[42]
DON	WLRS	62.5 µg/kg–12.5 mg/kg	62.5 µg/kg	spiked maize wheat	3-AcDON 929% 3DON-Glc 23%	[44]
DON	DON-Chip	0.01–20 µg/g	4.7 ng/g	food, feed	n.d.	[45]
ZON DON	NIR-based LFIA	0.012–0.33 ng/mL 0.082–6.7 ng/mL	0.55 µg/kg 3.8 µg/kg	maize	AFB1 <1% FB1 <1% OTA <1% T-2 <1%	[46]
DON OTA AFB1	Microfluidic immunoassay		10 ng/mL 40 ng/mL 0.1 ng/mL	spiked corn feed	OTA, AFB1 n.s. DON, AFB1 n.s. OTA, DON n.s.	[47]

Table 1. Cont.

Mycotoxin	Method	Detection Range	LOD	Matrix	Selectivity/cross Reactivity	Reference
FB1		0.5–10 µg/kg	10 µg/kg		α-ZEL 70.6%	
ZEN		0.25–5 µg/kg	2.5 µg/kg		Zeranol 32%	
T-2	LFIA	0.3–1 µg/kg	1.0 µg/kg	maize	HT-2 37%	[48]
DON		1–20 µg/kg	10 µg/kg		3-AcDON 347%	
AFB1		0.25–0.5 µg/kg	0.5 µg/kg		15-AcDON 34%	
					AFM1 45%	

Deoxynivalenol (DON), 15-acetyl-deoxynivalenol (15-AcDON), 3-acetyl-deoxynivalenol (3-AcDON), Deoxynivalenol 3-glucoside (3DON-Glc), Zearalenone (ZON), α-zearalenol (α-ZEL), β-zearalenol (β-ZEL) α-zearalanol (Zeranol), Ochratoxin A (OTA), Ochratoxin B (OTB), Aflatoxin B1 (AFB1), Aflatoxin B2 (AFB2), Aflatoxin M1 (AFM1), HT-2-glucoside (HT-2Glc), Fumonisin B1 (FB1), Fumonisin B2 (FB2), T-2 glucoside (T2-G), signal is not significant (n.s.), no data (n.d.), surface plasmon resonance (SPR), Imaging surface plasmon resonance (iSPR), optical waveguide lightmode spectroscopy (OWLS), planar waveguide (PW), white light reflectance spectroscopy (WLRS), near-infrared fluorescence-based lateral flow immunosensor (NIR-based LFIA).

2.1.2. Label-Based Optical Immunosensors

Jiang et al. [45] presented a paper-based microfluidic device (DON-Chip) for DON determination. In the competitive immunoassay, AuNPs were used for labelling. For signal reading, a low-powered digital microscope connecting to a computer's USB port was used for image acquisition and signal analysis to enable on-site determination. Detection of DON in aqueous extracts of food and feed was carried out by DON-chip, and the results were compared by those obtained by commercial DON ELISA, which showed linear correlation. The LOD of DON was 4.7 ng/g, and the linear working range was between 0.01–20 µg/g. For simultaneous determination of ZON and DON, Jin et al. [46] developed a novel dual near-infrared fluorescence-based lateral flow immunosensor (NIR-based LFIA). On the nitrocellulose membrane, DON and ZON conjugated to BSA were immobilised in the same test line. The anti-ZON and anti-DON antibodies were labelled by near-infrared dyes with distinct fluorescence characteristics as detection reagents. With the optimised sensor, the ZON and DON content of maize samples were determined with a LOD of 0.55 µg/kg and 3.8 µg/kg, respectively. The assay took 20 min to perform, providing a fast and sensitive tool for simultaneous determination of two mycotoxins (Figure 2).

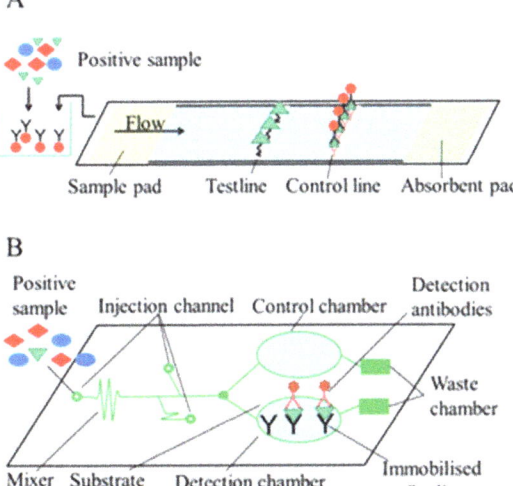

Figure 2. Operating principles of label-based optical immunosensors. (**A**) Paper-based microfluidic device; (**B**) microfluidic capillary chip.

A multiplexed microfluidic capillary chip with smartphone detection for DON, OTA, and AFB1 determination was demonstrated [47]. A competitive immunoassay format was used to detect mycotoxins simultaneously, where mycotoxin-BSA conjugates were immobilised on a polydimethylsiloxane (PDMS) surface. Toxins present in the sample compete with the toxins immobilised on the surface for the binding site of the polyclonal antibodies conjugated with horseradish peroxidase. After that, hydrogen peroxide as a substrate and tetramethylbenzidine (TMB) as a chromophore were added, and the colorimetric signal was detected by a smartphone and analysed in ImageJ software. The assay could be performed in less than 10 min with a LOD of 10 ng/mL for DON, making the assay capable of fast, on-site analysis. Another smartphone-based sensor was developed by Liu et al. [48] using a dual fluorescence or colour detection mode device integrated with two lateral flow immunoassays for multiplex mycotoxin (DON, ZON) determination in cereals. When fluorescence detection was applied, the assays were more sensitive, but recoveries from maize for both formats were the same.

2.2. Electrochemical Immunosensors

In the electrochemical biosensors, the reaction between the target molecule and the recognition element by using electrochemical dyes or enzymatic reactions generates changes in the signal for conductance or impedance, measurable current, or change accumulation, which can be quantified by voltammetric, potentiometric, amperometric, or conductometric techniques [49] (Figure 3). The use of electrochemical biosensors is very common due to their high sensitivity, selectivity, low cost, simplicity, and in some cases their miniaturisation, portability, and integration into automated devices [50–52]. In the last decade, the use of screen-printed electrodes (SPE) in electrochemical biosensor development has received great attention because they can be made of different materials and shapes and can be modified with a wide variety of nanomaterials, such as carbon nanotubes, graphene, and metallic nanoparticles as gold, silver, and magnetic nanoparticles coupled with different biological recognition elements (DNA, RNA, aptamers, enzymes, antibodies) [53–59] (Figure 3A,B).

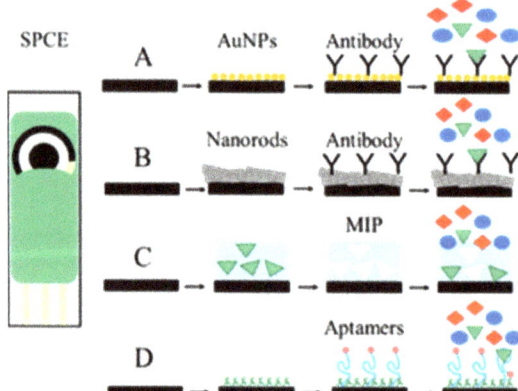

Figure 3. Structure principles of electrochemical sensors. (**A**) Gold nanoparticles (AuNPs); (**B**) nanorods, nanotubes (Au, C, etc.); (**C**) molecular imprinting polymers (MIP); (**D**) aptamers.

An electrochemical immunosensor to determine ZON in maize using modified screen-printed carbon electrodes (SPCE) was developed by Riberi et al. [60]. On the surface of the SPCE modified with multi-walled carbon nanotubes/polyethyleneimine dispersions and AuNPs, ZON polyclonal antibodies were immobilised. A competitive immunoassay was used for ZON determination where ZON presented in the sample, and a horseradish peroxidase (HRP)-labelled ZON conjugate competed for the limited amount of polyclonal antibodies immobilised on the surface. After that, hydrogen peroxide was added, and a steady-state current was obtained, which was proportional to the amount of ZON in the samples and was detected at a potential of -0.3 V by amperometry. The biosensors showed good stability during at least four days. The calibration curve was linear in the ZON concentration range from 0.1 to 100 pg/mL.

A differential pulse voltammetry (DPV) detection-based immunosensor using disposable SPE was prepared for ZON determination by Goud et al. [61]. On the activated sensor surface, a ZON-BSA conjugate was immobilised by the EDC/NHS method. A competitive assay format was used for ZON determination, and alkaline phosphatase-labelled antibody and 1-naphthyl phosphate (1-NP) as a substrate was used to detect primary antibody binding to the surface. The produced 1-naphthol was detected via DPV, which allowed the determination of the ZON concentration of the sample. The LOD was 0.25 ng/mL, and the dynamic measuring range of ZON was 0.25–256 ng/mL.

A mesoporous silica-modified SPCE-based immunosensor was presented by Regiart et al. [62]. For the immunosensor anti-ZON antibodies were immobilised by GA on the surface of the modified electrode. During measurement, ZON presented in the sample was recognised and bound to the immobilised antibodies on the surface of the electrode. Then, to detect immunocomplex formation, HRP-conjugated anti-ZON antibodies were added, and hydrogen peroxide with 4-tert-butylcatechol (4-TBC) were used in a substrate and chromophore solution. The HRP enzyme catalyzes the oxidation of 4-TBC to 4-tert-butylbenzoquinone. The enzymatic product was detected by amperometry at -100 mV. The measured current was proportional to the concentration of ZON present in the sample. The linear measuring range of ZON detection was 1.88–45 ng/mL, and the LOD was 0.57 ng/mL in *Amaranthus cruentus* seeds.

An electrochemical immunosensor fabricated on indium tin oxide (ITO)-coated glass was introduced by Lu et al. [63] for multiple mycotoxin determination. A dual-channel three-electrode sensor consisted of two working electrodes that were modified with AuNPs and functionalised with anti-FB1 and anti-DON antibodies and a Ag/AgCl pseudo-reference electrode etched on the ITO-coated glass and was integrated with a microfluidic channel. The binding of the toxin present in the sample to the antibody immobilised on the working electrode produced an electrochemical signal, which was detected by DPV. With this immunosensor set-up, a LOD of 97 pg/mL and 35 pg/mL could be achieved, and linear ranges of detection were 0.3–140 ng/mL and 0.2–60 ng/mL for FB1 and DON, respectively.

The statistical parameters of the measurements, the cross reactivity, and the matrix analysed of electrochemical immunosensors for DON and ZON detection are summarized in Table 2.

Table 2. Statistics of measuring parameters, cross reactivity, and the matrix analysed of electrochemical immunosensors for DON and ZON detection.

Mycotoxin	Method	Detection Range	LOD	Matrix	Selectivity	Reference
ZON	Amperometry	0.1 to 100 pg/mL	0.15 pg/mL	spiked maize	n.d.	[60]
ZON	DPV	0.25–256 ng/mL	0.25 ng/mL	spiked beer, wine	AFB1 AFM1 85–90% OTA OTB	[61]
ZON	Amperometry	1.88–45 ng/mL	0.57 ng/mL	*Amaranthus cruentus* seeds	n.d.	[62]
FB1 DON	DPV	0.3–140 ng/mL 0.2–60 ng/mL	97 pg/mL 35 pg/mL	spiked corn sample	n.d.	[63]

Deoxynivalenol (DON), Zearalenone (ZON), Fumonisin B1 (FB1), Aflatoxin B1 (AFB1), Aflatoxin M1 (AFM1), Ochratoxin A (OTA), Ochratoxin B (OTB), differential pulse voltammetry (DPV), no data (n.d.).

2.3. Piezoelectric Immunosensors

Quartz crystal microbalance (QCM) is a piezoelectric effect-based mass measuring system. The QCM sensor is made of a quartz crystal disk cut to a specific orientation with respect to the crystal axes and sandwiched between two metal electrodes (usually gold) that can be made to oscillate at a defined frequency by applying alternating voltage. Its resonant frequency depends on the thickness of the crystal (Figure 4). The thinner the applied crystal, the higher its resonant frequency and sensitivity. QCM monitors the mass or thickness of the adlayers on the surface of the quartz crystal. The main advantages of QCM are high sensitivity, high stability, fast response, and low cost. It also provides label-free detection capabilities for biosensor applications. However, QCM faces some disadvantages, as its performance significantly depends on the temperature and other environmental parameters, and its sensitivity falls short of the requirements when measuring low molecular weight substances [64]. In order to fulfill the requirements of high sensitivity regarding mycotoxin detection (as they are low molecular weight compounds, so they cannot generate sufficient frequency changes) piezoelectric biosensors need to apply competitive inhibition immunoassay formats, or the signal has to be amplified by applying secondary antibodies or nanoparticles.

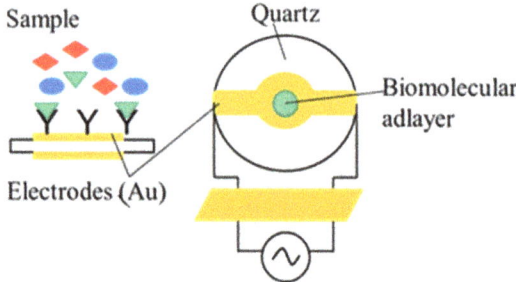

Figure 4. Structure principle of piezoelectric immunosensors.

Although there are several examples of piezoelectric immunosensors for mycotoxin determination in the recent scientific literature [1,65–69], there have been very few developments for the piezoelectric determination of ZON and DON. Very recently a portable, label-free QCM immunosensor was introduced by Liu et al. [70] for ZON determination in different food matrices. In the sensor, ZON-ovalbumin conjugate was immobilised with EDC/NHS on the surface of the mercaptodecylic acid-modified chip. The frequency response caused by the specific binding of anti-ZON antibody (100 μg/mL) on the chip surface was detected in the presence or absence of ZON. A high sensitivity of ZON determination with a LOD as low as 0.37 ng/mL was obtained, with excellent selectivity and stability. The effectiveness of the sensor was verified in spiked corn, wheat flour, soy sauce, and milk samples, and satisfactory recoveries were attained. The sensor could be reused six times without any significant attenuation of frequency of the sensor chip (below 10%) and could be stored for fifteen days without significant signal loss. The sensor allowed quick ZON determination since it took five minutes to measure a sample.

Nolan et al. [71] developed a mass-sensitive microarray biosensor working under the same principle as QCM for multiplex mycotoxin determination. The sensor consisted of 4×16 mass-sensitive transducer pixels. Each pixel consisted of a zinc oxide piezoelectric layer sandwiched between two electrodes where the top electrode was coated with silicon dioxide with a thin gold layer on the top where mycotoxin conjugates were immobilized, and the entire set-up was mounted on the top of an acoustic mirror. With the optimised sensor, simultaneous determination of T2-toxin, ZON, and FB1 were examined. To assess sensitivity, IC_{50} values were calculated. Sensitivity of the multiplex assay were 6.1 ng/mL,

3.6 ng/mL, and 2.4 ng/mL, and the working range of the assay for T2, FB1, and ZON were 1.5–24.4 ng/mL, 0.9–14.3 ng/mL, and 0.6–9.6 ng/mL, respectively.

3. Sensors Based on Artificial Recognition Elements

MIPs are synthetic polymers that can be used to form an artificial receptor for the target analyte. They are synthesised by polymerisation of a monomer with a cross-linking agent in the presence of the target analyte. Upon cross-linking, a cavity is formed around the template, and after its removal, a recognition site appears for the target analyte. The formed polymer can be used as a recognition element in affinity-based sensors. MIPs are cheaper, have higher reusability, and are more resistant to pH and to ionic strength compared to antibodies; therefore, their use in sensor development is beneficial [72,73]. Aptamers are single-stranded nucleic acid (DNA or RNA) molecules with a high affinity to the target molecule. They are fabricated by an in vitro selection and amplification technology (SELEX) [74]. During several selection rounds, only those oligonucleotides are selected and enriched from the huge oligonucleotide library, which can bind with very high affinity to the specific molecular target. It can be stated that the affinity of aptamers can be as good as those of antibodies and in some cases, even better. In addition to that, aptamers are more stable and flexible and can be chemically modified, allowing their immobilisation in sensors.

3.1. Aptasensors

The use of aptamers over antibodies has been an emerging trend in the field of biosensor development in the last decades. Aptamers are synthetic, short, single-stranded nucleic acids with a high affinity to the target molecule. Due to their small size, high affinity, high stability, and specificity, they offer many advantages over conventional antibodies as recognition elements. Having such high affinity, aptamer-based homogeneous and heterogeneous sensors have emerged as a promising tool among the biosensors (Figure 3D). Fluorescent, colorimetric, and electrochemical detection methods are commonly used in these sensor systems. A fluorometric aptamer-based method was developed for simultaneous determination of ZON and FB1 using gold nanorods (AuNRs) and upconversion nanoparticles (UCNPs) [75]. In the sensor, UCNPs were modified with aptamers for ZON and FB1. The functionalised UCNPs were attached with their corresponding complementary nucleic acid (cDNA) sequences. To the AuNPs, different cDNAs for ZON and FB1 were attached, and the AuNPs and the UCNPs were assembled together. In the presence of ZON and FB1 in the sample, the biocomplex of UCNPs-AuNRs will be unstable, and the UCNP part separates from the complex, resulting in the recovery of fluorescence signals. Under 980-nm laser excitation, ZON was detected at 606 nm and FB1 at 753 nm. The LODs of the assay for ZON and FB1 were 1 pg/mL and 3 fg/mL, respectively, with average recoveries from spiked maize samples of 90 to 107%.

Similarly, a fluorescent aptasensor created through UCNPs was presented for ZON determination in corn and beer [76]. A ZON-specific aptamer was used as a recognition probe, while the complementary strand was adopted as a signal probe. In the sensor, ZON aptamer was immobilised on the surface of the amino-modified magnetic nanoparticles, while cDNA was immobilised on the surface of UCNPs and were mixed together to form the duplex structure. When ZON is present in the sample, the ZON-aptamer dissociates from the complex and binds to ZON; therefore, a decrease in the fluorescence intensity occurs. For excitation, a 980 nm laser light was used, and ZON was detected at 543 nm. In this sensing platform, a linear response of 0.05–100 ng/mL was obtained between the fluorescence signal and ZON levels with a LOD of 0.126 µg/kg in corn and 0.007 ng/mL for beer, demonstrating that the developed aptasensor offered a novel approach for ZON analysis in food. Li et al. [77] presented an aptasensor for ZON determination in maize samples that was based on fluorescence resonance energy transfer (FRET) between fluorescent UCNPs modified with aptamer as donors and graphene oxide modified with carboxyl groups as acceptor. When UCNPs and functionalised graphene oxide were at a close distance (less than 10 nm), fluorescence quenching was noticed. As the aptamers prefer to bind to their corresponding mycotoxins, in the presence of ZON, the formation of aptamers change, so aptamer modified-UCNPs are far away from the surface of the functionalised graphene oxide. The presented sensor had a wide working range (0.005–100 ng/mL), good stability (28 days), and the results showed that the aptamer-UCNP-functionalised graphene oxide probe provided a rapid, accurate, and simple to use system for ZON detection.

Azri et al. [78] fabricated an electrochemical label-free competitive aptasensor for ZON determination. The sensor had a working range of 0.01 to 1000 ng/mL ZON concentration with a LOD of 0.017 ng/mL. With the established aptasensor, ZON concentrations of maize grain extracts were determined. For ZON determination, He et al. [79] described a voltammetric aptasensor based on the use of porous platinum nanotubes/AuNPs and thionine-labelled graphene oxide for signal amplification. The working range of the aptasensor was 0.5 pg/mL to 0.5 µg/mL for ZON with a LOD of 0.17 pg/mL.

Recently, an aptasensor for ultrasensitive detection of ZON by using $CoSe_2$ nanocrystal /AuNRs, 3D structured DNA-PtNi@Co-metal-organic framework networks, and nicking enzyme as signal amplification system was proposed [80]. In the sensor DPV detection method was used for ZON determination. Comparing to other ZON methods, the aptasensor possessed outstanding sensitivity (LOD = 1.37 fg/mL) and wider linear range (10.0 fg/mL to 10.0 ng/mL). In addition, no additional substrate was needed compared to conventional enzymatic amplification by substrate cycling. Ong et al. [81] described a novel aptasensor for DON determination where they used iron nanoflorets graphene nickel (INFGN) as a transducer. The INFGN enabled a feasible bio-capturing due to its large surface area where the hydroxyl groups act as linkers. The biomolecular interaction in the sensor results in conductivity changes determined by current-voltage measurement using a picoammeter. The sensor showed good stability, it retained 30.65% of its activity after 48 h, and provided highly sensitive and selective detection of DON at a LOD of 2.11 pg/mL. Another research group used the 3D sakura-shaped copper (II) ions@L-glutamic acid nano-metal-organic coordination polymers (MOCPs) for the first time to develop an electrochemical aptasensor for ultrasensitive detection of ZON. Cronoamperometry was used for ZON determination. Under optimal conditions, dynamic range of 1 fg/mL to 100 ng/mL ZON was obtained with a LOD of 0.45 fg/mL [82].

Han et al. [83] presented a co-reduced molybdenum disulphide and gold nanoparticles ($rMoS_2$-Au)-based electrochemical aptasensor for ZON and FB1 simultaneous detection. For sensor fabrication on the surface of the reduced molybdenum disulphide and AuNPs, coated glassy carbon electrode ZON and FB1 aptamers were conjugated. The corresponding cDNA sequences and thionine and 6-(ferrocenyl)hexanethiol as probes for ZON and FB1 detection were immobilised on AuNPs, which were bound to the aptamers through the complementary base pairing. In the presence of ZON and FB1, the labelled corresponding cDNAs are replaced by the target molecule, resulting in signals proportional to the concentrations of the analytes. Differential pulse voltammetry was used to detect the concentrations of the mycotoxins. The aptasensor allowed ZON and FB1 determination in the range of 1×10^{-3}–10 ng/mL and 1×10^{-3}–1×10^2 ng/mL, respectively. The sensor possesses the LOD of 5×10^{-4} ng/mL. The performance of the aptasensor was successfully demonstrated in real maize samples with satisfactory recoveries.

The statistical parameters of the measurements, the cross reactivity, and the matrix analysed of aptasensors for DON and ZON detection are summarized in Table 3.

Table 3. Statistics of measuring parameters, cross reactivity, and the matrix analysed of aptasensors for DON and ZON detection.

Mycotoxin	Method	Detection Range	LOD	Matrix	Selectivity	Reference
ZON FB1	Fluorometric method	0.05–100 µg/L 0.01–100 ng/L	0.01 µg/L 0.003 ng/L	spiked corn sample	AFB1, OTA, PAT, OTB n.s.	[75]
ZON	Upconversion fluorescence	0.005–100 ng/mL	0.0018 ng/mL	maize	AFB1, AFB2, OTA, DON, FB1 ≈Low n.d.	[77]
ZON	Fluorescense	0.05–100 µg/L	0.126 µg/kg	spiked corn	AFB1, AFB2, OTA, FB1, FB2, α-ZEL, β-ZEL <13%	[76]
ZON	Square wave voltammetry	0.01–1000 ng/mL	0.017 ng/mL	spiked maize	α-ZEL, β-ZEL, ZON-14-Glc, DON, FB1 ≈high n.d.	[78]
ZON	Voltammetry	0.5 pg/mL–0.5 µg/mL	0.17 pg/mL	spiked maize	DON, AFB1, PAT ≈Low n.d.	[79]
ZON	DPV	10.0 fg/mL– 10.0 ng/mL	1.37 fg/mL	spiked maize	DON, OTA, AFB1, PAT, FB1 n.s.	[80]
DON	Voltammerty	1 pg/mL–1 ng/mL	2.11 pg/mL	spiked rice	OTA, ZON <14%	[81]
ZON	Cronoamperometry	1 fg/mL to 100 ng/ml	0.45 fg/mL	spiked beer	T-2, OTA, FB1, AFB1 n.d.	[82]
ZON FB1	DPV	0.001–10 ng/mL 0.001–100 ng/mL	0.0005 ng/mL	maize	α-ZEL, FB2, AFB1, DON, T-2, OTA n.d.	[83]

Deoxynivalenol (DON), Zearalenone (ZON), α-zearalenol (α-ZEL), β-zearalenol (β-ZEL), Zearalenone-14-Glucoside (ZON-14-Glc), Ochratoxin A (OTA), Ochratoxin B (OTB), Aflatoxin B1 (AFB1), Aflatoxin B2 (AFB2), Aflatoxin M1 (AFM1), Fumonisin B1 (FB1), Fumonisin B2 (FB2), Patulin (PAT), differential pulse voltammetry (DPV), signal is not significant (n.s.), no data (n.d.).

3.2. Molecularly Imprinted Polymer Sensors

In recent years, MIPs are widely used primarily in the SPR biosensor technique. Comparing to antibodies, MIPs are more resistant to harsh regeneration conditions and are less likely to lose their binding capability. Although there are several methods to prepare MIPs for sensor applications, the most common method is the in situ polymerisation directly onto the sensor surface (Figure 3C). Choi et al. [84] developed an SPR sensor for ZON determination using MIPs as recognition elements. On the gold sensor surface, a molecularly imprinted polypyrrole film was prepared by electropolymerisation in the presence of ZON as a template. The sensor had a linear response in the range of 0.3–3000 ng/mL for ZON, and the LOD was 0.3 ng/g in corn samples. They also prepared a similar MIP-based SPR sensor for the determination of DON in which the linear measuring range was between 0.1–100 ng/mL. The selectivity of the MIP layer for 3- and 15-acetyl-DON was found to be 19% and 44%, respectively [85].

Sergeyeva et al. [86] developed a novel sensor for ZON detection in cereals suitable for field application. A ZON-selective urethane-acrylate MIP membrane was used to form the sensor, and the natural fluorescence of ZON was analysed by a Spotxel®Reader smartphone application. In the direct sensing mode, the LOD of ZON was 126 µg/kg, but the competitive sensing mode allowed a sensitivity improvement to a LOD of 1.26 µg/kg.

4. Conclusions

Quick, easy to use, and sensitive determination of mycotoxins are extremely important in the food and feed industry because the use of mycotoxin-contaminated commodities poses health risks to the consumers and to livestock as well. The application of biosensors could be an expedient alternative over advanced instrumental chromatographic techniques, as they offer cost-effective, rapid, portable, on-site determination possibilities of mycotoxins. Although developments of several immunosensors for mycotoxin determination have been reported in the scientific literature, they are mainly focused on aflatoxin and ochratoxin as target analytes, but much less attention has been paid to the determination of ZON and DON, and the reports dealing with masked mycotoxins are unduly rare. For the detection of small molecular mass analytes, substantial advances have occurred in the fields of electrochemical and optical immunosensing. Efforts for both types of these sensors are aimed to improve biosensor characteristics, including sensitivity, selectivity, fast response, and low cost; therefore, incorporation of nanomaterials (nanoparticles, nanorods, nanotubes, nanowires) into biosensors are being widely studied. The advantages of using nanoparticles are that they either increase the sensor surface area suitable for biomolecule immobilisation or enhance the signal derived from the immunocomplex formation. It has been found that nanomaterials applied in biosensors as signal amplification tags can improve sensitivity and can reduce the LOD by several orders of magnitude. The use of the favourable properties of nanomaterials in the determination of mycotoxins via immunosensors is particularly important, as these analytes are low molecular weight substances; therefore, their detection is challenging. Another emerging trend in biosensor development is the application of aptamers and MIPs as synthetic receptors in biosensor fabrication. During the past decade, the focus of the attention has turned towards the development of aptasensors due to the stability, selectivity, and sensitivity of these oligonucleotide-type artificial recognition elements. Despite new achievements, areas demanding more research still exist, particularly in the fields of masked mycotoxins and multiplex mycotoxin determination.

Author Contributions: All the authors participated in the preparation of the manuscript. All authors have read and agreed to the published version of the manuscript.

Funding: This research was funded by the Hungarian National Research, Development, and Innovation Office, projects TKP2020-NKA 24 "Tématerületi kiválóság program" in the Thematic Excellence Programme 2020–2021, and NVKP_16-1-2016-0049 "In situ, complex water quality monitoring by using direct or immunofluorimetry and plasma spectroscopy".

Institutional Review Board Statement: Not applicable.

Informed Consent Statement: Not applicable.

Conflicts of Interest: The authors declare no conflict of interest.

References

1. Ricciardi, C.; Castagna, R.; Ferrante, I.; Frascella, F.; Marasso, S.L.; Ricci, A.; Canavese, G.; Lorè, A.; Prelle, A.; Gullino, M.L.; et al. Development of a microcantilever-based immunosensing method for mycotoxin detection. *Biosens. Bioelectron.* **2013**, *40*, 233–239. [CrossRef]
2. CAST. Mycotoxins: Risk in plant, animal and human systems. In *Task Force Report-139*; Council for agricultural Science and Technology: Ames, IA, USA, 2003; ISBN -1887383220.
3. RASSF–Food and Feed Safety Alerts. Available online: https://ec.europa.eu/food/food/rasff-food-and-feed-safety-alerts_en (accessed on 23 June 2021).
4. Bretz, M.; Beyer, M.; Cramer, B.; Knecht, A.; Humpf, H.-U. Thermal Degradation of the *Fusarium* Mycotoxin Deoxynivalenol. *J. Agric. Food Chem.* **2006**, *54*, 6445–6451. [CrossRef]
5. Olopade, B.K.; Oranusi, S.U.; Nwinyi, O.C.; Gbashi, S.; Njobeh, P.B. Occurrences of Deoxynivalenol, Zearalenone and some of their masked forms in selected cereals from Southwest Nigeria. *NFS J.* **2021**, *23*, 24–29. [CrossRef]
6. Golge, O.; Kabak, B. Occurrence of deoxynivalenol and zearalenone in cereals and cereal products from Turkey. *Food Control* **2020**, *110*, 106982. [CrossRef]
7. Döll, S.; Dänicke, S. The Fusarium toxins deoxynivalenol (DON) and zearalenone (ZON) in animal feeding. *Prev. Vet. Med.* **2011**, *102*, 132–145. [CrossRef]
8. Eskola, M.; Kos, G.; Elliott, C.T.; Hajslova, J.; Mayar, S.; Krska, R. Worldwide contamination of food-crops with mycotoxins: Validity of the widely cited 'FAO estimate' of 25%. *Crit. Rev. Food Sci. Nutr.* **2020**, *60*, 2773–2789. [CrossRef] [PubMed]
9. Becker-Algeri, T.A.; Castagnaro, D.; De Bortoli, K.; De Souza, C.; Drunkler, D.A.; Badiale-Furlong, E. Mycotoxins in Bovine Milk and Dairy Products: A Review. *J. Food Sci.* **2016**, *81*, R544–R552. [CrossRef]
10. Cressey, P.; Pearson, A.; Baoumgren, A. Mycotoxins. In *Contaminants in Animal Feed. New Zealand Food Safety Technical Paper No: 2020/21*; Ministry for Primary Industries: Wellington, New Zealand, 2020; pp. 26–33.
11. Commission Recommendation 2006/576/EC of 17 August 2006 on the presence of deoxynivalenol, zearalenone, ochratoxin A, T-2 and HT-2 and fumonisins in products intended for animal feeding. *OJ* **2006**, *L229*, 7–9.
12. Valenta, H. Chromatographic methods for the determination of ochratoxin A in animal and human tissues and fluids. *J. Chromatogr. A* **1998**, *815*, 75–92. [CrossRef]

13. Lai, X.; Liu, R.; Ruan, C.; Zhang, H.; Liu, C. Occurrence of aflatoxins and ochratoxin A in rice samples from six provinces in China. *Food Control* **2015**, *50*, 401–404. [CrossRef]
14. Zhang, L.; Dou, X.-W.; Zhang, C.; Logrieco, A.F.; Yang, M.-H. A Review of Current Methods for Analysis of Mycotoxins in Herbal Medicines. *Toxins* **2018**, *10*, 65. [CrossRef] [PubMed]
15. Pascale, M.; De Girolamo, A.; Lippolis, V.; Stroka, J.; Mol, H.G.J.; Lattanzio, V.M.T. Performance Evaluation of LC-MS Methods for Multimycotoxin Determination. *J. AOAC Int.* **2019**, *102*, 1708–1720. [CrossRef] [PubMed]
16. Woo, S.Y.; Ryu, S.Y.; Tian, F.; Lee, S.Y.; Park, S.B.; Chun, H.S. Simultaneous Determination of Twenty Mycotoxins in the Korean Soybean Paste Doenjang by LC-MS/MS with Immunoaffinity Cleanup. *Toxins* **2019**, *11*, 594. [CrossRef] [PubMed]
17. De Santis, B.; Debegnach, F.; Gregori, E.; Russo, S.; Marchegiani, F.; Moracci, G.; Brera, C. Development of a LC-MS/MS Method for the Multi-Mycotoxin Determination in Composite Cereal-Based Samples. *Toxins* **2017**, *9*, 169. [CrossRef] [PubMed]
18. Kim, D.-H.; Hong, S.-Y.; Kang, J.W.; Cho, S.M.; Lee, K.R.; An, T.K.; Lee, C.; Chung, S.H. Simultaneous Determination of Multi-Mycotoxins in Cereal Grains Collected from South Korea by LC/MS/MS. *Toxins* **2017**, *9*, 106. [CrossRef] [PubMed]
19. Oueslati, S.; Berrada, H.; Juan-Garcia, A.; Mañes, J.; Juan, C. Multiple Mycotoxin Determination on Tunisian Cereals-Based Food and Evaluation of the Population Exposure. *Food Anal. Methods* **2020**, *13*, 1271–1281. [CrossRef]
20. Rodríguez-Carrasco, Y.; Moltó, J.C.; Mañes, J.; Berrada, H. Development of microextraction techniques in combination with GC-MS/MS for the determination of mycotoxins and metabolites in human urine. *J. Sep. Sci.* **2017**, *40*, 1572–1582. [CrossRef] [PubMed]
21. Alshannaq, A.; Yu, J.-H. Occurrence, Toxicity, and Analysis of Major Mycotoxins in Food. *Int. J. Environ. Res. Public Health* **2017**, *14*, 632. [CrossRef]
22. Shotwell, O.L.; Goulden, M.L.; Bennett, G.A. Determination of Zearalenone in Corn: Collaborative Study. *J. Assoc. Off. Anal. Chem.* **1976**, *59*, 666–670. [CrossRef]
23. Eppley, R.M.; Trucksess, M.W.; Nesheim, S.; Thorpe, C.W.; Pohland, A.E.; Applegate, S.L.; Bean, G.A.; Chang, H.; Chatel, R.; Van Deteghem, C.; et al. Thin Layer Chromatographic Method for Determination of Deoxynivalenol in Wheat: Collaborative Study. *J. Assoc. Off. Anal. Chem.* **1986**, *69*, 37–40. [CrossRef]
24. Syahir, A.; Usui, K.; Tomizaki, K.-Y.; Kajikawa, K.; Mihara, H. Label and Label-Free Detection Techniques for Protein Microarrays. *Microarrays* **2015**, *4*, 228–244. [CrossRef]
25. Damborský, P.; Švitel, J.; Katrlík, J. Optical biosensors. *Essays Biochem.* **2016**, *60*, 91–100. [CrossRef] [PubMed]
26. Peltomaa, R.; Glahn-Martínez, B.; Benito-Peña, E.; Moreno-Bondi, M.C. Optical Biosensors for Label-Free Detection of Small Molecules. *Sensors* **2018**, *18*, 4126. [CrossRef]
27. Piliarik, M.; Vaisocherová, H.; Homola, J. Surface Plasmon Resonance Biosensing. *Methods Mol. Biol.* **2009**, *503*, 65–88. [CrossRef]
28. Englebienne, P.; Van Hoonacker, A.; Verhas, M. Surface plasmon resonance: Principles, methods and applications in biomedical sciences. *J. Spectrosc.* **2003**, *17*, 372913. [CrossRef]
29. Man, Y.; Liang, G.; Li, A.; Pan, L. Recent Advances in Mycotoxin Determination for Food Monitoring via Microchip. *Toxins* **2017**, *9*, 324. [CrossRef] [PubMed]
30. Karczmarczyk, A.; Dubiak-Szepietowska, M.; Vorobii, M.; Rodriguez-Emmenegger, C.; Dostalek, J.; Feller, K.-H. Sensitive and rapid detection of aflatoxin M1 in milk utilizing enhanced SPR and p(HEMA) brushes. *Biosens. Bioelectron.* **2016**, *81*, 159–165. [CrossRef]
31. Karczmarczyk, A.; Reiner-Rozman, C.; Hageneder, S.; Dubiak-Szepietowska, M.; Dostalek, J.; Feller, K.-H. Fast and sensitive detection of ochratoxin A in red wine by nanoparticle-enhanced SPR. *Anal. Chim. Acta* **2016**, *937*, 143–150. [CrossRef]
32. Sun, L.; Wu, L.; Zhao, Q. Aptamer based surface plasmon resonance sensor for aflatoxin B1. *Microchim. Acta* **2017**, *184*, 2605–2610. [CrossRef]
33. Rehmat, Z.; Mohammed, W.S.; Sadiq, M.B.; Somarapalli, M.; Anal, A.K. Ochratoxin A detection in coffee by competitive inhibition assay using chitosan-based surface plasmon resonance compact system. *Colloids Surf. B Biointerfaces* **2019**, *174*, 569–574. [CrossRef] [PubMed]
34. Wei, T.; Ren, P.; Huang, L.; Ouyang, Z.; Wang, Z.; Kong, X.; Li, T.; Yin, Y.; Wu, Y.; He, Q. Simultaneous detection of aflatoxin B1, ochratoxin A, zearalenone and deoxynivalenol in corn and wheat using surface plasmon resonance. *Food Chem.* **2019**, *300*, 125176. [CrossRef]
35. Joshi, S.; Segarra-Fas, A.; Peters, J.; Zuilhof, H.; Van Beek, T.A.; Nielen, M.W.F. Multiplex surface plasmon resonance biosensing and its transferability towards imaging nanoplasmonics for detection of mycotoxins in barley. *Analyst* **2016**, *141*, 1307–1318. [CrossRef]
36. Hossain, Z.; Maragos, C.M. Gold nanoparticle-enhanced multiplexed imaging surface plasmon resonance (iSPR) detection of Fusarium mycotoxins in wheat. *Biosens. Bioelectron.* **2018**, *101*, 245–252. [CrossRef]
37. Hossain, Z.; McCormick, S.P.; Maragos, C.M. An Imaging Surface Plasmon Resonance Biosensor Assay for the Detection of T-2 Toxin and Masked T-2 Toxin-3-Glucoside in Wheat. *Toxins* **2018**, *10*, 119. [CrossRef]
38. Hu, W.; Chen, H.; Zhang, H.; He, G.; Li, X.; Zhang, X.; Liu, Y.; Li, C.M. Sensitive detection of multiple mycotoxins by SPRi with gold nanoparticles as signal amplification tags. *J. Colloid Interface Sci.* **2014**, *431*, 71–76. [CrossRef] [PubMed]
39. Adányi, N.; Majer-Baranyi, K.; Székács, A. Evanescent field effect-based nanobiosensors for agro-environmental and food safety. In *Nanobiosensors*; Grumezescu, A.M., Ed.; Elsevier: Cambridge, MA, USA, 2017; pp. 429–474. [CrossRef]

40. Majer-Baranyi, K.; Székács, A.; Szendrő, I.; Kiss, A.; Adányi, N. Optical waveguide lightmode spectroscopy technique–based immunosensor development for deoxynivalenol determination in wheat samples. *Eur. Food Res. Technol.* **2011**, *233*, 1041–1047. [CrossRef]
41. Székács, I.; Adányi, N.; Szendrő, I.; Székács, A. Direct and Competitive Optical Grating Immunosensors for Determination of *Fusarium* Mycotoxin Zearalenone. *Toxins* **2021**, *13*, 43. [CrossRef]
42. Nabok, A.; Al-Jawdah, A.M.; Gémes, B.; Takács, E.; Székács, A. An Optical Planar Waveguide-Based Immunosensors for Determination of *Fusarium* Mycotoxin Zearalenone. *Toxins* **2021**, *13*, 89. [CrossRef]
43. Koukouvinos, G.; Tsialla, Z.; Petrou, P.; Misiakos, K.; Goustouridis, D.; Moreno, A.U.; Fernandez-Alba, A.R.; Raptis, I.; Kakabakos, S.E. Fast simultaneous detection of three pesticides by a White Light Reflectance Spectroscopy sensing platform. *Sens. Actuators B Chem.* **2017**, *238*, 1214–1223. [CrossRef]
44. Anastasiadis, V.; Raptis, I.; Economou, A.; Kakabakos, S.E.; Petrou, P.S. Fast Deoxynivalenol Determination in Cereals Using a White Light Reflectance Spectroscopy Immunosensor. *Biosensors* **2020**, *10*, 154. [CrossRef] [PubMed]
45. Jiang, Q.; Wu, J.; Yao, K.; Yin, Y.; Gong, M.M.; Yang, C.; Lin, F. Paper-Based Microfluidic Device (DON-Chip) for Rapid and Low-Cost Deoxynivalenol Quantification in Food, Feed, and Feed Ingredients. *ACS Sens.* **2019**, *4*, 3072–3079. [CrossRef]
46. Jin, Y.; Chen, Q.; Luo, S.; He, L.; Fan, R.; Zhang, S.; Yang, C.; Chen, Y. Dual near-infrared fluorescence-based lateral flow immunosensor for the detection of zearalenone and deoxynivalenol in maize. *Food Chem.* **2021**, *336*, 127718. [CrossRef] [PubMed]
47. Machado, J.M.D.; Soares, R.R.G.; Chu, V.; Conde, J.P. Multiplexed capillary microfluidic immunoassay with smartphone data acquisition for parallel mycotoxin detection. *Biosens. Bioelectron.* **2018**, *99*, 40–46. [CrossRef] [PubMed]
48. Liu, Z.; Hua, Q.; Wang, J.; Liang, Z.; Li, J.; Wu, J.; Shen, X.; Lei, H.; Li, X. A smartphone-based dual detection mode device integrated with two lateral flow immunoassays for multiplex mycotoxins in cereals. *Biosens. Bioelectron.* **2020**, *158*, 112178. [CrossRef] [PubMed]
49. Bard, A.J.; Faulkner, L.R.; Leddy, J.; Zoski, C.G. *Electrochemical Methods: Fundamentals and Applications*; Wiley: New York, NY, USA, 1980.
50. AlHamoud, Y.; Yang, D.; Kenston, S.S.F.; Liu, G.; Liu, L.; Zhou, H.; Ahmed, F.; Zhao, J. Advances in biosensors for the detection of ochratoxin A: Bio-receptors, nanomaterials, and their applications. *Biosens. Bioelectron.* **2019**, *141*, 111418. [CrossRef]
51. Radi, A.-E.; Eissa, A.; Wahdan, T. Molecularly Imprinted Impedimetric Sensor for Determination of Mycotoxin Zearalenone. *Electroanalysis* **2020**, *32*, 1788–1794. [CrossRef]
52. Evtugyn, G.; Hianik, T. Electrochemical Immuno- and Aptasensors for Mycotoxin Determination. *Chemosensors* **2019**, *7*, 10. [CrossRef]
53. Arduini, F.; Micheli, L.; Moscone, D.; Palleschi, G.; Piermarini, S.; Ricci, F.; Volpe, G. Electrochemical biosensors based on nanomodified screen-printed electrodes: Recent applications in clinical analysis. *TrAC Trends Anal. Chem.* **2016**, *79*, 114–126. [CrossRef]
54. Goud, K.Y.; Kailasa, S.K.; Kumar, V.; Tsang, Y.F.; Lee, S.E.; Gobi, K.V.; Kim, K.-H. Progress on nanostructured electrochemical sensors and their recognition elements for detection of mycotoxins: A review. *Biosens. Bioelectron.* **2018**, *121*, 205–222. [CrossRef] [PubMed]
55. Le, V.T.; Vasseghian, Y.; Dragoi, E.-N.; Moradi, M.; Khaneghah, A.M. A review on graphene-based electrochemical sensor for mycotoxins detection. *Food Chem. Toxicol.* **2021**, *148*, 111931. [CrossRef] [PubMed]
56. Shoala, T. Carbon nanostructures: Detection, controlling plant diseases and mycotoxins. In *Micro and Nano Technologies*; Abd-Elsalam, K.A., Ed.; Elsevier: Cambridge, MA, USA, 2020; pp. 261–277. [CrossRef]
57. Rhouati, A.; Bulbul, G.; Latif, U.; Hayat, A.; Li, Z.-H.; Marty, J.L. Nano-Aptasensing in Mycotoxin Analysis: Recent Updates and Progress. *Toxins* **2017**, *9*, 349. [CrossRef]
58. Zhang, X.; Wang, Z.; Xie, H.; Sun, R.; Cao, T.; Paudyal, N.; Fang, W.; Song, H. Development of a Magnetic Nanoparticles-Based Screen-Printed Electrodes (MNPs-SPEs) Biosensor for the Quantification of Ochratoxin A in Cereal and Feed Samples. *Toxins* **2018**, *10*, 317. [CrossRef]
59. Kailasa, S.K.; Park, T.J.; Singhal, R.K.; Basu, H. Nanoparticle-integrated electrochemical devices for identification of mycotoxins. In *Handbook of Nanomaterials in Analytical Chemistry*; Hussain, C.M., Ed.; Elsevier: Cambridge, MA, USA, 2020; pp. 275–296. [CrossRef]
60. Riberi, W.I.; Tarditto, L.V.; Zon, M.A.; Arévalo, F.; Fernández, H. Development of an electrochemical immunosensor to determine zearalenone in maize using carbon screen printed electrodes modified with multi-walled carbon nanotubes/polyethyleneimine dispersions. *Sens. Actuators B Chem.* **2018**, *254*, 1271–1277. [CrossRef]
61. Goud, K.Y.; Kumar, V.S.; Hayat, A.; Gobi, K.V.; Song, H.; Kim, K.-H.; Marty, J.L. A highly sensitive electrochemical immunosensor for zearalenone using screen-printed disposable electrodes. *J. Electroanal. Chem.* **2019**, *832*, 336–342. [CrossRef]
62. Regiart, M.; Fernández, O.; Vicario, A.; Villarroel-Rocha, J.; Sapag, K.; Messina, G.A.; Raba, J.; Bertolino, F.A. Mesoporous immunosensor applied to zearalenone determination in Amaranthus cruentus seeds. *Microchem. J.* **2018**, *141*, 388–394. [CrossRef]
63. Lu, L.; Gunasekaran, S. Dual-channel ITO-microfluidic electrochemical immunosensor for simultaneous detection of two mycotoxins. *Talanta* **2019**, *194*, 709–716. [CrossRef] [PubMed]
64. Tuantranont, A.; Wisitsora-At, A.; Sritongkham, P.; Jaruwongrungsee, K. A review of monolithic multichannel quartz crystal microbalance: A review. *Anal. Chim. Acta* **2011**, *687*, 114–128. [CrossRef]
65. Chauhan, R.; Singh, J.; Solanki, P.R.; Basu, T.; O'Kennedy, R.; Malhotra, B.D. Electrochemical piezoelectric reusable immunosensor for aflatoxin B1 detection. *Biochem. Eng. J.* **2015**, *103*, 103–113. [CrossRef]

66. Chauhan, R.; Solanki, P.R.; Singh, J.; Mukherjee, I.; Basu, T.; Malhotra, B. A novel electrochemical piezoelectric label free immunosensor for aflatoxin B1 detection in groundnut. *Food Control* **2015**, *52*, 60–70. [CrossRef]
67. Chauhan, R.; Singh, J.; Solanki, P.R.; Manaka, T.; Iwamoto, M.; Basu, T.; Malhotra, B. Label-free piezoelectric immunosensor decorated with gold nanoparticles: Kinetic analysis and biosensing application. *Sens. Actuators B* **2016**, *222*, 804–814. [CrossRef]
68. Karczmarczyk, A.; Haupt, K.; Feller, K.-H. Development of a QCM-D biosensor for Ochratoxin A detection in red wine. *Talanta* **2017**, *166*, 193–197. [CrossRef]
69. Spinella, K.; Mosiello, L.; Palleschi, G.; Vitali, F. Development of a QCM (Quartz Crystal Microbalance) Biosensor to Detection of Mycotoxins. In *Sensors and Microsystems. Lecture Notes in Electrical Engineering*; Di Natale, C., Ferrari, V., Ponzoni, A., Sberveglieri, G., Ferrari, M., Eds.; Springer: Cham, Switzerland, 2014; Volume 268, pp. 195–198. [CrossRef]
70. Liu, S.; Liu, X.; Pan, Q.; Dai, Z.; Pan, M.; Wang, S. A Portable, Label-Free, Reproducible Quartz Crystal Microbalance Immunochip for the Detection of Zearalenone in Food Samples. *Biosensors* **2021**, *11*, 53. [CrossRef]
71. Nolan, P.; Auer, S.; Spehar, A.; Oplatowska-Stachowiak, M.; Campbell, K. Evaluation of Mass Sensitive Micro-Array biosensors for their feasibility in multiplex detection of low molecular weight toxins using mycotoxins as model compounds. *Talanta* **2021**, *222*, 121521. [CrossRef] [PubMed]
72. Uygun, Z.O.; Uygun, H.D.E.; Ermis, N.; Canbay, E. Molecularly Imprinted Sensors—New Sensing Technologies. In *Biosensors: Micro and Nanoscale Applications*; Rinken, T., Ed.; IntechOpen: London, UK, 2015. [CrossRef]
73. Naseri, M.; Mohammadniaei, M.; Sun, Y.; Ashley, J. The Use of Aptamers and Molecularly Imprinted Polymers in Biosensors for Environmental Monitoring: A Tale of Two Receptors. *Chemosensors* **2020**, *8*, 32. [CrossRef]
74. Hianik, T. Aptamer-Based Biosensors. In *Encyclopedia of Interfacial Chemistry*; Wandelt, K., Ed.; Elsevier: Cambridge, MA, USA, 2018; Volume 7.1, pp. 11–19. [CrossRef]
75. He, D.; Wu, Z.; Cui, B.; Jin, Z.; Xu, E. A fluorometric method for aptamer-based simultaneous determination of two kinds of fusarium mycotoxins zearalenone and fumonisin B1 making use of gold nanorods and upconversion nanoparticles. *Microchim. Acta* **2020**, *187*, 254. [CrossRef] [PubMed]
76. Wu, Z.; Xu, E.; Chughtai, M.F.; Jin, Z.; Irudayaraj, J. Highly sensitive fluorescence sensing of zearalenone using a novel aptasensor based on upconverting nanoparticles. *Food Chem.* **2017**, *230*, 673–680. [CrossRef]
77. Li, Y.; Li, Y.; Zhang, D.; Tan, W.; Shi, J.; Li, Z.; Liu, H.; Yu, Y.; Yang, L.; Wang, X.; et al. A fluorescence resonance energy transfer probe based on functionalized graphene oxide and upconversion nanoparticles for sensitive and rapid detection of zearalenone. *LWT* **2021**, *147*, 111541. [CrossRef]
78. Azri, F.A.; Eissa, S.; Zourob, M.; Chinnappan, R.; Sukor, R.; Yusof, N.A.; Raston, N.H.A.; Alhoshani, A.; Jinap, S. Electrochemical determination of zearalenone using a label-free competitive aptasensor. *Microchim. Acta* **2020**, *187*, 266. [CrossRef]
79. He, B.; Yan, X. An amperometric zearalenone aptasensor based on signal amplification by using a composite prepared from porous platinum nanotubes, gold nanoparticles and thionine-labelled graphene oxide. *Microchim. Acta* **2019**, *186*, 383. [CrossRef]
80. He, B.; Yan, X. Ultrasensitive electrochemical aptasensor based on CoSe2/AuNRs and 3D structured DNA-PtNi@Co-MOF networks for the detection of zearalenone. *Sens. Actuators B Chem.* **2020**, *306*, 127558. [CrossRef]
81. Ong, C.C.; Sangu, S.S.; Illias, N.M.; Gopinath, S.C.B.; Saheed, M.S.M. Iron nanoflorets on 3D-graphene-nickel: A 'Dandelion' nanostructure for selective deoxynivalenol detection. *Biosens. Bioelectron.* **2020**, *154*, 112088. [CrossRef]
82. Ji, X.; Yu, C.; Wen, Y.; Chen, J.; Yu, Y.; Zhang, C.; Gao, R.; Mu, X.; He, J. Fabrication of pioneering 3D sakura-shaped metal-organic coordination polymers Cu@L-Glu phenomenal for signal amplification in highly sensitive detection of zearalenone. *Biosens. Bioelectron.* **2019**, *129*, 139–146. [CrossRef]
83. Han, Z.; Tang, Z.; Jiang, K.; Huang, Q.; Meng, J.; Nie, D.; Zhao, Z. Dual-target electrochemical aptasensor based on co-reduced molybdenum disulfide and Au NPs (rMoS2-Au) for multiplex detection of mycotoxins. *Biosens. Bioelectron.* **2020**, *150*, 111894. [CrossRef] [PubMed]
84. Choi, S.-W.; Chang, H.-J.; Lee, N.; Kim, J.-H.; Chun, H.S. Detection of Mycoestrogen Zearalenone by a Molecularly Imprinted Polypyrrole-Based Surface Plasmon Resonance (SPR) Sensor. *J. Agric. Food Chem.* **2009**, *57*, 1113–1118. [CrossRef] [PubMed]
85. Choi, S.-W.; Chang, H.-J.; Lee, N.; Chun, H.S. A Surface Plasmon Resonance Sensor for the Detection of Deoxynivalenol Using a Molecularly Imprinted Polymer. *Sensors* **2011**, *11*, 8654–8664. [CrossRef] [PubMed]
86. Sergeyeva, T.; Yarynka, D.; Dubey, L.; Dubey, I.; Piletska, E.; Linnik, R.; Antonyuk, M.; Ternovska, T.; Brovko, O.; Piletsky, S.; et al. Sensor Based on Molecularly Imprinted Polymer Membranes and Smartphone for Detection of *Fusarium* Contamination in Cereals. *Sensors* **2020**, *20*, 4304. [CrossRef] [PubMed]

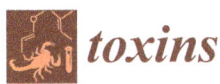

Article

Occurrence of Zearalenone and Its Metabolites in the Blood of High-Yielding Dairy Cows at Selected Collection Sites in Various Disease States

Wojciech Barański [1], Magdalena Gajęcka [2,*], Łukasz Zielonka [2], Magdalena Mróz [2], Ewa Onyszek [3], Katarzyna E. Przybyłowicz [4], Arkadiusz Nowicki [1], Andrzej Babuchowski [3] and Maciej T. Gajęcki [2]

[1] Department of Animal Reproduction with Clinic, Faculty of Veterinary Medicine, University of Warmia and Mazury in Olsztyn, Oczapowskiego 13, 10-718 Olsztyn, Poland; wojbar@uwm.edu.pl (W.B.); arkadiusz.nowicki@uwm.edu.pl (A.N.)
[2] Department of Veterinary Prevention and Feed Hygiene, Faculty of Veterinary Medicine, University of Warmia and Mazury in Olsztyn, Oczapowskiego 13, 10-718 Olsztyn, Poland; lukaszz@uwm.edu.pl (Ł.Z.); magdzia.mroz@gmail.com (M.M.); gajecki@uwm.edu.pl (M.T.G.)
[3] Institute of Dairy Industry Innovation Ltd., Kormoranów 1, 11-700 Mrągowo, Poland; ewa.onyszek@iipm.pl (E.O.); andrzej.babuchowski@iipm.pl (A.B.)
[4] Department of Human Nutrition, Faculty of Food Sciences, University of Warmia and Mazury in Olsztyn, Słoneczna 45F, 10-719 Olsztyn, Poland; katarzyna.przybylowicz@uwm.edu.pl
* Correspondence: mgaja@uwm.edu.pl; Tel.: +48-89-523-3773; Fax: +48-89-523-3618

Abstract: Zearalenone (ZEN) and its metabolites, alpha-zearalenol (α-ZEL) and beta-zearalenol (β-ZEL), are ubiquitous in plant materials used as feed components in dairy cattle diets. The aim of this study was to confirm the occurrence of ZEN and its selected metabolites in blood samples collected from different sites in the hepatic portal system (posthepatic–external jugular vein EJV; prehepatic–abdominal subcutaneous vein ASV and median caudal vein MCV) of dairy cows diagnosed with mastitis, ovarian cysts and pyometra. The presence of mycotoxins in the blood plasma was determined with the use of combined separation methods involving immunoaffinity columns, a liquid chromatography system and a mass spectrometry system. The parent compound was detected in all samples collected from diseased cows, whereas α-ZEL and β-ZEL were not identified in any samples, or their concentrations were below the limit of detection (LOD). Zearalenone levels were highest in cows with pyometra, where the percentage share of average ZEN concentrations reached 44%. Blood sampling sites were arranged in the following ascending order based on ZEN concentrations: EJV (10.53 pg/mL, 44.07% of the samples collected from this site), ASV (14.20 pg/mL, 49.59% of the samples) and MCV (26.67 pg/mL, 67.35% of the samples). The results of the study indicate that blood samples for toxicological analyses should be collected from the MCV (prehepatic vessel) of clinically healthy cows and/or cows with subclinical ZEN mycotoxicosis. This sampling site increases the probability of correct diagnosis of subclinical ZEN mycotoxicosis.

Keywords: zearalenone; mastitis; ovarian cysts; pyometra; hepatic portal system; dairy cows

Key Contribution: Zearalenone metabolites were not detected in the blood plasma of cows with healthy ruminal microbiota. When the rumen contents containing ZEN reach the intestines, the mycotoxin is transported to the liver by the prehepatic circulation.

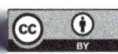

1. Introduction

Zearalenone (ZEN) is a resorcinic acid lactone produced by fungi of the genus *Fusarium*, which, due to its structural similarity to 17β-estradiol and affinity to estrogen receptors [1], is classified as mycoestrogens. In mammals, ZEN binds to estrogen receptors that display tropism for female reproductive cells. Zearalenone poses a health risk for dairy cows because it is highly stable in contaminated animal feedstuffs and difficult to degrade through heating and other physical treatments [2].

High-yielding dairy cows are highly susceptible to metabolic diseases such as milk fever, ketosis and rumen acidosis, which are frequently accompanied by subclinical and clinical symptoms of udder infection and decreased reproductive performance. Metabolic disorders are most frequently observed in three critical periods [3]: (i) dry period, (ii) parturition, and (iii) first 100 days of lactation. These periods are characterized by an increased risk of udder inflammation and aseptic diffuse inflammation of the laminar corium, which are indicative of compromised innate immunity, decreased acquired immunity to infectious factors [4], and higher susceptibility to undesirable substances, including secondary metabolites of molds such as ZEN and its metabolites.

In dairy cows, susceptibility to mycotoxins is largely determined by the degree to which these substances are eliminated by ruminal microbiota before they are assimilated by the body [5]. Very few mycotoxins are resistant to microbial detoxification in the rumen, and they cause typical symptoms of poisoning with toxic metabolites. Silage and other stored feedstuffs can contain mycotoxins that possess antibacterial properties and modify ruminal microbiota. These compounds can compromise the detoxification capacity of rumen microorganisms. The rumen contents contaminated with mycotoxins may be absorbed in the duodenum, leading to certain mycotoxin concentrations in dairy cows. The clinical symptoms of mycotoxin poisoning are generally non-specific, and they include metabolic and hormonal disorders accompanied by inflammatory states caused by a weakened immune response [4]. During transition periods, cows are particularly susceptible to mycotoxicosis because the presence of molds and/or mycotoxins in cattle diets further deepens the negative energy balance [3].

In dairy cows, the risk of exposure to ZEN can be assessed directly by identifying mycotoxins in the feed matrix [6], or indirectly by analyzing the respective biomarkers in biological fluids and tissues. Feed matrices are widely applied to evaluate the risk [7] resulting from e.g., the presence of ZEN and its metabolites. However, this approach has several limitations. The feed production process and the health status of animals may affect the bioavailability of ZEN and its metabolites in feed and, consequently, increase the risk of exposure in dairy cows. In addition, mycotoxins are not evenly distributed in the feed matrix, and feed intake is difficult to estimate accurately. Since ZEN is transmitted by numerous vectors (green fodder, roughage and concentrated fodder or water), the levels of this mycotoxin and its metabolites can be more reliably quantified in blood samples (indirect analysis).

Our observations show that during clinical activities, field veterinarians need to be aware of some simple information about mycotoxins: (i) mycotoxins are very often found in small amounts in the plant material used for feed production; (ii) not every laboratory has equipment for detecting the presence of very small amounts (these may be values below the sensitivity of the method); (iii) mycotoxin contamination may occur during the vegetation of feed crops, and the mycotoxins are then evenly distributed throughout the plant material; (iv) the feed may become contaminated with mycotoxins during the storage of the final product (concentrated feed) and then the distribution of eg ZEN may be pinpointed in the feed; (v) the accumulation in the macro-organism of low doses of mycotoxins (below the NOAEL value) taken in the feed takes a very long time, making it impossible to trace the mycotoxin vector; and (iv) ZEN is mycoestrogen and its presence in the mammalian body is immediately noted in the form of endocrine system dysfunction and the resulting perturbations in estrogen-dependent tissues.

In cattle, mycotoxicoses are diagnosed based on the presence of clinical symptoms of infertility or hormonal disorders during exposure to high ZEN doses. However, the influence of very low, measurable concentrations of ZEN on the health status of dairy cows has never been investigated. Such mycotoxin concentrations are frequently encountered in plant materials that are used in the production of feed for dairy cattle [6–8].

Mycotoxins exert various effects on the health status of animals exposed to their different doses [9,10]. The symptoms and health consequences (toxicological) of exposure to high doses of most mycotoxins have been relatively well researched and described [10]. Prolonged exposure to low monotonic doses of mycotoxins is usually well tolerated by monogastric animals [11], which suggests that these compounds can meet the animals' life needs, or exert protective [8,12–15] or therapeutic effects [16]. In ruminants, exposure and digestion processes are similar to those observed in monogastric animals when the rumen contents pass into the intestines. Therefore, the clinical presentation of ZEN mycotoxicosis is also similar [14].

During exposure to low mycotoxin doses, the dose-response relationship has been also undermined by the low dose hypothesis. The above applies particularly to hormonally active chemical compounds [17], including mycoestrogens such as ZEN and its metabolites which disrupt the functioning of the hormonal system, even when ingested in small quantities [18]. This ambiguous dose-response relationship does not justify direct analyses or meta-analyses of the risk (clinical symptoms or the results of laboratory analyses) associated with low dose stimulation and high dose inhibition, which is consistent with the hormesis paradigm [19]. The concept of the lowest identifiable dose which produces counter-intuitive effects is becoming increasingly popular in biomedical sciences [20]. The relevant mechanisms should be investigated to support rational decision-making [8,21]. Such decisions involve the selection of blood sampling sites which are most adequate for assessing the risk of mycotoxin exposure in dairy cows. The main routes of blood inflow and outflow to/from the liver should be examined taking into account the availability of blood vessels and the extent of natural (hepatic) detoxification. Topographic anatomy of anastomoses between the portal venous system (*vena portae*) with the major veins [22], including the external jugular vein (EJV, *v. jugularis externa*-posthepatic), the abdominal subcutaneous vein (ASV, *v. epigastrica cranialis superficialis*-prehepatic) and the median caudal vein (MCV, *v. caudalis mediana*-prehepatic) should be analyzed to confirm the reliability and consistency of the results [4].

The aim of the study was to confirm the occurrence of ZEN and its selected metabolites in the blood of high-yielding dairy cows and selected collection sites (external jugular vein, abdominal subcutaneous vein and median caudal vein) in various disease states (Mastitis, ovarian cysts and Pyometra), in natural conditions.

2. Results

2.1. Clinical Observations

Clinical signs of ZEN mycotoxicosis were not observed during the experiment (such as reduced growth rate and milk yield, and causes significant economic cost to the dairy industry). However, cows may have been exposed to natural sources of ZEN in plant materials. Cattle diets probably contained very small amounts of the mycotoxin that approximated the minimal anticipated biological effect level (MABEL). Zearalenone transmission vector/vectors could not be identified with full certainty.

2.2. Concentrations of Zearalenone in Peripheral Blood

Alpha-ZEL and β-ZEL were not detected in blood samples, or their concentrations were below the limit of detection (LOD).

Highly significant ($p \leq 0.01$) differences in ZEN concentrations (Figure 1) were observed only in blood samples collected from the MCV. These differences were noted between cows with pyometra compared to blood samples from cows with mastitis (difference of 18.20 pg/mL), cows with ovarian cysts (difference of 21.21 pg/mL) or asymptomatic cows (difference of 26.23 pg/mL). Regardless of the sampling site, ZEN levels were highest in cows displaying clinical symptoms of pyometra. In cows with mastitis and pyometra, ZEN concentrations were lowest in blood sampled from the EJV (5.70 pg/mL and 10.53 pg/mL, respectively) and highest in samples collected from the MCV (8.47 pg/mL and 26.67 pg/mL, respectively. For ovarian cysts, the trend was the opposite between collection sites (from 7.63 pg/mL at EJV to 5.46 pg/mL at MCV).

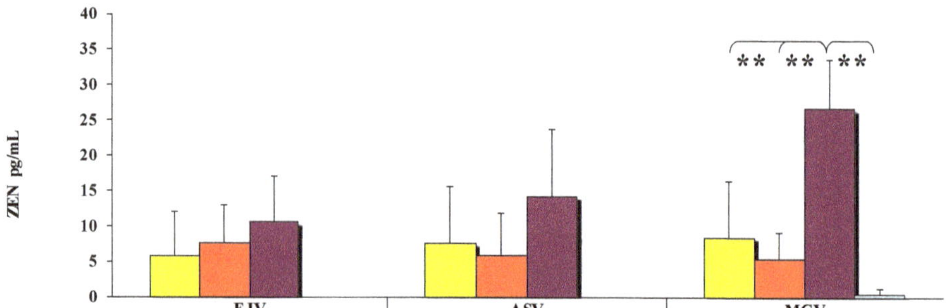

	EJV		ASV		MCV	
Mastitis	5.71	± 6.23	7.57	± 8.07	8.47	± 7.89
Ovarian cysts	7.63	± 5.26	5.86	± 6.02	5.46	± 3.74
Pyometra	10.53	± 6.49	14.21	± 9.59	26.67	± 6.92
Asymptomatic	0	± 0.0	0	± 0.0	0.44	± 0.77

Figure 1. Mean values ($\bar{x}$) and standard deviation (SD) of ZEN concentrations (pg/mL) in peripheral blood sampled from different sites: (1) external jugular vein (EJV, *v. jugularis externa*-posthepatic); (2) abdominal subcutaneous vein (ASV, *v. epigastrica cranialis superficialis*-prehepatic); (3) median caudal vein (MCV, *v. caudalis mediana*-prehepatic) of cows diagnosed with mastitis, ovarian cysts and pyometra, and asymptomatic cows. Limit of detection (LOD) > values below the limit of detection were regarded as equal to 0. Differences were regarded as statistically significant at ** $p \leq 0.01$.

At the same time, it was found that the mean highest ZEN value (number of samples: the sum of the ZEN concentration values in these samples) was obtained in samples taken from median caudal vein (which accounted for 57%), compared to the other sampling sites (Figure 2).

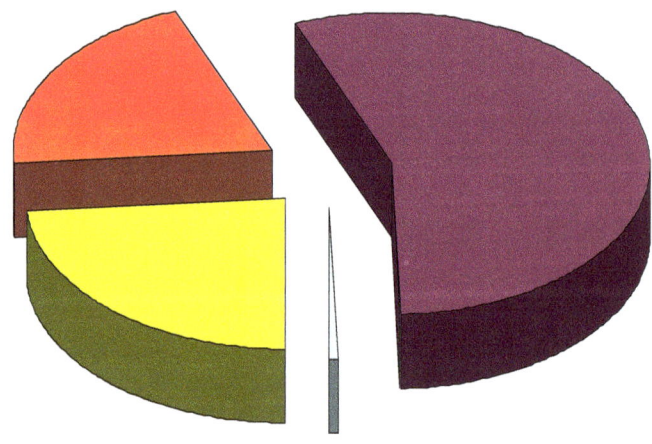

☐ Mastitis ■ Ovarian cysts ■ Pyometra ☐ Asymptomatic

Figure 2. Percentage share of the average ZEN concentrations in blood sampled from cows diagnosed with mastitis, ovarian cysts and pyometra and from asymptomatic cows in the monitored herd.

A comparison of ZEN concentrations in samples of peripheral blood (Figure 3) collected from diseased cows revealed significant differences ($p \leq 0.05$) only in the blood of cows with pyometra. The difference between the samples collected from the EJV and the MCV was determined at 16.16 pg/mL. In cows diagnosed with mastitis and ovarian cysts,

ZEN concentrations were highly similar (no significant differences) and very low relative to those noted in cows with pyometra.

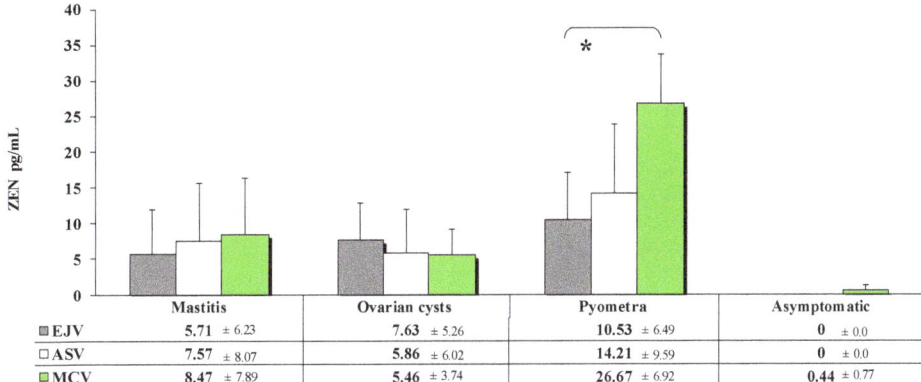

Figure 3. Mean values ($\bar{x}$) and standard deviation (SD) of ZEN concentrations (pg/mL) in peripheral blood of cows collected in various disease states (Mastitis; Ovarian cysts; Pyometra; Asymptomatic) at different collection sites [external jugular vein (EJV-*v. jugularis externa*-posthepatic); abdominal subcutaneous vein (ASV-*v. epigastrica cranialis superficialis*-prehepatic); oraz median caudal vein (MCV-*v. caudalis mediana*-prehepatic)]. Limits of detection (LOD) > values below the limit of detection were regarded as equal to 0. Statistically significant difference was determined at * $p \leq 0.05$.

The data presented in Figure 3; Figure 4 show that the highest values of the ZEN level were recorded in Pyometra cows, where the percentage share of the mean values of ZEN concentrations was 44.08%.

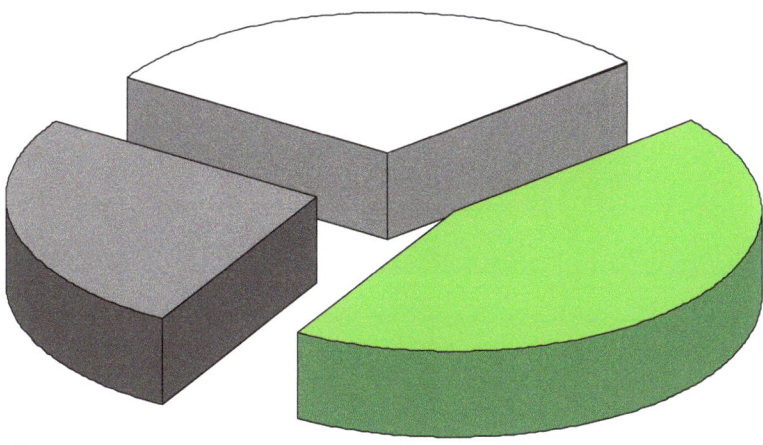

Figure 4. Percentage share of average ZEN concentrations in blood samples collected from different sites (*external jugular vein*-EJV-posthepatic; *abdominal subcutaneous vein*-ASV-prehepatic; *median caudal vein*-MCV-prehepatic) in the monitored herd of dairy cows.

The share of individual blood sampling sites in the values of the ZEN level indicates an upward trend, starting with *external jugular vein* (10.53 ng/mL, which constituted 44.13% in this collection site), through the obtained values in *abdominal subcutaneous vein* (14.20 ng/mL, which was 51.39% at this point of samples), and ending with the concentration values obtained in blood samples collected in *median caudal vein* (26.67 ng/mL, which constituted 65.68% at this point of collection).

3. Discussion

It is generally believed that ruminants are less susceptible to the harmful effects of mycotoxins than monogastric animals because some mycotoxins are degraded by ruminal microbiota [23]. Despite the above, mycotoxins can induce subclinical conditions in dairy cows [24].

The results of the present study should be interpreted in view of the following observations: (i) the feed administered to dairy cows was probably contaminated with very low doses of ZEN [5]; (ii) this is the first study of the type; therefore, the present findings cannot be compared with published data and have to be interpreted by extrapolation.

According to Fushimi et al. [25], very low levels of ZEN in feed do not affect reproductive performance, but they affect anti-Müllerian hormone levels in the blood [26,27] which play an important role in folliculogenesis and are most highly expressed in the granulosa cells of preantral follicles, mostly in the antral stage [28,29]. These hormones inhibit follicle stimulating hormone (FSH)-induced growth and development of the remaining primary follicles and the selection of the dominant follicle [30–32].

In cows, β-ZEL is identified more frequently than α-ZEL in the intestinal contents contaminated with low doses of ZEN, which implies that detoxification processes are predominant during exposure to very low ZEN doses. It should also be noted that: (i) ZEN could be utilized as a substrate that regulates (inversely) the expression of genes encoding HSDs (Hydroxysteroid Dehydrogenases) which act of molecular switches for the modulation of steroid hormone prereceptors [33–35]; (ii) enterohepatic recirculation occurs before ZEN and its metabolites are biotransformed and eliminated; and (iii) in vitro studies have demonstrated that ZEN metabolites are detected within 15 min to 1 h after ingestion, which indicates that this mycotoxin is rapidly metabolized by ruminal microbiota [5,23]. In the present study, the latter observation was confirmed in asymptomatic cows.

These hypotheses (alone or in combination) could explain the differences in the concentrations of ZEN and its metabolites in the peripheral blood of dairy cows exposed to low doses of the mycotoxin. However, these differences could be also attributed to unknown factors that cause rumen inflammations, thus increasing the risk of absorption of toxic compounds, such as lipopolysaccharides (major risk factors) and/or mycotoxins, through the rumen wall [23]. According to Dänicke et al. [4,36], low ruminal pH (which compromises the buffering capacity of the rumen, [23]) inhibits the biotransformation of parent compounds such as ZEN and metabolite synthesis, which could explain the absence of ZEN metabolites in the examined blood samples (Figures 1 and 2). The cited authors also argued that in ruminants, ZEN (parent compound) can be transported to the postruminal digestive tract at unchanged levels and cause mycotoxicosis [37] or digestive disorders contributing to feed-borne diseases such as mastitis, ovarian cysts and pyometra [3]. The above could be explained by a higher rumen passage rate which decreases ruminal pH, thus decreasing the proportion of Gram-positive bacteria and increasing the population of Gram-negative bacteria. These processes occur mainly during the transition period which is accompanied by vast changes in the metabolic processes of cows due to energy, mineral and vitamin deficiencies.

In the present study, ZEN and its metabolites were not detected in asymptomatic cows (Figures 1 and 3), which could be attributed to the rapid biotransformation of mycotoxins by ruminal microbiota or very low concentrations of ZEN in unspecified feed transmission vectors [6]. Similar results were reported in vitro by Debevere et al. [23] who observed that the biotransformation of ZEN to α-ZEL and β-ZEL (only in the rumen) is highly limited at normal ruminal pH.

Zearalenone metabolites were not detected in diseased cows (Figures 1 and 3). However, trace amounts of the parent compound were identified in the blood, probably because ZEN is not completely metabolized in the rumen. This mycotoxin is transported to successive intestinal segments in unmodified form, and it reaches peripheral organs with the blood and enters the prehepatic circulation that ends in the portal vein (*vena portae*) which supplies blood to the liver [4,22]. The evaluated herd was probably exposed to ZEN for a long period of time or continuously. In laboratory analyses, ZEN is very often detected in maize silage, green fodder and hay [6,37], which indicates that this mycotoxin is present in feed throughout the year. The present results point to dysfunctions of ruminal microbiota or the liver, a unique immunological site that protects the body against mycotoxins. These defense mechanisms can participate in the development of tolerance [38] or initiate a separate immune response [4].

Subclinical disease states caused by mycotoxins should be analyzed in greater detail in high-yielding dairy cows. Disease states can be also caused by saprophytic or conditionally pathogenic microorganisms (bacterial lipopolysaccharides) which contribute to comorbidities, including mycotoxicosis [23]. The etiological factors of disease include an increase in the rumen passage rate caused by increased concentrate intake or the postnatal period (as a result of the physiological loss of the fetus), as well as metabolic disorders such as subacute rumen acidosis resulting from changes ("shift") in ruminal microbiota [39]. Mycotoxins are less effectively detoxified in the rumen, and they are transported to the intestinal lumen [5]. Zearalenone reaches the intestines and unpaired organs in the abdominal cavity, and it is carried by the prehepatic circulation to the hepatic portal vein and the liver. As a result, substances absorbed from the digestive tract can be more accurately controlled [22].

The above observations were confirmed by ZEN levels in blood samples collected from the MCV of cows with pyometra. These samples were characterized by the highest concentrations of ZEN (Figures 2–4). After ingestion, ZEN reaches the proximal and, subsequently, distal segments of the intestines, and it is transported to the liver by prehepatic vessels where it detoxifies from undesirable or dangerous substances as part of the functional circulation. The described hypothesis was also validated by the percentage share of average ZEN concentrations in blood samples collected from diseased cows. In blood sampled from cows with pyometra, the above parameter was determined at 57% (Figure 2), whereas in the remaining (posthepatic) sampling sites, ZEN concentrations (Figures 1 and 3) and their percentage share (Figures 2 and 4) were much lower because the analyzed mycotoxin had already been detoxified in the liver.

4. Materials and Methods

All experimental procedures were consistent with Polish regulations defining the conditions and methods of animal experimentation (opinion No. 01/2010/D issued on 21 December, 2016-by the Local Ethics Committee for Animal Experimentation of the University of Warmia and Mazury in Olsztyn, Poland).

4.1. Experimental Animals and Feed

The animals were kept in a barn with access to pasture. Blood for toxicological analyses was sampled from cows clinically diagnosed with mastitis (9 animals), ovarian cysts (6 animals), pyometra (5 animals) and from 9 asymptomatic cows (with no clinical symptoms).

The research lasted one year, and it involved 150 dairy cows that were free of clinical symptoms of ZEN mycotoxicosis. The milk yield (herd average) at the end of the last farming year was 9700 L per lactation 305 days (there was an upward trend). All cows are fed the fodder at the bunk feeding based on the average yield of the production group.

There are 3 production groups in the herd: (1)—the most efficient (approximately the first 150 days of lactation); (2)—from day 151 to the end of lactation; (3)—dry cows. The tested dairy cows health problems occurred only in Group 1. Groups 1 and 2 receive an additional amount of total mixed ration (TMR) at the feeding station, depending on their individual performance. Group 3 only receives feed at the bunk feeding. Total mixed ration for dairy cows for all animals in the barn was supplied by the same producer. TMR was administered twice a day, at 6:00 a.m. and 5:00 p.m., in a powdery form. The TMR composition declared by the manufacturer is presented in Table 1.

Table 1. Declared total mixed ration for caws.

The Feed Materials Used	
Maize, rapeseed extraction meal, soybean meal, wheat bran, triticale, distillation dried cereal and corn, dried and molasses beet pulp, sunflower meal, wheat mix, beetroot molasses, decoction of sugar beet molasses, rumen-protected fatty acid salts of plant origin, calcium carbonate, sodium chloride and niacin.	
Ingredients	Composition [1] Declared by the Manufacturer (%)
Barley middling's	36.5
Triticale middling's	18.5
Cornmeal	18.0
Post-extraction rapeseed meal	7.0
Post-extraction soybean meal	9.0
Protein concentrate R-056	9.0
Vitamin-mineral supplements [1]	2.0

[1] Composition of the vitamin-mineral supplements per kg: vitamin A—17,500.00 IU; vitamin D3—5000.00 IU; vitamin E (alpha-tocopherol)—100 mg; B3 (niacin)—400 mg; biotin—400.00 µg; iron (iron sulfate) —110 mg; manganese (manganese sulfate)—125 mg; zinc (zinc sulfate)—125 mg; copper ($CuSO_4 \cdot 5H_2O$)—20 mg; vitamin iodine (potassium iodide)—1.8 mg; selenium (sodium selenate)—0.35 mg; Seldox antioxidatum (BHA-E320, BHT-E321, Ethoxyquin E324)—0.95 mg; flavoring substances—0.5 g.

In addition to the presented TMR composition, the manufacturer also declared the share of components in TMRs for dairy cows, as shown in Table 2.

Table 2. Declared total analytical components in total mixed ration for caws.

Components	Analytical Components–Manufacturer's Declared Composition (%)
Crude protein	19.00
Crude fiber	6.50
Raw oils and fats	4.10
Crude ash	6.20
Sugar	7.50
Total calcium	0.80
Total phosphorus	0.60
General sodium	0.30
Total magnesium	0.30

The approximate chemical composition of the silage to dairy cows (Table 3) was determined using the NIRS™ DS2500 F Feed Analyzer (FOSS, Hillerød, Denmark) which is a monochromatic NIR reflectance and transflectance analyzer with scanning range of 850–2500 nm.

Table 3. The results of the silage analysis in g/kg dry metter.

Indicators	Haylage	Maize Silage
Dry matter	231.05	434.24
pH	6.19	4.52
Ammonia fraction	11.95	10.93
Crude protein	198.25	80.17
Crude fiber	285.09	180.49
Ash	99.12	47.20
Sugar	-	11.17
Starch	-	302.20

Table 3. Cont.

Indicators	Haylage	Maize Silage
Neutral Detergent Fiber (NDF)	504.62	386.37
Acid Detergent Fiber (ADF)	310.75	217.58
Acid Detergent Lignine (ADL)	10.17	22.52
Crude fat	32.50	29.99
Straw.mat org VOS	682.64	688.52
Neutral Detergent Insoluble Crude Protein (NDICP)	38.19	21.92
Acid Detergent Insoluble Crude Protein (ADICP)	9.18	7.53
Lactic acid	52.91	55.63
Volatile Fatty Acids (VFA)	248.88	133.69
Acetic acid	18.30	14.76
Butyric acid	3.05	-

4.2. Blood Sampling

In each cow, blood was sampled from three sites in the hepatic portal system [22]: (1) external jugular vein (EJV, *v. jugularis externa*-posthepatic); (2) abdominal subcutaneous vein (ASV, *v. epigastrica cranialis superficialis*-prehepatic); (3) median caudal vein (MCV, *v. caudalis mediana*-prehepatic). Blood samples of 10 mL each were collected from each site into vials containing 0.5 mL of heparin solution. The samples were centrifuged at 3000 rpm for 20 min at a temperature of 4 °C. The separated plasma was stored at −18 °C until sample analysis for the presence of ZEN (according to the schedule of the monitoring program).

4.3. Extraction Recovery

The standard addition (fortification) method was used to evaluate the recovery in this study. Non-contaminated sample matrix (blood serum) were enriched by three mycotoxins (ZEN, α-ZEL, β-ZEL) at low (5 pg/mL) medium (10 pg/mL) and high (20 pg/mL) concentrations and pretreated using the methodology outlined in Section 4.4. After analysis, the extraction recovery (ER) method was calculated as: ER = A/B × 100; where A is the slope of the fortified sample after extraction and B is the slope of the fortified sample before extraction. Recovery after extraction from fortified samples ranged from 90% to 102%, suggesting that the pretreatment method met the requirement for mycotoxin determination.

4.4. Mycotoxin Extraction

Zearalenone, α-ZEL and β-ZEL were extracted from the blood plasma with the use of immunoaffinity columns (Zearala-TestTM Zearalenone Testing System, G1012, VICAM, Watertown, MA, USA). All extraction procedures were conducted in accordance with the manufacturers' instructions. The eluates were placed in a water bath with a temperature of 50 °C, and the solvent was evaporated in a stream of nitrogen. Dry residues were combined with 0.5 mL of 99.8% methanol to dissolve the mycotoxins. The procedure were monitored with the use of external standards (Cayman Chemical 1180 East Ellsworth Road Ann Arbor, Michigan 48108 USA, ZEN-catalog number 11353; Batch 0593470-1; α-ZEN-catalog number 16549; Batch 0585633-2; β-ZEN-catalog number 19460; Batch 0604066-7), and the results were validated by mass spectrometry.

4.5. Chromatographic Analysis of ZEN and Its Metabolites

The concentrations of ZEN and its metabolites, α-ZEL and β-ZEL, were determined by the Institute of Dairy Industry Innovation in Mrągowo. Zearalenone and its metabolites were quantified in the blood plasma with the use of combined separation methods involving immunoaffinity columns (Zearala-TestTM Zearalenone Testing System, G1012, VICAM, Watertown, MA, USA), Agilent 1260 liquid chromatography (LC) system, and a mass spectrometry (MS, Agilent 6470) system. The prepared samples will be analyzed with the use of the Zorbax rapid resolution chromatographic column (2.1 × 50 mm; 1.8 micron Agilent Eclipse Plus C18) in gradient mode. The mobile phase will contain 0.1% (v/v)

formic acid in water (solvent A) and 0.1% (v/v) formic acid in acetonitrile (solvent B). Gradient conditions will be as follows: initially, 20% B that increases to 100% B in 4.0 min and back to 20% B in 0.1 min.

Mycotoxin concentrations were determined with an external standard and were expressed in ppt (pg/mL). Matrix-matched calibration standards were applied in the quantification process to eliminate matrix effects that can decrease sensitivity. Calibration standards were dissolved in matrix samples based on the procedure that was used to prepare the remaining samples. A signal-to-noise ratio of 3:1 will be used to estimate the limits of detection (LOD) for ZEN, α-ZEL and β-ZEL. The LOQ will be estimated as the triple LOD value.

4.6. Mass Spectrometric Conditions

The mass spectrometer was operate with ESI in the negative ion mode. The MS/MS parameters were opimized for each compoud. The linearity was tested by a calibration curve including six levels. Table 4 shows the optimized analysis conditions for the mycotoxins tested.

Table 4. Optimized conditions for mycotoxins tested.

Analyte	Precursor	Quantification Ion	Confirmation Ion	LOD (ng mL^{-1})	LOQ (ng mL^{-1})	Linearity (%R^2)
ZEN	317.1	273.3	187.1	0.03	0.1	0.999
α-ZEL	319.2	275.2	160.1	0.3	0.9	0.997
β-ZEL	319.2	275.2	160.1	0.3	1	0.993

4.7. Statistical Analysis

Statistical analyses were performed by the Department of Discrete Mathematics and Theoretical Computer Science, Faculty of Mathematics and Computer Science of the University of Warmia and Mazury in Olsztyn. Plasma concentrations of ZEN and its metabolites were determined in asymptomatic cows and in three groups of experimental cows: (1) with clinically diagnosed mastitis, (2) with clinically diagnosed ovarian cysts, and (3) with clinically diagnosed pyometra. In each cow, blood was sampled from three different sites. The results were expressed as means ($\bar{x}$) with standard deviation (SD). In both cases, the differences between mean values were determined by one-way ANOVA. If significant differences were noted between groups, the differences between paired means were determined in Tukey's multiple comparison test. If all values were below LOD (mean and variance equal zero) in any group, the values in the remaining groups were analyzed by one-way ANOVA (if the number of the remaining groups was higher than two), and the means in these groups were compared against zero by Student's t-test. Differences between groups were determined by Student's t-test. The results were regarded as highly significant at $p < 0.01$ (**) and as significant at $0.01 < p < 0.05$ (*). Data were processed statistically in Statistica v.13 (TIBCO Software Inc., Silicon Valley, CA, USA, 2017).

5. Conclusions

The results of this study suggest that blood samples for toxicological analyses should be collected from the MCV (prehepatic vessel) of clinically healthy cows and/or cows displaying subclinical symptoms of disease (ZEN mycotoxicosis). Blood sampled from the MCV improves the reliability of diagnosis of subclinical ZEN mycotoxicosis.

Author Contributions: W.B., M.G., Ł.Z. and M.T.G. designed the experiments. Data were analyzed and interpreted by W.B., M.G, M.M., E.O. and K.E.P. The manuscript was drafted and critically read by W.B., M.G., Ł.Z., A.N., A.B. and M.T.G. The manuscript was revised, read and approved by all authors. All authors have read and agreed to the published version of the manuscript.

Funding: The project was financially supported by the Minister of Science and Higher Education under the program entitled "Regional Initiative of Excellence" for the years 2019-2022 (project No. 010/RID/2018/19; amount of funding PLN 12,000,000).

Institutional Review Board Statement: Not applicable.

Informed Consent Statement: Not applicable.

Data Availability Statement: Not applicable.

Conflicts of Interest: The authors declare no conflict of interest.

References

1. Gajęcka, M.; Dabrowski, M.; Otrocka-Domagała, I.; Brzuzan, P.; Rykaczewska, A.; Cieplińska, K.; Barasińska, M.; Gajęcki, M.T.; Zielonka, Ł. Correlations between exposure to deoxynivalenol and zearalenone and the immunohistochemical expression of estrogen receptors in the intestinal epithelium and the *m*RNA expression of selected colonic enzymes in pre-pubertal gilts. *Toxicon* **2020**, *173*, 75–93. [CrossRef]
2. Zhang, W.; Zhang, L.; Jiang, X.; Liu, X.; Li, Y.; Zhang, Y. Enhanced adsorption removal of aflatoxin B_1, zearalenone and deoxynivalenol from dairy cow rumen fluid by modified nano-montmorillonite and evaluation of its mechanism. *Anim. Feed Sci. Tech.* **2020**, *259*, 114366. [CrossRef]
3. McGuffey, R.K. A 100-Year Review: Metabolic modifiers in dairy cattle nutrition. *J. Dairy Sci.* **2017**, *100*, 10113–10142. [CrossRef] [PubMed]
4. Dänicke, S.; Bannert, E.; Tesch, T.; Kersten, S.; Frahm, J.; Bühler, S.; Sauerwein, H.; Görs, S.; Kahlert, S.; Rothkötter, H.J.; et al. Oral exposure of pigs to the mycotoxin deoxynivalenol does not modulate the hepatic albumin synthesis during a LPS-induced acute-phase reaction. *Innate. Immun.* **2020**, *26*, 716–732. [CrossRef] [PubMed]
5. Gruber-Dorninger, C.; Faas, J.; Doupovec, B.; Aleschko, M.; Stoiber, C.; Höbartner-Gußl, A.; Schöndorfer, K.; Killinger, M.; Zebeli, Q.; Schatzmayr, D. Metabolism of zearalenone in the rumen of dairy cows with and without application of a zearalenone-degrading enzyme. *Toxins* **2021**, *13*, 84. [CrossRef] [PubMed]
6. Muñoz-Solano, B.; González-Peñas, E. Mycotoxin determination in animal feed: An LC-FLD method for simultaneous quantification of aflatoxins, ochratoxins and zearelanone in this matrix. *Toxins* **2020**, *12*, 374. [CrossRef] [PubMed]
7. Mahato, D.K.; Devi, S.; Pandhi, S.; Sharma, B.; Maurya, K.K.; Mishra, S.; Dhawan, K.; Selvakumar, R.; Kamle, M.; Mishra, A.K.; et al. Occurrence, impact on agriculture, human health, and management strategies of zearalenone in food and feed: A review. *Toxins* **2021**, *13*, 92. [CrossRef] [PubMed]
8. Rykaczewska, A.; Gajęcka, M.; Dąbrowski, M.; Wiśniewska, A.; Szcześniewska, J.; Gajęcki, M.T.; Zielonka, Ł. Growth performance, selected blood biochemical parameters and body weight of pre-pubertal gilts fed diets supplemented with different doses of zearalenone (ZEN). *Toxicon* **2018**, *152*, 84–94. [CrossRef]
9. Rykaczewska, A.; Gajęcka, M.; Onyszek, E.; Cieplińska, K.; Dąbrowski, M.; Lisieska-Żołnierczyk, S.; Bulińska, M.; Babuchowski, A.; Gajęcki, M.T.; Zielonka, Ł. Imbalance in the blood concentrations of selected steroids in prepubertal gilts depending on the time of exposure to low doses of zearalenone. *Toxins* **2019**, *11*, 561. [CrossRef]
10. Zachariasova, M.; Dzumana, Z.; Veprikova, Z.; Hajkovaa, K.; Jiru, M.; Vaclavikova, M.; Zachariasova, A.; Pospichalova, M.; Florian, M.; Hajslova, J. Occurrence of multiple mycotoxins in European feeding stuffs, assessment of dietary intake by farm animals. *Anim. Feed Sci. Tech.* **2014**, *193*, 124–140. [CrossRef]
11. Gajęcka, M.; Zielonka, Ł.; Gajęcki, M. Activity of zearalenone in the porcine intestinal tract. *Molecules* **2017**, *22*, 18. [CrossRef] [PubMed]
12. Dunbar, B.; Patel, M.; Fahey, J.; Wira, C. Endocrine control of mucosal immunity in the female reproductive tract: Impact of environmental disruptors. *Mol. Cell. Endocrinol.* **2012**, *354*, 85–93. [CrossRef]
13. Frizzell, C.; Ndossi, D.; Verhaegen, S.; Dahl, E.; Eriksen, G.; Sørlie, M.; Ropstad, E.; Muller, M.; Elliott, C.T.; Connolly, L. Endocrine disrupting effects of zearalenone, alpha- and beta-zearalenol at the level of nuclear receptor binding and steroidogenesis. *Toxicol. Lett.* **2011**, *206*, 210–217. [CrossRef]
14. Kolle, S.N.; Ramirez, T.; Kamp, H.G.; Buesen, R.; Flick, B.; Strauss, V.; van Ravenzwaay, B. A testing strategy for the identification of mammalian, systemic endocrine disruptors with particular focus on steroids. *Regul. Toxicol. Pharm.* **2012**, *63*, 259–278. [CrossRef]
15. Cieplińska, K.; Gajęcka, M.; Dąbrowski, M.; Rykaczewska, A.; Zielonka, Ł.; Lisieska-Żołnierczyk, S.; Bulińska, M.; Gajęcki, M.T. Time-dependent changes in the intestinal microbiome of gilts exposed to low zearalenone doses. *Toxins* **2019**, *11*, 296. [CrossRef] [PubMed]
16. Marchais-Oberwinkler, S.; Henn, C.; Moller, G.; Klein, T.; Negri, M.; Oster, A.; Spadaro, A.; Werth, R.; Wetzel, M.; Xu, K.; et al. 17β-Hydroxysteroid dehydrogenases (17β-HSDs) as therapeutic targets: Protein structures, functions, and recent progress in inhibitor development. *J. Steroid. Biochem.* **2011**, *125*, 66–82. [CrossRef]
17. Vandenberg, L.N.; Colborn, T.; Hayes, T.B.; Heindel, J.J.; Jacobs, D.R.; Lee, D.-H.; Shioda, T.; Soto, A.M.; vom Saal, F.S.; Welshons, W.V.; et al. Hormones and endocrine-disrupting chemicals: Low-dose effects and nonmonotonic dose responses. *Endoc. Rev.* **2012**, *33*, 378–455. [CrossRef] [PubMed]

18. Kowalska, K.; Habrowska-Górczyńska, D.E.; Piastowska-Ciesielska, A. Zearalenone as an endocrine disruptor in humans. *Environ. Toxicol. Phar.* **2016**, *48*, 141–149. [CrossRef] [PubMed]
19. Grenier, B.; Applegate, T.J. Modulation of intestinal functions following mycotoxin ingestion: Meta-analysis of published experiments in animals. *Toxins* **2013**, *5*, 396–430. [CrossRef] [PubMed]
20. Calabrese, E.J. Hormesis: Path and progression to significance. *Int. J. Mol. Sci.* **2018**, *19*, 2871. [CrossRef] [PubMed]
21. Hickey, G.L.; Craig, P.S.; Luttik, R.; de Zwart, D. On the quantification of intertest variability in ecotoxicity data with application to species sensitivity distributions. *Environ. Toxicol. Chem.* **2012**, *31*, 1903–1910. [CrossRef]
22. Hebel, M.; Niedzielski, D. Computed tomography in the diagnosis of portal vascular anastomosis in dogs. *Wet. Prakt.* **2017**, *4*, 1–4.
23. Debevere, S.; Cools, A.; De Baere, S.; Haesaert, G.; Rychlik, M.; Croubels, S.; Fievez, V. In vitro rumen simulations show a reduced disappearance of deoxynivalenol, nivalenol and enniatin B at conditions of rumen acidosis and lower microbial activity. *Toxins* **2020**, *12*, 101. [CrossRef] [PubMed]
24. Sotnichenko, A.; Pantsov, E.; Shinkarev, D.; Okhanov, V. Hydrophobized reversed-phase adsorbent for protection of dairy cattle against lipophilic toxins from diet. efficiensy in vitro and in vivo. *Toxins* **2019**, *11*, 256. [CrossRef]
25. Fushimi, Y.; Takagi, M.; Monniaux, D.; Uno, S.; Kokushi, E.; Shinya, U.; Kawashima, C.; Otoi, T.; Deguchi, E.; Fink-Gremmels, J. Effects of dietary contamination by zearalenone and its metabolites on serum anti-Müllerian hormone: Impact on the reproductive performance of breeding cows. *Reprod. Domest. Anim.* **2015**, *50*, 834–839. [CrossRef]
26. He, J.; Wei, C.; Li, Y.; Liu, Y.; Wang, Y.; Pan, J.; Liu, J.; Wu, Y.; Cui, S. Zearalenone and alpha-zearalenol inhibit the synthesis and secretion of pig follicle stimulating hormone via the non-classical estrogen membrane receptor GPR30. *Mol. Cell. Endocrinol.* **2018**, *461*, 43–54. [CrossRef] [PubMed]
27. Sharma, R.P.; Schuhmacher, M.; Kumar, V. Review on crosstalk and common mechanisms of endocrine disruptors: Scaffolding to improve PBPK/PD model of EDC mixture. *Environ. Int.* **2017**, *99*, 1–14. [CrossRef]
28. Ida, T.; Fujiwara, H.; Taniguchi, Y.; Kohyama, A. Longitudinal assessment of anti-Müllerian hormone after cesarean section and influence of bilateral salpingectomy on ovarian reserve. *Contraception* **2021**. [CrossRef] [PubMed]
29. Xu, H.; Zhang, M.; Zhang, H.; Alpadi, K.; Wang, L.; Li, R.; Qiao, J. Clinical applications of serum anti-müllerian hormone measurements in both males and females: An update. *Innovation* **2021**, *2*, 100091. [CrossRef]
30. Gajęcka, M. The effect of low-dose experimental zearalenone intoxication on the immunoexpression of estrogen receptors in the ovaries of pre-pubertal bitches. *Pol. J. Vet. Sci.* **2012**, *15*, 685–691. [CrossRef]
31. Liu, X.L.; Wu, R.Y.; Sun, X.F.; Cheng, S.F.; Zhang, R.Q.; Zhang, T.Y.; Zhang, X.F.; Zhao, Y.; Shen, W.; Li, L. Mycotoxin zearalenone exposure impairs genomic stability of swine follicular granulosa cells in vitro. *Int. J. Biol. Sci.* **2018**, *14*, 294–305. [CrossRef] [PubMed]
32. Zheng, W.; Feng, N.; Wang, Y.; Noll, L.; Xu, S.; Liu, X.; Lu, N.; Zou, H.; Gu, J.; Yuan, Y.; et al. Effects of zearalenone and its derivatives on the synthesis and secretion of mammalian sex steroid hormones: A review. *Food Chem. Toxicol.* **2019**, *126*, 262–276. [CrossRef]
33. Gajęcka, M.; Woźny, M.; Brzuzan, P.; Zielonka, Ł.; Gajęcki, M. Expression of CYPscc and 3β-HSD mRNA in bitches ovary after long-term exposure to zearalenone. *Bull. Vet. Inst. Puławy* **2011**, *55*, 777–780.
34. Engeli, R.T.; Rohrer, S.R.; Vuorinen, A.; Herdlinger, S.; Kaserer, T.; Leugger, S.; Schuster, D.; Odermatt, A. Interference of paraben compounds with estrogen metabolism by inhibition of 17β-hydroxysteroid dehydrogenases. *Int. J. Mol. Sci.* **2017**, *18*, 2007.
35. Bayala, B.; Zoure, A.A.; Baron, S.; de Joussineau, C.; Simpore, J.; Lobaccaro, J.M.A. Pharmacological modulation of steroid activity in hormone-dependent breast and prostate cancers: Effect of some plant extract derivatives. *Int. J. Mol. Sci.* **2020**, *21*, 3690. [CrossRef]
36. Dänicke, S.; Matthäus, K.; Lebzien, P.; Valenta, H.; Stemme, K.; Ueberschär, K.-H.; Razzazi-Fazeli, E.; Böhm, J.; Flachowsky, G. Effects of Fusarium toxin-contaminated wheat grain on nutrient turnover, microbial protein synthesis and metabolism of deoxynivalenol and zearalenone in the rumen of dairy cows. *J. Anim. Physiol. Anim. Nutr.* **2005**, *89*, 303–315. [CrossRef] [PubMed]
37. Marczuk, J.; Obremski, K.; Lutnicki, K.; Gajęcka, M.; Gajęcki, M. Zearalenone and deoxynivalenol mycotoxicosis in dairy cattle herds. *Pol. J. Vet. Sci.* **2012**, *15*, 365–372. [CrossRef] [PubMed]
38. Benagiano, M.; Bianchi, P.; D'Elios, M.M.; Brosens, I.; Benagiano, G. Autoimmune diseases: Role of steroid hormones. *Best. Pract. Res. Cl. Ob.* **2019**, *60*, 24–34. [CrossRef]
39. Khafipour, E.; Li, S.; Plaizier, J.C.; Krause, D.O. Rumen microbiome composition determined using two nutritional models of subacute ruminal acidosis. *Appl. Environ. Microbiol.* **2009**, *75*, 7115–7124. [CrossRef]

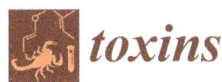

Article

Concentration of Zearalenone, Alpha-Zearalenol and Beta-Zearalenol in the Myocardium and the Results of Isometric Analyses of the Coronary Artery in Prepubertal Gilts

Magdalena Gajęcka [1,*], Michał S. Majewski [2], Łukasz Zielonka [1], Waldemar Grzegorzewski [3,4], Ewa Onyszek [5], Sylwia Lisieska-Żołnierczyk [6], Jerzy Juśkiewicz [7], Andrzej Babuchowski [5] and Maciej T. Gajęcki [1]

[1] Department of Veterinary Prevention and Feed Hygiene, Faculty of Veterinary Medicine, University of Warmia and Mazury in Olsztyn, Oczapowskiego 13/29, 10-718 Olsztyn, Poland; lukaszz@uwm.edu.pl (Ł.Z.); gajecki@uwm.edu.pl (M.T.G.)
[2] Department of Pharmacology and Toxicology, Faculty of Medical Sciences, University of Warmia and Mazury in Olsztyn, Warszawska 30, 10-082 Olsztyn, Poland; michal.majewski@uwm.edu.pl
[3] Institute of Biology and Biotechnology, College of Natural Sciences, University of Rzeszów, Pigonia 1, 35-310 Rzeszow, Poland; wgrzegorzewski@ur.edu.pl
[4] Interdisciplinary Center for Preclinical and Clinical Research, Department of Biotechnology, Institute of Biol-ogy and Biotechnology, College of Natural Sciences, University of Rzeszów, Pigonia 1, 35-310 Rzeszow, Po-land
[5] Dairy Industry Innovation Institute Ltd., Kormoranów 1, 11-700 Mrągowo, Poland; ewa.onyszek@iipm.pl (E.O.); andrzej.babuchowski@iipm.pl (A.B.)
[6] Independent Public Health Care Centre of the Ministry of the Interior and Administration, and the Warmia and Mazury Oncology Centre in Olsztyn, Wojska Polskiego 37, 10-228 Olsztyn, Poland; lisieska@wp.pl
[7] Department of Biological Function of Foods, Institute of Animal Reproduction and Food Research, Division of Food Science, Tuwima 10, 10-748 Olsztyn, Poland; j.juskiewicz@pan.olsztyn.pl
* Correspondence: mgaja@uwm.edu.pl

Abstract: The carry-over of zearalenone (ZEN) to the myocardium and its effects on coronary vascular reactivity in vivo have not been addressed in the literature to date. Therefore, the objective of this study was to verify the hypothesis that low ZEN doses (MABEL, NOAEL and LOAEL) administered per os to prepubertal gilts for 21 days affect the accumulation of ZEN, α-ZEL and β-ZEL in the myocardium and the reactivity of the porcine coronary arteries to vasoconstrictors: acetylcholine, potassium chloride and vasodilator sodium nitroprusside. The contractile response to acetylcholine in the presence of a cyclooxygenase (COX) inhibitor, indomethacin and / or an endothelial nitric oxide synthase (e-NOS) inhibitor, L-NAME was also studied. The results of this study indicate that the carry-over of ZEN and its metabolites to the myocardium is a highly individualized process that occurs even at very low mycotoxin concentrations. The concentrations of the accumulated ZEN metabolites are inversely proportional to each other due to biotransformation processes. The levels of vasoconstrictors, acetylcholine and potassium chloride, were examined in the left anterior descending branch of the porcine coronary artery after oral administration of ZEN. The LOAEL dose clearly decreased vasoconstriction in response to both potassium chloride and acetylcholine ($P < 0.05$ for all values) and increased vasodilation in the presence of sodium nitroprusside ($P = 0.021$). The NOAEL dose significantly increased vasoconstriction caused by acetylcholine ($P < 0.04$), whereas the MABEL dose did not cause significant changes in the vascular response. Unlike higher doses of ZEN, 5 µg/kg had no negative influence on the vascular system.

Keywords: zearalenone; low doses; carry-over; myocardium; vascular reactivity

Key Contribution: The concentrations of ZEN and its metabolites in the myocardium decreased proportionally to the applied dose; and they were comparable with the levels determined in the blood. The ZEN dose and the time of exposure limit the increase in the concentrations of selected metabolites in the myocardium. Zearalenone and its metabolites target the smooth muscles of porcine coronary arteries. The analyzed mycotoxin regulates the synthesis of nitric oxide and modulates its bioavailability.

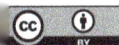

1. Introduction

Zearalenone and its metabolites, á-zearalenol (á-ZEL) and â-zearalenol (â-ZEL), are commonly encountered in plant materials [1]. Since their structure resembles that of estradiol, mycotoxins contribute to reproductive disorders [2–4]. Alpha-zearalenol is the main ZEN metabolite that affects pigs. Other animal species (such as broiler chickens, cows and sheep) are more susceptible to β-ZEL whose metabolic activity is lower [5]. The activity of ZEN is determined by biotransformation processes in plants [6] and animals [7], the immune status [8–10] of the reproductive system (during puberty, reproductive cycle and pregnancy—due to changes in steroid hormones concentrations) [11–13] and the digestive system of animals exposed to this mycotoxin [3,4,14,15].

Different doses of mycotoxins exert various effects [4,15]. Both the symptoms and health (toxicological) effects of high doses of most mycotoxins have been extensively studied [16]. Animals can tolerate long-term exposure to low monotonic doses of mycotoxins [3,17] which actually may serve vital life needs [9,18–21] or therapeutic purposes [22]. However, low mycotoxin doses may also have a negative impact on health [23]. A low dose [24] was defined in our previous clinical studies [15,25,26] based on the presence or absence of clinical symptoms of ongoing ZEN mycotoxicosis (e.g., changes in estradiol, progesterone or testosterone levels [4], changes in blood biochemical parameters and body weight [15,17] or quantitative and qualitative changes in the intestinal microbiome [3,26]). Three doses were identified based on the results of our previous research and other authors' findings: the lowest observed adverse effect level (LOAEL, >10 μg ZEN/kg BW) [3,12,27] dose which causes clinical symptoms [28]; the highest no observed adverse effect level (NOAEL, 10 μg ZEN/kg BW) [29] dose, also referred to as the maximum safe starting dose [24], which does not cause clinical symptoms (subclinical states); and the minimal anticipated biological effect level (MABEL, <10 μg ZEN/kg BW) dose, namely the lowest measurable dose [24] or the effective in vivo dose that positively interacts with the host organism in various stages of life, and produces measurable effects without any side effects [24].

The dose-response relationship has been undermined by the low-dose hypothesis, especially with respect to chemical compounds exhibiting hormonal activity [30] such as ZEN-type mycoestrogen and its metabolites, which are endocrine disruptors (EDs) even when administered in low doses [13]. The dose-response relationship does not permit a direct analysis / meta-analysis of the risk (clinical symptoms or the results of laboratory tests) resulting from the transition from high to low doses [31]. The concept of the lowest identifiable dose, namely a dose that produces an effect contrary to the expected outcome, is gaining increasing popularity in biomedical sciences. The associated mechanisms have to be investigated to support decision making in selected processes [15,32].

Substances that can contribute to both maintaining and disrupting homeostasis have challenged the traditional concepts in toxicology, particularly "the dose makes the poison" adage. Zearalenone and its metabolites (ZELs) have been found to evoke different responses when administered in low doses to mammals [3], which has also been reported by Knutsen et al. [23]. According to the Scientific Panel on Contaminants in the Food Chain (CONTAM), the impact of ZEN on the health status of animals needs to re-evaluated, taking into account the responses of different animal species to the lowest detectable doses of ZEN (LOAEL, NOAEL, MABEL) [23,33,34] found in feed, including both the parent compound and its derivatives [15].

Our previous research revealed that ZEN accelerates eryptosis, namely the apoptosis of red blood cells. Due to its mechanism of action [15,35], ZEN increases intracellular Ca^{2+} [35–37] levels, induces oxidative stress and decreases energy resources [38]. These responses are linked with the pathogenesis of anemia and microcirculatory disorders. Microcirculatory disorders are observed in various tissues during exposure to ZEN, as manifested by numerous extravasations and the presence of vessels with dilated lumina and multiple extravasations [20,39] in prepubertal female mammals. The observed changes prompted the hypothesis that ZEN and/or its metabolites can act as vasodilators in the presence of vasoconstrictors [40,41]. Therefore, the objective of this study was to determine whether exposure to low doses of ZEN (MABEL, NOAEL—the highest dose and LOAEL—one of the lowest doses) administered per os to prepubertal gilts for 21 days reach the myocardium and induces changes in reactivity in response to vasoconstrictors (acetylcholine and potassium chloride) and vasodilators (sodium nitroprusside) in the left anterior descending branch of the coronary artery.

2. Results

2.1. Experimental Feed

The feed analyzed in this experiment did not contain any mycotoxins, or its mycotoxin content was below the sensitivity of the method (VBS). The concentrations of modified and masked mycotoxins were not analyzed.

2.2. Clinical Observations

Experimental animals did not exhibit the clinical signs of ZEN mycotoxicosis were not observed during the experiment. However, changes in specific tissues or cells were frequently noted in analyses of selected serum biochemical profiles, genotoxicity of cecal water, selected steroid concentrations and intestinal microbiota parameters in samples collected from the same animals and in analyses of the animals' growth performance. The results of these analyses were presented in our previous studies [3,4,15,25,26].

2.3. Concentrations of Zearalenone and Its Metabolites in the Heart Muscle

In general, the concentrations of ZEN and its metabolites in the myocardium of prepubertal gilts did not differ significantly between analytical dates or experimental groups (Table 1).

Table 1. The carry-over factor and the mean ($\bar{x}$) concentrations of ZEN and its metabolites (α-ZEL and β-ZEL) (ng/g) in the myocardium of prepubertal gilts.

Weeks of Exposure	Feed Intake [kg/day]	Total doses of ZEN in Groups Respectively [µg/kg BW]	Group E1 [ng/g] (%)	Carry-over Factor	Group E2 [ng/g]/(%)	Carry-over Factor	Group E3 [ng/g]/(%)	Carry-over Factor
				Zearalenone				
D1	0.8	80.5/161.9/242.7	0.691 ± 0.635 (100%)	8×10^{-6}	2.275 ± 2.22 (86.69%)	14×10^{-6}	1.387 ± 1.93(78.22%)	17×10^{-6}
D2	1.1	101.01/196.9/298.2	0.977 ± 0.579 (73.62%)	9×10^{-6}	2.621 ± 1.499 (91.48%)	13×10^{-6}	4.89 ± 4.405(93.42%)	16×10^{-6}
				α-ZEL				
D1	not applicable	not applicable	0.0 ± 0.0 (0%)	0	0.316 ± 0.061 (12.04%)	19×10^{-7}	0.353 ± 0.104(19.9%)	14×10^{-7}
D2	not applicable	not applicable	0.146 ± 0.143 (11%)	14×10^{-7}	0.167 ± 0.146 (5.82%)	1×10^{-6}	0.312 ± 0.213(5.96%)	1×10^{-6}
				β-ZEL				
D1	not applicable	not applicable	0.0 ± 0.0 (0%)	0	0.033 ± 0.029 (1.25%)	2×10^{-7}	0.033 ± 0.004(1.86%)	1×10^{-7}
D2	not applicable	not applicable	0.204 ± 0.046 (15.37%)	2×10^{-6}	0.077 ± 0.017 **(2.68%)	4×10^{-7}	0.032 ± 0.004 **(0.61%)	1×10^{-7}

Abbreviation: D1—exposure day 7; D2—exposure day 21. Experimental groups: Group E1—5 µg ZEN/kg BW; Group E2—10 µg ZEN/kg BW; Group E3—15 µg ZEN/kg BW. LOD > values below the limit of detection were expressed as 0. The results were regarded as highly significant at $P < 0.01$ (**).

Highly significant difference in the concentrations of β-ZEL was noted on D2 (exposure day 21) between group E1 (5 µg ZEN/kg BW) (0.204 ng/g—highest value) vs. groups E2 (10 µg ZEN/kg BW) and E3 (15 µg ZEN/kg BW) (difference of 0.127 and 0.172 ng/g, respectively). On the remaining days of the experiment, relatively high but not statistically significant differences were observed between mean values ($\bar{x}$). On D1 (exposure day 7), ZEN levels were lowest in group E1 and highest in E2, i.e., they were inversely proportional to the administered dose. The concentrations of ZEN metabolites were proportional to the applied dose. The proportionality of ZEN and α-ZEL concentrations relative to the administered dose was maintained in the apex of the heart on D2. In contrast, β-ZEL concentrations were highest in group E1, lower in group E2 and lowest in group E3.

Carry-Over Factor

The carry-over factor (CF) was calculated to determine the release of ZEN and its metabolites from the gastrointestinal tract and their absorption and, possibly, distribution [4] to, e.g., the myocardium of prepubertal gilts. The CF values for ZEN (Table 1) in the myocardium were determined in the range of 8×10^{-6} in group E1 on D1 to 16×10^{-6} in group E3 on D2. The CF values for α-ZEL ranged from 0.0 in group E1 to 14×10^{-7} in group E2 on D1, and from 1×10^{-6} in groups E2 and E3 to 14×10^{-7} in group E1 on D2 (ZEN 5). The CF for β-ZEL ranged from 0.0 in group E1 to 2×10^{-7} in group E2 on D1, and from 1×10^{-7} in group E3 to 2×10^{-6} in group E1 on D2. These values were proportionally lower than the values noted in other tissues (not in the heart muscle) during exposure to higher doses of ZEN [17,21,42–44].

2.4. Vascular Reactivity Analyses

Porcine coronary arteries (PCAs) contracted in response to KCl within the concentration range of 2.5 to 30 mM (Figure 1A–D). The calculated D1$_{AUC}$ values were: $\frac{E1}{control} = 1.61$, $P < 0.05$; $\frac{E2}{control} = 1.84$, $P < 0.01$; $\frac{E3}{control} = 0.54$, $P < 0.001$, meanwhile D2$_{AUC}$ ratio was: $\frac{E1}{control} = 1.38$, $P = 0.6$, $\frac{E2}{control} = 1.00$, $P = 0.9$, $\frac{E3}{control} = 0.39$, $P < 0.001$ (Figure 1B). A significant difference in the contractile response on $\frac{D2}{D1} AUC$ was noted only in E2 vessels (0.53-fold, $P < 0.01$), but not in the control (0.97-fold, $P = 0.8$), E1 (0.83-fold, $P = 0.6$) and E3 (0.70-fold, $P = 0.15$).

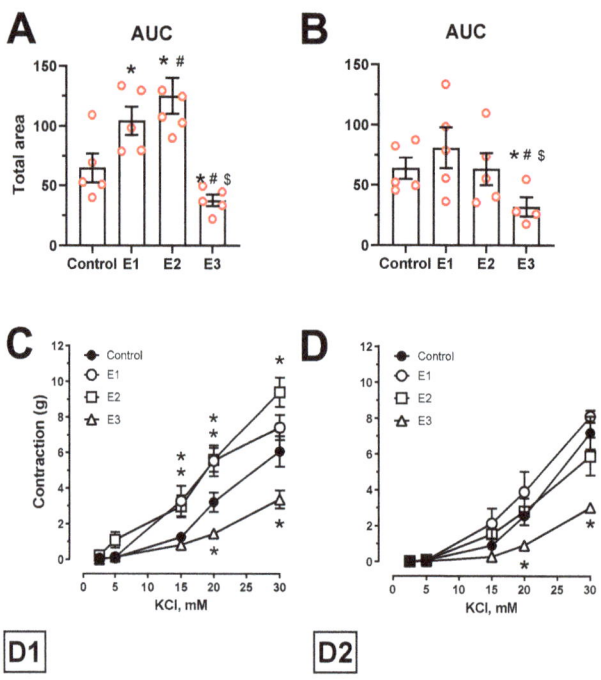

Figure 1. The effect of varying doses of ZEN (E1 = 5, E2 = 10, E3 = 15 µg ZEN/kg BW) on the cumulative contraction to KCl (2.5 to 30 mM) on exposure days D1 (7th day) (**A,C**) and D2 (21st day) (**B,D**). The results (means ± SEM) are expressed as AUC (**A,B**) and as a cumulative concentration-response curve in as grams of tension of porcine coronary arteries (**C,D**). $n = 5$. * $P < 0.05$ vs. control, # $P < 0.05$ vs. E1, $ $P < 0.05$ vs. E2 (two-way ANOVA, followed by Tukey's post-hoc test). Decreased contractile-response to KCl was observed in group E3 figure in D1 and D2 only. The effect of E1 and E2 was temporary and was limited to a shorter exposure (D1).

Acetylcholine concentrations of 10^{-7} to 10^{-5} M induced significant contraction of porcine coronary arteries (Figure 2A–D and Table 2). The calculated $D1_{AUC}$ values were based on the AUC (Figure 2A): $\frac{E1}{control} = 0.57$, $P < 0.01$; $\frac{E2}{control} = 1.33$, $P < 0.05$; $\frac{E3}{control} = 0.27$, $P < 0.001$ and $D2_{AUC}$: $\frac{E1}{control} = 0.49$, $P < 0.001$; $\frac{E2}{control} = 1.15$, $P < 0.6$; $\frac{E3}{control} = 0.25$, $P < 0.001$ (Figure 2B). No significant differences in the $\frac{D2}{D1} AUC$ ratio was observed on the control (0.98-fold), E1 (0.83-fold), E2 (0.85-fold) and E3 (0.91-fold), all P values ≥ 0.8.

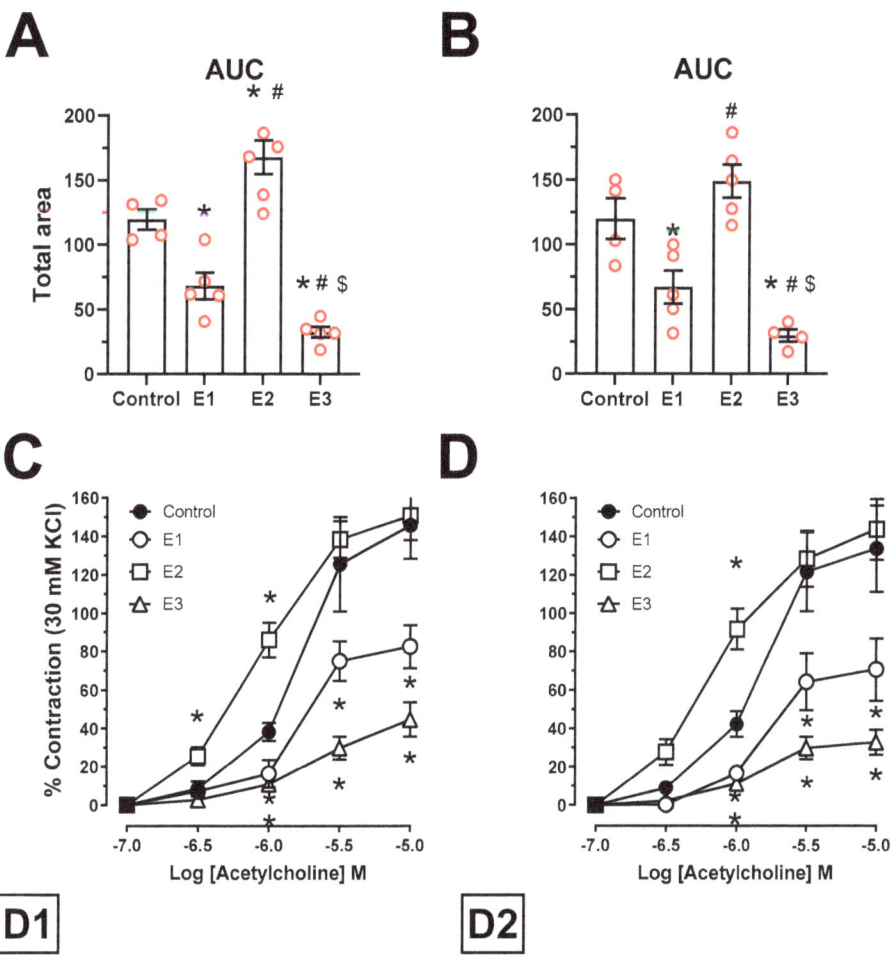

Figure 2. The effect of varying doses of ZEN (E1 = 5, E2 = 10, E3 = 15 µg ZEN/kg BW) on the cumulative contractions to acetylcholine on exposure day D1 (7th day) (**A**,**C**) and D2 (21st day) (**B**,**D**). The results (means ± SEM) are expressed as AUC (**A**,**B**) and as a cumulative concentration-response curve of the percentage inhibition of the contraction induced by 30 mM KCl of porcine coronary arteries (**C**,**D**). n = 5. * $P < 0.05$ vs. control, # $P < 0.05$ vs. E1, $ $P < 0.05$ vs. E2 (two-way ANOVA, followed by Tukey's post-hoc test). Both E1 and E3 decreased the contractile-response to acetylcholine in D1 and in D2. E2 modulated the response in D1 and this was not observed after longer exposure (in D2).

Table 2. Changes in vasoconstriction induced by acetylcholine and changes in vasodilatation induced by sodium nitroprusside (%) in porcine coronary arteries (expressed by AUC, E_{max} and pD_2 values).

	Control			Group E1			Group E2			Group E3		
	AUC	E_{max} (%)	pD_2	AUC	E_{max} (%)	pD_2	AUC	E_{max} (%)	pD_2	AUC	E_{max} (%)	pD_2
D_1ACh	122.6 ± 15.01	147.8 ± 11.33	5.801 ± 0.077	69.93 ± 11.20*	82.87 ± 7.853*	5.788 ± 0.103	162.6 ± 14.58*	155.1 ± 10.69	6.087 ± 0.074	32.73 ± 6.205*	51.08 ± 13.19*	5.606 ± 0.210
D_2ACh	119.8 ± 19.10	135 ± 15.39	5.859 ± 0.112	58.29 ± 13.33*	70.89 ± 10.28*	5.831 ± 0.149	137.6 ± 9.264	111.3 ± 10.30	6.263 ± 0.101*	29.81 ± 5.434*	33.13 ± 4.47*	5.876 ± 0.129
D_1SNP	137.5 ± 10.36	76.9 ± 5.03	5.469 ± 0.2543	116.3 ± 21.18	67.74 ± 9.994	5.605 ± 0.433	128.6 ± 14.23	89.5 ± 5.012	5.217 ± 0.153	134.3 ± 12.20	97.78 ± 7.674	4.952 ± 0.175
D_2SNP	101.6 ± 18.32	79.99 ± 6.529	5.171 ± 0.175	74.25 ± 11.65*	60.12 ± 8.205*	4.833 ± 0.273	110.5 ± 13.74	93.53 ± 5.480	4.963 ± 0.116	141.7 ± 12.62*	97.78 ± 7.674*	4.952 ± 0.175

Abbreviations: AUC, area under the dose-response curve; E_{max}, maximal response values; pD_2, drug concentration exhibiting 50% of the Emax expressed as the negative log molar; SNP, sodium nitroprusside. Values are expressed as mean ± S.E.M. *$P < 0.05$ vs. the control group (one-way ANOVA, followed by Tukey's post-hoc test).

Sodium nitroprusside (10^{-7}–10^{-4} M) caused a concentration-dependent relaxation of PCAs (Figure 3A,B and Table 2), with the onset at 10^{-7} M and maximal response at 10^{-4} M (Figure 3C,D). The calculated $D1_{AUC}$ values were: $\frac{E1}{control} = 0.85$, $P = 0.5$; $\frac{E2}{control} = 0.94$, $P = 0.8$; $\frac{E3}{control} = 1.03$, $P = 0.9$ $D2_{AUC}$: $\frac{E1}{control} = 0.73$, $P < 0.05$; $\frac{E2}{control} = 1.09$, $P = 0.8$; $\frac{E3}{control} = 1.39$, $P < 0.01$ (Figure 3B). A significant difference in the $\frac{D2}{D1}AUC$ was noted in E1 (0.64-fold, $P < 0.05$). This was not observed for the control (0.74-fold, $P = 0.6$), E2 (0.86-fold, $P = 0.8$) and E3 (0.948-fold, $P = 0.9$).

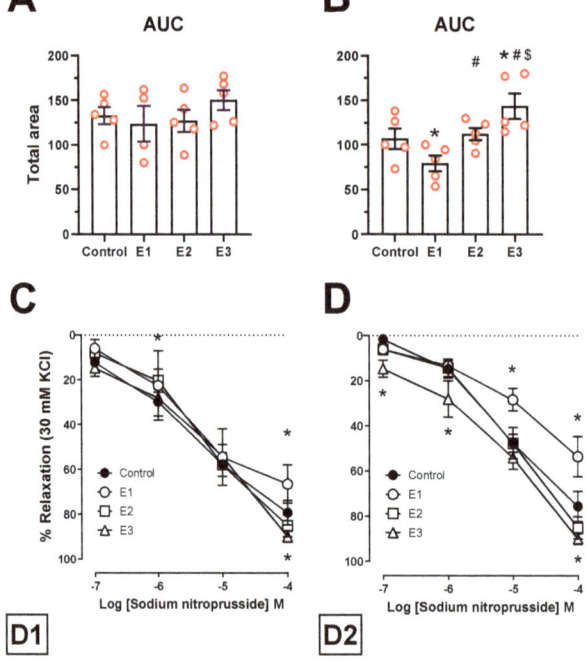

Figure 3. The effect of different doses of ZEN (E1 = 5, E2 = 10, E3 = 15 µg ZEN/kg BW) on the cumulative contractions to sodium nitroprusside (SNP) on exposure day D1 (7th day) (**A,C**) and D2 (21st day) (**B,D**). The results (means ± SEM) are expressed as AUC (**A,B**) and as a cumulative concentration-response curve of the percentage inhibition of the contraction induced by 30 mM KCl of porcine coronary arteries (**C,D**). $n = 5$. * $P < 0.05$ vs. control, # $P < 0.05$ vs. E1, $ $P < 0.05$ vs. E2 (two-way ANOVA, followed by Tukey's post-hoc test). An enhanced relaxant-response was observed in the E3 group in D2 only. In the E1 group decreased response was observed in term of longer exposure (D2).

The calculated AUC, Emax (%) and pD2 for acetylcholine and sodium nitroprusside are presented in Table 2.

Neither L-NAME (4.4×10^{-5} M) nor indomethacin (4.4×10^{-6} M) had a significant effect on baseline vascular tone (data not presented). Indomethacin did not affect arterial sensitivity to acetylcholine in control PCA (0.80, $P > 0.3$), but it decreased the response in E1 (0.55, $P < 0.001$) and E2 (0.74, $P < 0.01$), and potentiated the response in E3 (2.39, $P < 0.0001$; Figure 4). L-NAME increased the sensitivity of the PCA to acetylcholine in all studied groups: control (1.36, $P < 0.05$), E1 (2.48, $P < 0.001$), E2 (1.29, $P < 0.01$) and E3 (3.39, $P < 0.001$). Only in E3, preincubation with both indomethacin + L-NAME increased arterial sensitivity to acetylcholine 5.11-fold ($P < 0.001$) vs. control conditions. The above was not observed in the control group (1.06, $P = 0.3$), E1 (0.87, $P = 0.8$) or group E2 (1.22, $P = 0.4$).

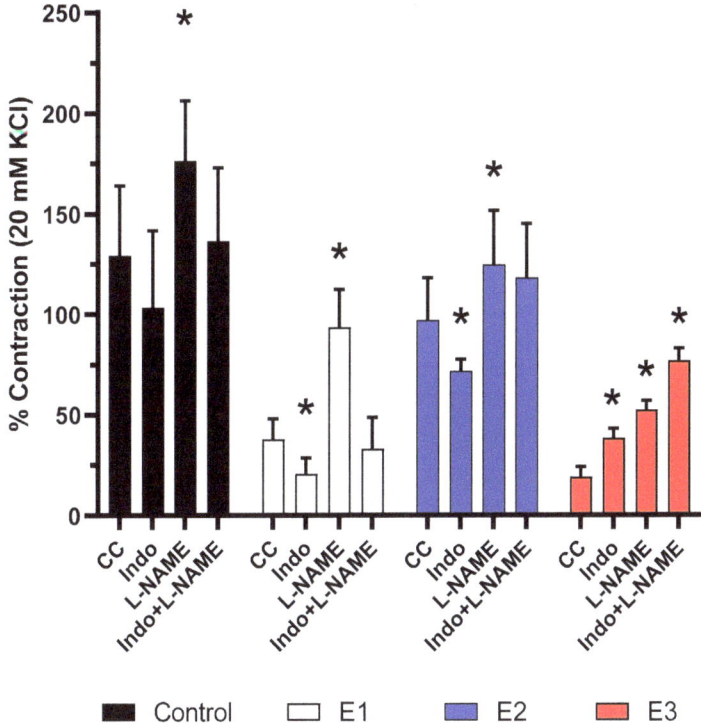

Figure 4. The effect of nitric oxide synthase inhibitor (L-NAME, 4.4×10^{-5} M), cyclooxygenase inhibitor (indomethacin, 4.4×10^{-6} M) on acetylcholine-induced contraction of the porcine coronary arteries. The results (means ± SEM) are expressed as percentage inhibition of the contraction induced by 30 mM KCl. $n = 5$. * $P < 0.05$ vs. control conditions (CC), (two-way ANOVA, followed by Tukey's post-hoc test). Acetylcholine-induced concentration was potentiated in the presence of both Indo+L-NAME in the E3 group, but not in the E1 group and E2 group.

3. Discussion

An analysis of the physiological condition of prepubertal gilts indicates that ZEN acts as both an undesirable substance and an endocrine disruptor (ED) [4]. Even when ingested at MABEL, NOAEL (highest) and LOAEL (very low) doses, ZEN significantly increases the concentrations of selected hormones and causes hyperestrogenism, i.e., supraphysiological hormone levels [4,15,42], in prepubertal gilts. Zearalenone is also characterized by a non-monotonic dose-response curve (according to the principle of hormesis [43]). Therefore, the results of research studies investigating the effects of different ZEN doses on tissues [44,45], cells [46] and cell organelles [47] are difficult to compare.

3.1. Zearalenone and Its Metabolites in the Heart Muscle

In the present study, the carry-over of ZEN and its metabolites in the myocardium of prepubertal gilts was highly individualized (absence of significant differences due to high variation in SD values) (Table 1). The presence of ZEN and a steady increase in its concentrations, proportional to the administered dose, were noted in the myocardium of gilts in groups E1 and E2 on D1. Zearalenone levels were much lower in group E3 on D1, which is partially consistent with previous findings [44]. Similar conclusions were drawn by Gajęcka et al. [17] from a study of female wild boars. The concentrations of α-ZEL (rising trend) and β-ZEL in the myocardium were inversely proportional to each other, which, in our opinion, is a normal response [4]. The bioavailability of ZEN and its metabolites in the myocardium is affected by biotransformation processes in prepubertal females. Interestingly, the distribution of ZEN and metabolite concentrations in the myocardium was similar to the values reported in blood by Rykaczewska et al. [4]. In contrast to the results reported by Yan et al. [44], ZEN metabolites were not detected on D1 (or were below the sensitivity of the method), which could be due to the low supply of endogenous steroid hormones. According to other studies [48,49], a deficiency of ovarian hormones in mammals leads to pressure overload, thus compromising cardiac function. Supplementation with 17β-estradiol [50] or mycoestrogen can reverse these effects or alter the profile of estrogen hormones (by modulating feminization) [4,51]. It should also be stressed that the 7th day of exposure (D1) marks the end of adaptive processes, in particular adaptive immunity [52]. These substances could also be used as substrates that regulate the expression of genes encoding hydroxysteroid dehydrogenase [3], a molecular switch that enables the modulation of steroid hormone prereceptors. These processes were most visible in group E1, where only the parent mycotoxin was detected (100%). In the remaining groups, the presence of metabolites was noted, and their concentrations increased proportionally to the applied dose. The observations made in group E1 (MABEL dose) indicate that prepubertal females utilize even the smallest amounts of estrogen-like substances (what are they zearalenone and its metabolites—[44]) to compensate for endogenous estrogen deficiency (inducing supraphysiological hormonal levels in prepubertal females—[4]), which can increase cardiac automaticity [53].

On D2, ZEN concentrations increased proportionally to the administered dose and were higher than on D1. In group E1, the proportions of both metabolites (%) were higher than in groups E2 and E3 (group E1: ZEN—73.62%, α-ZEL—11%, β-ZEL—15.37%; group E2: 91.48%, 5.82% and 2.68%, respectively; group E3: 93.42%, 5.96% and 0.61%, respectively). Similar to D1, the concentrations of α-ZEL (rising trend) and β-ZEL in the myocardium were inversely proportional to each other. The levels of α-ZEL were higher, whereas β-ZEL levels were lower in groups E2 and E3. This could result from the saturation of myocardial tissue with ZEN and its metabolites, e.g., active estrogen receptors [54] as well as other factors that influence the demand for ZEN and ZEN-like mycotoxins over time of exposure [55]. Unlike in the current experiment, Yan et al. [44] did not detect ZEN, but identified both ZEN metabolites in samples of heart muscle tissue. However, the cited study was conducted in vitro, and the animals' age or sex were not specified, which makes it impossible to directly compare the above results with our findings.

The carry-over of ZEN, an exogenous estrogen-like substance, from the porcine gastrointestinal tract to myocardial tissue via the blood was also analyzed by calculating the CF. The CF values for myocardial tissue in prepubertal gilts have never been determined in the literature, in particular during exposure to three low, monotonic doses of ZEN for 21 consecutive days. Even a cursory analysis of CF values indicates that the accumulation of ZEN and its metabolites was much lower in the myocardium than in the blood [4]. Mycotoxin concentrations ranged from 1×10^{-1} to 1×10^{-3} in the blood, and from 0 (only in group E1 on D1 for both metabolites) to 1×10^{-7} (in the remaining groups on both D1 and

D2) in the myocardium. These observations suggest that differences in carry-over decrease the accumulation of ZEN and its metabolites in the myocardium [48]. These differences are very difficult to explain. Based on the existing knowledge and the extrapolation of previous results, it could be suggested that by disrupting endocrine processes, EDs exert specific effects on cells and tissues [4,51,56] and modulate the structure and functions of the heart muscle [48]. Most importantly, EDs can induce different responses, depending on the dose, exposure duration and the stage of growth and development in mammals [15], in particular females.

Therefore, it can be hypothesized that low doses of undesirable substances (including ZEN) exert minor or much smaller effects on myocardial homeostasis, compared with other cells and tissues in the studied animals due to much lower availability.

3.2. Isometric Tension Analyses

The vasodilatory and vasoconstrictive properties of isolated porcine coronary arteries with an intact endothelium, which regulate vascular smooth muscle contraction, were also analyzed in the study. The blood vessels in various organs and species may respond differently to agonists and antagonists. Potassium chloride and acetylcholine induce vasocontraction, whereas sodium nitroprusside induces vasodilation in porcine coronary arteries (PCAs).

The KCl-induced contraction of the PCAs was enhanced in groups E1 and E2 on D1. However, a decreased response was noted in group E3. On D2, KCl-induced vasoconstriction did not differ in groups E1 and E2, but it decreased further in group E3. These results indicate that the sensitivity of smooth muscles of PCAs to K^+ is highly dependent on the concentrations of ZEN in the diet and the duration of exposure to this mycotoxin.

Acetylcholine-induced contraction decreased in group E3, which is similar to the response observed for KCl, so this effect might not be entirely dependent on the muscarinic receptors. Surprisingly, decreased response was also observed in group E1 but not in group E2. Acetylcholine's effect on vascular tension is dependent on muscarinic receptors [57], which suggests that ZEN is able to modulate the function of these receptors.

Sodium nitroprusside is a donor of exogenous nitric oxide with the endothelium-independent effect. In this study, the sensitivity of PCAs to the nitric oxide was increased in group E3 after prolonged exposure. Surprisingly, arterial sensitivity to nitric oxide decreased in group E1, which suggests that the sensitivity of smooth muscles to nitric oxide changes in response to dietary ZEN, which is endothelium-independent mechanism. These results also indicate that smooth muscles of PCA are targeted by ZEN and its metabolites, and that ZEN my regulate the mechanism(s) of nitric oxide synthesis, which is dose- and time-dependent. Further investigation is needed to examine the mechanism(s) underlying different responses to ZEN and their potential dependence on the endothelium.

The analysis of the effects of COX and e-NOS inhibitors shed a new light on the properties of ZEN. COX inhibitors potentiated ACh-induced vasoconstriction only in group E3. This response decreased in groups E1 and E2, whereas no significant changes were found in the control group. These findings suggest that ACh-induced vasoconstriction in group E3 was at least partly dependent on the net vasodilator effect of prostanoids, whereas the decreased response in groups E1 and E2 was dependent on the vasoconstrictor effect of prostanoids. e-NOS inhibitors increased vasoconstriction in all groups (C, E1, E2 and E3), which indicates that nitric oxide plays a key role in vascular tone regulation of PCA. However, this effect was more pronounced in groups E3 (3.39-fold) and E1 (2.48-fold) than in group E2 (1.29-fold) and the control (1.36-fold), which suggests that ZEN is able to modulate the bioavailability or sensitivity of nitric oxide. When both COX and e-NOS are blocked, mechanisms other than prostanoids and nitric oxide are engaged in vascular tone regulation. These mechanisms are regulated by hormonal changes and, possibly, ZEN. Acetylcholine's effects were potentiated in the presence of COX and e-NOS inhibitors in group E3, but not in groups E1 or E2.

These results indicate that a different mechanism is responsible for the net vasoconstrictor effect which was upregulated only in group E3. The vasodilator effect of prostanoids (PGI_2) and nitric oxide was upregulated by the administered ZEN dose. The endothelium-derived hyperpolarizing factor (EDHF) could be yet another mechanism of vascular control. The major routes of EDHF regulation include the metabolism of arachidonic acid to epoxyeicosatrienoic acids (EETs), potassium channels, gap junctions and hydrogen peroxide [58]. However, further research is needed to clarify the exact mechanism(s), including EDHF, by which ZEN acts on PCA.

3.3. Conclusions

The following conclusion can be drawn from the present study: among ZEN doses analyzed both in vivo and in vitro, the presence of ZEN and its metabolites in the myocardium is found even at the MABEL dose and could be a safe dose for the myocardium regardless of the time of exposure. Meanwhile LOAEL highly affects the functioning of the porcine coronary arteries.

4. Materials and Methods

4.1. In Vivo Study

4.1.1. General Information

All experimental procedures involving animals were carried out in compliance with Polish regulations setting forth the terms and conditions of animal experimentation (Opinions No. 12/2016 and 45/2016/DLZ of the Local Ethics Committee for Animal Experimentation of 27 April 2016 and 30 November 2016).

4.1.2. Experimental Animals and Feed

The in vivo experiment was conducted at the Department of Veterinary Prevention and Feed Hygiene of the Faculty of Veterinary Medicine at the University of Warmia and Mazury in Olsztyn on 40 clinically healthy prepubertal gilts with initial BW of 14.5 ± 2 kg. The animals were housed in pens, and they had free access to water. Throughout the experiment, gilts in all groups received the same feed. The animals were randomly divided into three experimental groups (group E1, group E2 and group E3; n = 10) and a control group (group C, n = 10). Group E1 gilts were orally administered ZEN (SIGMA-ALDRICH Z2125-26MG USA) at 5 μg ZEN/kg BW, group E2 gilts received 10 μg ZEN/kg BW and group E3 gilts—15 μg ZEN/kg BW.

Analytical samples of ZEN were dissolved in 96 μl of 96% ethanol (SWW 2442-90, Polskie Odczynniki SA, Poland) in doses appropriate for different BW. Feed saturated with different doses of ZEN in an alcohol solution was placed in gel capsules. Before administration to the animals, the capsules were stored at room temperature before administration to evaporate the alcohol. In the experimental groups, ZEN was administered daily in gel capsules before morning feeding. The animals were weighed every week, and the results were used to adjust mycotoxin doses on an individual basis. Feed was the carrier, and control group gilts received the same gel capsules, but without mycotoxins.

The feed offered to all groups of experimental animals was supplied by the same producer. Throughout the experiment, feed was provided ad libitum in loose form, twice daily (at 8:00 a.m. and 5:00 p.m.). The manufacturer's declared composition of the complete diet is shown in Table 3.

The proximate chemical composition of the diets fed to gilts in groups C, E1, E2 and E3 was evaluated with the use of the NIRS™ DS2500 F feed analyzer (FOSS, Hillerød, Denmark) which is a monochromator-based NIR reflectance and transflectance analyzer with a scanning range of 850–2500 nm.

Table 3. Declared composition of the complete diet.

Ingredient	Manufacturer's Declared Composition (%)
Soybean meal	16
Wheat	55
Barley	22
Wheat bran	4.0
Chalk	0.3
Zitrosan	0.2
Vitamin-mineral premix [1]	2.5

[1] Composition of the vitamin-mineral premix per kg: vitamin A—500,000 IU; iron—5000 mg; vitamin D3—100,000 IU; zinc—5000 mg; vitamin E (alpha-tocopherol)—2000 mg; manganese—3000 mg; vitamin K—150 mg; copper ($CuSO_4 \cdot 5H_2O$)—500 mg; vitamin B_1—100 mg; cobalt—20 mg; vitamin B—300 mg; iodine—40 mg; vitamin B_6—150 mg; selenium—15 mg; vitamin B_{12}—1500 µg; L-lysine—9.4 g; niacin—1200 mg; DL-methionine + cystine—3.7 g; pantothenic acid—600 mg; L-threonine—2.3 g; folic acid—50 mg; tryptophan—1.1 g; biotin—7500 µg; phytase + choline—10 g; ToyoCerin probiotic+calcium—250 g; antioxidant+mineral phosphorus and released phosphorus—60 g; magnesium—5 g; sodium and calcium—51 g.

4.1.3. Toxicological Analysis of Feed

Feed was analyzed for the presence of ZEN and DON. Mycotoxin content was determined by extraction on immunoaffinity columns (Zearala-TestTM Zearalenone Testing System, G1012, VICAM, Watertown, MA, USA; DON-TestTM DON Testing System, VICAM, Watertown, MA, USA) and in a high-performance liquid chromatography (HPLC) system (Hewlett Packard type 1100 and 1260) with a mass spectrometer (MS) and a chromatography column (Atlantis T3 3 µm 3.0 × 150 mm Column No. 186003723, Waters, AN Etten-Leur, Ireland). The mobile phase was an 80:10 mixture of water and acetonitrile with the addition of 2 mL of acetic acid per 1 L of the mix. The flow rate was 0.4 mL/min. The obtained values did not exceed the limit of quantification (LoQ) set at 2 ng/g for ZEN and 5 ng/g for DON. The analyzed compounds were quantified at the Department of Veterinary Prevention and Feed Hygiene, Faculty of Veterinary Medicine, University of Warmia and Mazury in Olsztyn [14].

4.1.4. Toxicological Analysis of the Apex of the Heart

Tissues Samples

Five prepubertal gilts from every group were euthanized on analytical dates 1 (D1-exposure day 7) and 2 (D2—exposure day 21) by intravenous administration of pentobarbital sodium (Fatro, Ozzano Emilia BO, Italy) and bleeding. Samples were collected from the myocardium (the apex of the heart) immediately after cardiac arrest and were rinsed with phosphate buffer. The collected samples were stored at a temperature of $-20\ °C$.

Extraction Procedure

The presence of ZEN, α-ZEL and β-ZEL in the apex of the heart was determined with the use of immunoaffinity columns (Zearala-TestTM Zearalenone Testing System, G1012, VICAM, Watertown, MA, USA). All extraction procedures were carried out in accordance with the recommendations of column manufacturers. After extraction, the eluents were placed in a water bath at a temperature of 50 °C and were evaporated in a stream of nitrogen. Dry residues were stored at $-20\ °C$ until chromatographic analysis. Next, 0.5 mL of 99% acetonitrile (ACN) was added to dry residues to dissolve the mycotoxin. The process was monitored with the use of internal standards, and the results were validated by mass spectrometry.

Chromatographic Quantification of ZEN and Its Metabolites

Zearalenone and its metabolites were quantified at the Institute of Dairy Industry Innovation in Mrągowo. The biological activity of ZEN, α-ZEL and β-ZEL in the myocardium was determined by combined separation methods, immunoaffinity chromatography (Zearala-TestTM Zearalenone Testing System, G1012, VICAM, Watertown, MA, USA), liquid chromatography (LC) (Agilent 1260 LC system) and mass spectrometry (MS). Samples were analyzed on a chromatographic column (Atlantis T3, 3 μm 3.0 × 150 mm, column No. 186003723, Waters, AN Etten-Leur, Ireland). The mobile phase was composed of 70% acetonitrile (LiChrosolvTM, No. 984 730 109, Merck-Hitachi, Mannheim, Germany), 20% methanol (LiChrosolvTM, No. 1.06 007, Merck-Hitachi, Mannheim, Germany) and 10% deionized water (MiliporeWater Purification System, Millipore S.A. Molsheim-France) with the addition of 2 mL of acetic acid per 1 L of the mixture. The column was flushed with 99.8% methanol (LIChrosolvTM, No. 1.06 007, Merck-Hitachi, Mannheim, Germany) to remove the bound mycotoxin. The eluents were placed in a water bath with a temperature of 50 °C, and the solvent was evaporated in a stream of nitrogen. Mycotoxin concentrations were determined with an external standard and were expressed in ppb (ng/mL). Matrix-matched calibration standards were applied in the quantification process to eliminate matrix effects that can decrease sensitivity. Calibration standards were dissolved in matrix samples based on the procedure that was used to prepare the remaining samples. The material for calibration standards was free of mycotoxins. The limits of detection (LOD) for ZEN, α-ZEL and β-ZEL were determined as the concentration at which the signal-to-noise ratio decreased to 3. The concentrations and percentage content of ZEN, α-ZEL and β-ZEL were determined in each group and on both analytical dates (Table 1).

Carry-Over Factor

Carry-over toxicity takes place when organisms exposed to low doses of mycotoxins survive. Mycotoxins can compromise tissue or organ functions [59] and modify their biological activity [4,15]. The carry-over factor (CF) was determined in the myocardium when the daily dose of ZEN (5 μg ZEN/kg BW, 10 μg ZEN/kg BW or 15 μg ZEN/kg BW) administered to each animal was equivalent to 560–6255 μg ZEN/kg of the complete diet, depending on daily feed intake. Mycotoxin concentrations in tissues were expressed in terms of the dry matter content of the samples.

The CF was calculated as follows:

$$carry-over\ factor = \frac{toxin\ concentration\ in\ tissue\ [ng/g]}{toxin\ concentration\ in\ diet\ [ng/g]} \quad (1)$$

Statistical Analysis

Data were processed statistically at the Department of Discrete Mathematics and Theoretical Computer Science, Faculty of Mathematics and Computer Science of the University of Warmia and Mazury in Olsztyn. The bioavailability of ZEN and its metabolites in the apex of heart was analyzed in group C and three experimental groups on two analytical dates. The results were expressed as means ($\bar{x}$) with standard deviation (SD). The following parameters were analyzed: (i) differences in the mean values for three ZEN doses (experimental groups) and the control group on both analytical dates, and (ii) differences in the mean values for specific ZEN doses (groups) on both analytical dates. In both cases, the differences between mean values were determined by one-way ANOVA. If significant differences were noted between groups, the differences between paired means were determined by Tukey's multiple comparison test. If all values were below LOD (mean and variance equal zero) in any group, the values in the remaining groups were analyzed by one-way ANOVA (if the number of the remaining groups was higher than two), and the means in these groups were compared against zero by Student's t-test. Differences between groups were determined by Student's t-test. The results were regarded as highly significant at $P < 0.01$ (**) and as significant at $0.01 < P < 0.05$ (*). Data were processed statistically using Statistica v.13 software (TIBCO Software Inc., Silicon Valley, CA, USA, 2017).

4.2. Laboratory Analyses

4.2.1. Sampling for In Vitro Analyses

Tissue samples for in vitro analyses were collected from the same animals as the tissues for the toxicological analysis. The animals were euthanized by intravenous administration of pentobarbital sodium (Fatro, Ozzano Emilia BO, Italy) and exsanguinated.

4.2.2. In Vitro Analysis

In vitro analyses were performed at the Department of Pharmacology and Toxicology of the Faculty of Medicine at the University of Warmia and Mazury in Olsztyn, Poland.

4.2.3. Drugs

Acetylcholine (ACh) chloride, sodium nitroprusside (SNP), bradykinin acetate salt, indomethacin, N^G-nitro-L-arginine methyl ester (L-NAME) and potassium chloride (KCl) (Chempur, Poland) were obtained from Sigma-Aldrich unless stated otherwise. Stock solutions (10 mM) of indomethacin and L-NAME were prepared in DMSO. These solutions were stored at $-20\ °C$, and appropriate dilutions were made in Krebs-Henseleit solution (KHS in mM: NaCl 120, KCl 4.76, $NaHCO_3$ 25, $NaH_2PO_4 \cdot H_2O$ 1.18, $CaCl_2$ 1.25, $MgSO_4 \cdot 7H_2O$ 1.18, glucose 5.5) on the day of the experiment. At these concentrations, DMSO did not alter the reactivity of coronary arteries.

4.2.4. Vascular Reactivity Analyses

Porcine hearts were transported on ice and rinsed with cold aerated KHS. The left anterior descending branches of the coronary artery (MID LAD, D1-D2 sections) were excised at room temperature (n = 5). The surrounding connective tissues were removed, the arteries were cut into 4 mm rings and suspended between two stainless-steel rods positioned in 5 mL tissue baths (Graz Tissue Bath System, Harvard Apparatus) filled with aerated (95% O_2 + 5% CO_2) KHS at 37 °C (pH 7.4). The resting tension of 1.5 g was applied and further readjusted every 15 min during a 60 min equilibration period before further analysis.

The viability of each porcine coronary artery was determined by contraction with 30 mM KCl before relaxation with 1 mM bradykinin. Rings that failed to produce an average contraction greater than or equal to 4.0 g when challenged with KCl and relaxation greater than or equal to 40% when treated with bradykinin were excluded from the study (approx. 10–20% of prepared rings). The rings were washed three times with fresh KHS, and baseline tension was readjusted before the examination.

After an initial equilibration period of 60 min, contractile responses elicited by either a cumulative concentration of KCl (2.5–30 mM) or a single maximum depolarizing concentration of KCl (30 mM) were assessed. The rings were also assessed for contractile responses generated by a cumulative concentration of acetylcholine (ACh: 0.1–10 µM). The cumulative concentrations of sodium nitroprusside (SNP: 0.1–100 µM) were assessed to determine the possible contribution of exogenous nitric oxide (NO) to relaxation responses on endothelium-intact rings that had been precontracted with submaximal concentrations of KCl (30 mM).

In experiments evaluating the influence of COX and e-NOS-inhibitors on contractile responses, indomethacin (4.4×10^{-6} M) and L-NAME (4.4×10^{-5} M) were added to the chambers 30 min before the arteries were constricted with acetylcholine. Each tissue was exposed to the contracting agent only once.

4.2.5. Statistical Analysis

Data were expressed as means $\pm$ SD (Standard Deviation), where n denoted the number of porcine hearts from which arterial rings were obtained. The contraction elicited by KCl was expressed in g of tension. ACh-induced contraction and SNP-induced relaxation were expressed as a percentage of the initial contraction elicited by 30 mM KCl. Dose-response curves were analyzed for the area under the curve, F_{max} and EC_{50} in GraphPad

Prism 9.0.2. Data were processed statistically by comparing the curves obtained in each experimental group with the control curve in two-way ANOVA, followed by Tukey's multiple comparisons test. Differences were regarded as significant at $P \leq 0.05$.

Author Contributions: The experiments were conceived and designed by M.G., M.S.M. and M.T.G. The experiments were performed by M.G., M.S.M., E.O. and Ł.Z. Data were analyzed and interpreted by M.G., M.S.M., W.G., J.J. and S.L.-Ż. The manuscript was drafted by M.G. and M.S.M. and critically edited by A.B., Ł.Z. and M.T.G. All authors have read and agreed to the published version of the manuscript.

Funding: The study was supported by the "Healthy Animal—Safe Food" Scientific Consortium of the Leading National Research Centre (KNOW) pursuant to a decision of the Ministry of Science and Higher Education No. 05-1/KNOW2/2015. The project was financially co-supported by the Minister of Science and Higher Education under the program entitled "Regional Initiative of Excellence" for the years 2019-2022, Project No. 010/RID/2018/19, amount of funding PLN 12,000,000.

Institutional Review Board Statement: Not applicable.

Informed Consent Statement: Not applicable.

Data Availability Statement: Not applicable.

Conflicts of Interest: The authors declare no conflict of interest.

References

1. Ropejko, K.; Twarużek, M. Zearalenone and Its Metabolites—General Overview, Occurrence, and Toxicity. *Toxins* **2021**, *13*, 35. [CrossRef] [PubMed]
2. Wielogórska, E.; Elliott, C.; Danaher, M.; Connolly, L. Validation and application of a reporter gene assay for the determination of estrogenic endocrine disruptor activity in milk. *Food Chem. Toxicol.* **2014**, *69*, 260–266. [CrossRef] [PubMed]
3. Gajęcka, M.; Zielonka, Ł.; Gajęcki, M. Activity of Zearalenone in the Porcine Intestinal Tract. *Molecules* **2016**, *22*, 18. [CrossRef]
4. Rykaczewska, A.; Gajęcka, M.; Onyszek, E.; Cieplińska, K.; Dąbrowski, M.; Lisieska-Żołnierczyk, S.; Bulińska, M.; Babuchowski, A.; Gajęcki, M.T.; Zielonka, Ł. Imbalance in the Blood Concentrations of Selected Steroids in Pre-pubertal Gilts Depending on the Time of Exposure to Low Doses of Zearalenone. *Toxins* **2019**, *11*, 561. [CrossRef]
5. Flores-Flores, M.E.; Lizarraga, E.; de Cerain, A.L.; González-Peñas, E. Presence of mycotoxins in animal milk: A review. *Food Control.* **2015**, *53*, 163–176. [CrossRef]
6. Broekaert, N.; Devreese, M.; De Baere, S.; De Backer, P.; Croubels, S. Modified Fusarium mycotoxins unmasked: From occurrence in cereals to animal and human excretion. *Food Chem. Toxicol.* **2015**, *80*, 17–31. [CrossRef]
7. Marin, D.E.; Pistol, G.; Neagoe, I.V.; Calin, L.; Taranu, I. Effects of zearalenone on oxidative stress and inflammation in weanling piglets. *Food Chem. Toxicol.* **2013**, *58*, 408–415. [CrossRef] [PubMed]
8. Martín, L.; Wood, K.; McEwen, P.; Smith, T.; Mandell, I.; Yannikouris, A.; Swanson, K. Effects of feeding corn naturally contaminated with Fusarium mycotoxins and/or a modified yeast cell wall extract on the performance, immunity and carcass characteristics of grain-fed veal calves. *Anim. Feed. Sci. Technol.* **2010**, *159*, 27–34. [CrossRef]
9. Dunbar, B.; Patel, M.; Fahey, J.; Wira, C. Endocrine control of mucosal immunity in the female reproductive tract: Impact of environmental disruptors. *Mol. Cell. Endocrinol.* **2012**, *354*, 85–93. [CrossRef]
10. Dąbrowski, M.; Obremski, K.; Gajęcka, M.; Gajęcki, M.T.; Zielonka, Ł. Changes in the Subpopulations of Porcine Peripheral Blood Lymphocytes Induced by Exposure to Low Doses of Zearalenone (ZEN) and Deoxynivalenol (DON). *Molecules* **2016**, *21*, 557. [CrossRef] [PubMed]
11. Alm, H.; Brüssow, K.-P.; Torner, H.; Vanselow, J.; Tomek, W.; Dänicke, S.; Tiemann, U. Influence of Fusarium-toxin contaminated feed on initial quality and meiotic competence of gilt oocytes. *Reprod. Toxicol.* **2006**, *22*, 44–50. [CrossRef]
12. Gajęcka, M.; Zielonka, Ł.; Gajęcki, M. The Effect of Low Monotonic Doses of Zearalenone on Selected Reproductive Tissues in Pre-Pubertal Female Dogs—A Review. *Molecules* **2015**, *20*, 20669–20687. [CrossRef]
13. Kowalska, K.; Habrowska-Górczyńska, D.E.; Piastowska-Ciesielska, A.W. Zearalenone as an endocrine disruptor in humans. *Environ. Toxicol. Pharmacol.* **2016**, *48*, 141–149. [CrossRef]
14. Gajęcki, M. The effect of experimentally induced *Fusarium* mycotoxicosis on selected diagnostic and morphological parameters of the porcine digestive tract. In Proceedings of the Final Report for the National Centre for Research and Development in Warsaw, Poland, Development Project NR12-0080-10 entitled, Warsaw, Poland, 30 November 2013; pp. 1–180.
15. Rykaczewska, A.; Gajęcka, M.; Dąbrowski, M.; Wiśniewska, A.; Szcześniewska, J.; Gajęcki, M.T.; Zielonka, Ł. Growth performance, selected blood biochemical parameters and body weights of pre-pubertal gilts fed diets supplemented with different doses of zearalenone (ZEN). *Toxicon* **2018**, *152*, 84–94. [CrossRef] [PubMed]

16. Zachariasova, M.; Dzumana, Z.; Veprikova, Z.; Hajkovaa, K.; Jiru, M.; Vaclavikova, M.; Zachariasova, A.; Pospichalova, M.; Florian, M.; Hajslova, J. Occurrence of multiple mycotoxins in European feedingstuffs, assessment of dietary intake by farm animals. *Anim. Feed. Sci. Technol.* **2014**, *193*, 124–140. [CrossRef]
17. Gajęcka, M.; Tarasiuk, M.; Zielonka, Ł.; Dąbrowski, M.; Gajęcki, M. Risk assessment for changes in the metabolic profile and body weights of pre-pubertal gilts during long-term monotonic exposure to low doses of zearalenone (ZEN). *Res. Veter. Sci.* **2016**, *109*, 169–180. [CrossRef]
18. Frizzell, C.; Ndossi, D.; Verhaegen, S.; Dahl, E.; Eriksen, G.S.; Sørlie, M.; Ropstad, E.; Muller, M.; Elliott, C.; Connolly, L. Endocrine disrupting effects of zearalenone, alpha- and beta-zearalenol at the level of nuclear receptor binding and steroidogenesis. *Toxicol. Lett.* **2011**, *206*, 210–217. [CrossRef]
19. Kolle, S.N.; Ramirez, T.; Kamp, H.G.; Buesen, R.; Flick, B.; Strauss, V.; Van Ravenzwaay, B. A testing strategy for the identification of mammalian, systemic endocrine disruptors with particular focus on steroids. *Regul. Toxicol. Pharmacol.* **2012**, *63*, 259–278. [CrossRef]
20. Gajęcka, M.; Zielonka, Ł.; Dabrowski, M.; Mróz, M.; Gajęcki, M. The effect of low doses of zearalenone and its metabolites on progesterone and 17β-estradiol concentrations in peripheral blood and body weights of pre-pubertal female Beagle dogs. *Toxicon* **2013**, *76*, 260–269. [CrossRef]
21. Zielonka, Ł.; Waśkiewicz, A.; Beszterda, M.; Kostecki, M.; Dabrowski, M.; Obremski, K.; Goliński, P.; Gajęcki, M. Zearalenone in the Intestinal Tissues of Immature Gilts Exposed per os to Mycotoxins. *Toxins* **2015**, *7*, 3210–3223. [CrossRef] [PubMed]
22. Marchais-Oberwinkler, S.; Henn, C.; Möller, G.; Klein, T.; Negri, M.; Oster, A.; Spadaro, A.; Werth, R.; Wetzel, M.; Xu, K.; et al. 17β-Hydroxysteroid dehydrogenases (17β-HSDs) as therapeutic targets: Protein structures, functions, and recent progress in inhibitor development. *J. Steroid Biochem. Mol. Biol.* **2011**, *125*, 66–82. [CrossRef]
23. EFSA Panel on Contaminants in the Food Chain (CONTAM); Knutsen, H.; Alexander, J.; Barregård, L.; Bignami, M.; Brüschweiler, B.; Ceccatelli, S.; Cottrill, B.; DiNovi, M.; Edler, L.; et al. Risks for animal health related to the presence of zearalenone and its modified forms in feed. *EFSA J.* **2017**, *15*, e04851. [CrossRef] [PubMed]
24. Schaller, T.H.; Snyder, D.J.; Spasojevic, I.; Gedeon, P.C.; Sanchez-Perez, L.; Sampson, J.H. First in human dose calculation of a single-chain bispecific antibody targeting glioma using the MABEL approach. *J. Immunother. Cancer* **2019**, *8*, e000213. [CrossRef]
25. Cieplińska, K.; Gajęcka, M.; Nowak, A.; Dąbrowski, M.; Łukasz, Z.; Gajęcki, M.T. The Genotoxicity of Caecal Water in Gilts Exposed to Low Doses of Zearalenone. *Toxins* **2018**, *10*, 350. [CrossRef]
26. Cieplińska, K.; Gajęcka, M.; Dąbrowski, M.; Rykaczewska, A.; Lisieska-Żołnierczyk, S.; Bulińska, M.; Zielonka, Ł.; Gajęcki, M.T. Time-Dependent Changes in the Intestinal Microbiome of Gilts Exposed to Low Zearalenone Doses. *Toxins* **2019**, *11*, 296. [CrossRef]
27. Stopa, E.; Babińska, I.; Zielonka, Ł.; Gajęcki, M.; Gajęcka, M. Immunohistochemical evaluation of apoptosis and proliferation in the mucous membrane of selected uterine regions in pre-pubertal bitches exposed to low doses of zearalenone. *Pol. J. Veter. Sci.* **2016**, *19*, 175–186. [CrossRef]
28. Alassane-Kpembi, I.; Pinton, P.; Oswald, I.P. Effects of Mycotoxins on the Intestine. *Toxins* **2019**, *11*, 159. [CrossRef] [PubMed]
29. Kramer, H.; Ham, W.V.D.; Slob, W.; Pieters, M. Conversion Factors Estimating Indicative Chronic No-Observed-Adverse-Effect Levels from Short-Term Toxicity Data. *Regul. Toxicol. Pharmacol.* **1996**, *23*, 249–255. [CrossRef]
30. Vandenberg, L.N.; Colborn, T.; Hayes, T.B.; Heindel, J.J.; Jacobs, D.R., Jr.; Lee, D.H.; Shioda, T.; Soto, A.M.; vom Saal, F.S.; Welshons, W.V.; et al. Hormones and Endocrine-Disrupting Chemicals: Low-Dose Effects and Nonmonotonic Dose Responses. *Endocr. Rev.* **2012**, *33*, 378–455. [CrossRef] [PubMed]
31. Grenier, B.; Applegate, T.J. Modulation of Intestinal Functions Following Mycotoxin Ingestion: Meta-Analysis of Published Experiments in Animals. *Toxins* **2013**, *5*, 396–430. [CrossRef] [PubMed]
32. Hickey, G.L.; Craig, P.S.; Luttik, R.; De Zwart, D. On the quantification of intertest variability in ecotoxicity data with application to species sensitivity distributions. *Environ. Toxicol. Chem.* **2012**, *31*, 1903–1910. [CrossRef]
33. Pastoor, T.P.; Bachman, A.N.; Bell, D.R.; Cohen, S.M.; Dellarco, M.; Dewhurst, I.C.; Doe, J.E.; Doerrer, N.G.; Embry, M.R.; Hines, R.N.; et al. A 21st century roadmap for human health risk assessment. *Crit. Rev. Toxicol.* **2014**, *44*, 1–5. [CrossRef]
34. Chain, E.P.O.C.I.T.F. Scientific Opinion on the risks for public health related to the presence of zearalenone in food. *EFSA J.* **2011**, *9*, 1–124. [CrossRef]
35. Gajęcka, M.; Przybylska-Gornowicz, B. The low doses effect of experimental zearalenone (ZEN) intoxication on the presence of Ca2+ in selected ovarian cells from pre-pubertal bitches. *Pol. J. Veter. Sci.* **2012**, *15*, 711–720. [CrossRef] [PubMed]
36. Qadri, S.M.; Bissinger, R.; Solh, Z.; Oldenborg, P.-A. Eryptosis in health and disease: A paradigm shift towards understanding the (patho)physiological implications of programmed cell death of erythrocytes. *Blood Rev.* **2017**, *31*, 349–361. [CrossRef]
37. Pyrshev, K.A.; Klymchenko, A.S.; Csúcs, G.; Demchenko, A.P. Apoptosis and eryptosis: Striking differences on biomembrane level. *Biochim. Biophys. Acta (BBA) Biomembr.* **2018**, *1860*, 1362–1371. [CrossRef] [PubMed]
38. Lang, E.; Lang, F. Mechanisms and pathophysiological significance of eryptosis, the suicidal erythrocyte death. *Semin. Cell Dev. Biol.* **2015**, *39*, 35–42. [CrossRef]
39. Gajęcka, M.; Rybarczyk, L.; Jakimiuk, E.; Zielonka, Ł.; Obremski, K.; Zwierzchowski, W.; Gajęcki, M. The effect of experimental long-term exposure to low-dose zearalenone on uterine histology in sexually immature gilts. *Exp. Toxicol. Pathol.* **2012**, *64*, 537–542. [CrossRef] [PubMed]

40. Gajęcka, M.; Stopa, E.; Tarasiuk, M.; Zielonka, Ł.; Gajęcki, M. The Expression of Type-1 and Type-2 Nitric Oxide Synthase in Selected Tissues of the Gastrointestinal Tract during Mixed Mycotoxicosis. *Toxins* **2013**, *5*, 2281–2292. [CrossRef] [PubMed]
41. Broadley, K.J.; Broadley, H.D. Non-adrenergic vasoconstriction and vasodilatation of guinea-pig aorta by β-phenylethylamine and amphetamine—Role of nitric oxide determined with L-NAME and NO scavengers. *Eur. J. Pharmacol.* **2018**, *818*, 198–205. [CrossRef]
42. Lawrenz, B.; Melado, L.; Fatemi, H. Premature progesterone rise in ART-cycles. *Reprod. Biol.* **2018**, *18*, 1–4. [CrossRef] [PubMed]
43. Calabrese, E.J. Hormesis: Path and Progression to Significance. *Int. J. Mol. Sci.* **2018**, *19*, 2871. [CrossRef] [PubMed]
44. Yan, Z.; Wang, L.; Wang, J.; Tan, Y.; Yu, D.; Chang, X.; Fan, Y.; Zhao, D.; Wang, C.; De Boevre, M.; et al. A QuEChERS-Based Liquid Chromatography-Tandem Mass Spectrometry Method for the Simultaneous Determination of Nine Zearalenone-Like Mycotoxins in Pigs. *Toxins* **2018**, *10*, 129. [CrossRef] [PubMed]
45. Zhou, J.; Ao, X.; Lei, Y.; Ji, C.; Ma, Q. Bacillus subtilis ANSB01G culture alleviates oxidative stress and cell apoptosis induced by dietary zearalenone in first-parity gestation sows. *Anim. Nutr.* **2020**, *6*, 372–378. [CrossRef]
46. Lee, H.-J.; Park, J.-H.; Oh, S.-Y.; Cho, D.-H.; Kim, S.; Jo, I. Zearalenone-Induced Interaction between PXR and Sp1 Increases Binding of Sp1 to a Promoter Site of the eNOS, Decreasing Its Transcription and NO Production in BAECs. *Toxins* **2020**, *12*, 421. [CrossRef]
47. Gajęcki, M.T.; Gajęcka, M.; Zielonka, Ł. Mycotoxins Occurence in Feed and Their Influence on Animal Health. In *Printed Edition of the Special Issue Published in Toxins*; Multidisciplinary Digital Publishing Institute: Basel, Switzerland, 2021; pp. 1–242. ISBN 978-3-03943-848-8.
48. Villarreal, F. In Pursuit of Understanding the Role of Estrogens in Regulating Cardiac Structure and Function. *JACC Basic Transl. Sci.* **2020**, *5*, 913–915. [CrossRef]
49. Firth, J.M.; Yang, H.-Y.; Francis, A.J.; Islam, N.; MacLeod, K.T. The Effect of Estrogen on Intracellular Ca2+ and Na+ Regulation in Heart Failure. *JACC Basic Transl. Sci.* **2020**, *5*, 901–912. [CrossRef] [PubMed]
50. Mahmoodzadeh, S.; Dworatzek, E. The Role of 17β-Estradiol and Estrogen Receptors in Regulation of Ca2+ Channels and Mitochondrial Function in Cardiomyocytes. *Front. Endocrinol.* **2019**, *10*, 310. [CrossRef] [PubMed]
51. Zielonka, Ł.; Gajęcka, M.; Lisieska-Żołnierczyk, S.; Dąbrowski, M.; Gajęcki, M.T. The Effect of Different Doses of Zearalenone in Feed on the Bioavailability of Zearalenone and Alpha-Zearalenol, and the Concentrations of Estradiol and Testosterone in the Peripheral Blood of Pre-Pubertal Gilts. *Toxins* **2020**, *12*, 144. [CrossRef]
52. Benagiano, M.; Bianchi, P.; D'Elios, M.M.; Brosens, I.; Benagiano, G. Autoimmune diseases: Role of steroid hormones. *Best Pract. Res. Clin. Obstet. Gynaecol.* **2019**, *60*, 24–34. [CrossRef]
53. Long, V.; Fiset, C. Contribution of estrogen to the pregnancy-induced increase in cardiac automaticity. *J. Mol. Cell. Cardiol.* **2020**, *147*, 27–34. [CrossRef]
54. Ueda, K.; Adachi, Y.; Liu, P.; Fukuma, N.; Takimoto, E. Regulatory Actions of Estrogen Receptor Signaling in the Cardiovascular System. *Front. Endocrinol.* **2020**, *10*, 909. [CrossRef]
55. Luisetto, M.; Naseer, A.; Nili, A.B.; Abdul, H.G.; Rasool, M.G.; Rehman, K.K.; Ahmadabadi, B.N.; Luca, C. Endogenus toxicology: Modern physio-pathological aspects and relationship with new therapeutic strategies. An integrative discipline incorporating concepts from different research discipline like Biochemistry, Pharmacology and Toxicology. *Arch. Cancer Sci. Ther.* **2019**, *3*, 1–24. [CrossRef]
56. Sharma, R.P.; Schuhmacher, M.; Kumar, V. Review on crosstalk and common mechanisms of endocrine disruptors: Scaffolding to improve PBPK/PD model of EDC mixture. *Environ. Int.* **2017**, *99*, 1–14. [CrossRef] [PubMed]
57. Gräser, T.; Leisner, H.; Vedernikov, Y.P.; Tiedt, N. The action of acetylcholine on isolated coronary arteries of different species. *Cor. Vasa* **1987**, *29*, 70–80. [PubMed]
58. Bryan, R.M.; You, J.; Golding, E.M.; Marrelli, S.P. Endothelium-derived Hyperpolarizing Factor. *Anesthesiology* **2005**, *102*, 1261–1277. [CrossRef]
59. Meerpoel, C.; Vidal, A.; Tangni, E.K.; Huybrechts, B.; Couck, L.; De Rycke, R.; De Bels, L.; De Saeger, S.; Broeck, W.V.D.; Devreese, M.; et al. A Study of Carry-Over and Histopathological Effects after Chronic Dietary Intake of Citrinin in Pigs, Broiler Chickens and Laying Hens. *Toxins* **2020**, *12*, 719. [CrossRef]

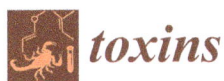

Study Protocol

Correlations between Low Doses of Zearalenone, Its Carryover Factor and Estrogen Receptor Expression in Different Segments of the Intestines in Pre-Pubertal Gilts—A Study Protocol

Magdalena Gajęcka [1,*], Magdalena Mróz [1], Paweł Brzuzan [2], Ewa Onyszek [3], Łukasz Zielonka [1], Karolina Lipczyńska-Ilczuk [4], Katarzyna E. Przybyłowicz [5], Andrzej Babuchowski [3] and Maciej T. Gajęcki [1]

[1] Department of Veterinary Prevention and Feed Hygiene, Faculty of Veterinary Medicine, University of Warmia and Mazury in Olsztyn, Oczapowskiego 13, 10-718 Olsztyn, Poland; magdzia.mroz@gmail.com (M.M.); lukaszz@uwm.edu.pl (Ł.Z.); gajecki@uwm.edu.pl (M.T.G.)

[2] Department of Environmental Biotechnology, Faculty of Environmental Sciences and Fisheries, University of Warmia and Mazury in Olsztyn, Słoneczna 45G, 10-719 Olsztyn, Poland; brzuzan@uwm.edu.pl

[3] Dairy Industry Innovation Institute Ltd., Kormoranów 1, 11-700 Mrągowo, Poland; ewa.onyszek@iipm.pl (E.O.); andrzej.babuchowski@iipm.pl (A.B.)

[4] Department of Epizootiology, Faculty of Veterinary Medicine, University of Warmia and Mazury in Olsztyn, Oczapowskiego 13/01, 10-718 Olsztyn, Poland; karolina.lipczynska@uwm.edu.pl

[5] Department of Human Nutrition, Faculty of Food Sciences, University of Warmia and Mazury in Olsztyn, Słoneczna 45F, 10-719 Olsztyn, Poland; katarzyna.przybylowicz@uwm.edu.pl

* Correspondence: mgaja@uwm.edu.pl

Abstract: Plant materials can be contaminated with *Fusarium* mycotoxins and their derivatives, whose toxic effects on humans and animals may remain subclinical. Zearalenone (ZEN), a low-molecular-weight compound, is produced by molds in crop plants as a secondary metabolite. The objective of this study will be to analyze the in vivo correlations between very low monotonic doses of ZEN (5, 10, and 15 µg ZEN/kg body weight—BW for 42 days) and the carryover of this mycotoxin and its selected metabolites from the intestinal contents to the intestinal walls, the *m*RNA expression of estrogen receptor alfa (ERα) and estrogen receptor beta (ERβ) genes, and the *m*RNA expression of genes modulating selected colon enzymes (CYP1A1 and GSTP1) in the intestinal mucosa of pre-pubertal gilts. An in vivo experiment will be performed on 60 clinically healthy animals with initial BW of 14.5 ± 2 kg. The gilts will be randomly divided into a control group (group C, $n = 15$) and three experimental groups (group ZEN5, group ZEN10, and group ZEN15; $n = 15$). Group ZEN5 will be administered *per os* 5 µg ZEN/kg BW (MABEL), group ZEN10—10 µg ZEN/kg BW (NOAEL), and group ZEN15—15 µg ZEN/kg BW (low LOAEL). In each group, five animals will be euthanized on analytical dates 1 (exposure day 7), 2 (exposure day 21), and 3 (exposure day 42). Samples for in vitro analyses will be collected from an intestinal segment resected from the following regions: the third (horizontal) part of the duodenum, jejunum, ileum, cecum, ascending colon, transverse colon, and descending colon. The experimental material will be collected under special conditions, and it will be transported to specialist laboratories where samples will be obtained for further analyses.

Keywords: zearalenone; digestive tract; carryover factor; ERs *m*RNA; CYP1A1 *m*RNA; GSTP1 *m*RNA; pre-pubertal gilts

Key Contribution: Low doses of ZEN probably determine the carryover of ZEN and its metabolites from the intestinal contents to the intestinal walls by significantly modulating the expression of ERs in the digestive tract of immature gilts in vivo and the involvement (expression effect) of intestinal enzymes in ZEN detoxification processes in the distal intestine.

Citation: Gajęcka, M.; Mróz, M.; Brzuzan, P.; Onyszek, E.; Zielonka, Ł.; Lipczyńska-Ilczuk, K.; Przybyłowicz, K.E.; Babuchowski, A.; Gajęcki, M.T. Correlations between Low Doses of Zearalenone, Its Carryover Factor and Estrogen Receptor Expression in Different Segments of the Intestines in Pre-Pubertal Gilts—A Study Protocol. *Toxins* **2021**, *13*, 379. https://doi.org/10.3390/toxins13060379

Received: 7 April 2021
Accepted: 25 May 2021
Published: 26 May 2021

Publisher's Note: MDPI stays neutral with regard to jurisdictional claims in published maps and institutional affiliations.

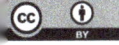

Copyright: © 2021 by the authors. Licensee MDPI, Basel, Switzerland. This article is an open access article distributed under the terms and conditions of the Creative Commons Attribution (CC BY) license (https://creativecommons.org/licenses/by/4.0/).

1. Introduction

A high percentage of plant-based raw materials used in feed production [1] may be contaminated with mycotoxins (undesirable substances), thus increasing the risk of poisoning in humans [2] and farm animals, particularly pigs [3]. The toxicological effects, health risks, and symptoms associated with exposure to high levels of mycotoxins, including zearalenone (ZEN), have been well documented [4–7]. According to the hormesis paradigm [8,9], health implications of exposure to low (measurable) doses of mycotoxins that are frequently encountered in feedstuffs are becoming increasingly important and need to be investigated. The dysfunctions caused by exposure to pure parent compounds [10–12] without metabolites or modified mycotoxins [9] constitute an interesting object of study in mammals.

Fusarium mycotoxins are absorbed primarily in the proximal part of the small intestine [3,13] due to considerable physiological differences between intestinal segments. Mycotoxins are transported to the blood, and blood analyses support noninvasive diagnoses of animal health [14] and the identification of new biomarkers of disease [15]. For instance, ZEN could be regarded as a pharmacodynamic biomarker [16] for determining, at least partially, the interactions between the mycotoxin and its target [17]. Zearalenone and its metabolites usually target cells [18], where they induce specific changes by regulating enzyme metabolism [9,19], gene expression [12], and by acting as ligands that bind to specific receptors in cell membranes and cell nuclei [20]. These mechanisms enable mycotoxins to participate in signal transduction, including in gastrointestinal tract tissues.

The existing body of knowledge [21] suggests that the side effects of exposure to low ZEN doses may be difficult to predict. This uncertainty results not only from the ingested dose but also from the time of exposure [15]. Low levels of mycotoxins can induce unexpected responses. For example, the presence of those undesirable substances may be "ignored" by the body or remain [22], in accordance with the theory of regulatory T-cells (T-regs) that states that they do not respond to a low number of infectious factors in the organism [23]. During prolonged exposure to ZEN administered *per os*, its absorption increases in the host organism [24], which is accompanied by a compensatory effect [25], where the activity of the analyzed parameters is initially suppressed and then returns to baseline values [26] despite ongoing exposure [10]. The above factors, the multidirectional effects of low doses of ZEN and its metabolites [21] in the porcine diet, as well as their ability to elicit specific responses in gilts require further scientific inquiry.

In our previous research [10–12], a low dose was defined [16] based on the presence or absence of clinical symptoms of ZEN mycotoxicosis. Three variants of mycotoxin doses were proposed based on our results and the findings of other authors: the lowest observed adverse effect level (LOAEL) dose (>10 µg ZEN/kg BW) [21,27,28] that induces clinical symptoms [3], the no observed adverse effects levels (NOAEL) dose (10 µg ZEN/kg BW), i.e., the highest dose that does not produce clinical symptoms (subclinical states) [29], and the minimal anticipated biological effect level (MABEL) dose (<10 µg ZEN/kg BW) [16], which is the smallest measurable dose (or the effective dose in vivo) that enters into positive interactions with the host in different life stages [7,10–12,16,30,31].

Since ZEN is a mycoestrogen, the existing dose–response paradigm can be superseded by the low-dose hypothesis [21], in particular with regard to hormonally active compounds [32]. This ambiguous dose–response relationship does not justify a simple and definitive translation of the risk associated with high doses to low doses [3,26] that are effective in vivo. The concept of a minimal dose has gained increasing popularity in biomedical sciences [14,16], and it is consistent with the main tenets of precision medicine [33]. This breakthrough concept accounts for individual variations as well as population characteristics to explain the holistic effects of a minimal dose. Such an approach expands the existing biological knowledge and examines individual variations (in livestock farming) in different areas of biological and medical sciences. Such analyses rely on specialist laboratory equipment to acquire comprehensive information about biomarkers (genes, gene expression products, and metabolites) [14,34]. However, a low dose can also be defined as a dose that delivers counterintuitive effects [8,16]. Therefore, the mechanisms of action associated with a low dose have to be understood to facilitate decision-making in quantitative and qualitative risk assessments [35,36].

Zearalenone metabolites are usually not detected during exposure to low doses of this mycotoxin. According to most studies, more α-ZEL than β-ZEL is produced during ZEN biotransformation in pigs, which are characterized by higher activity levels of 3α-HSD than that of other animal species [37]. However, this is not always the case, as demonstrated by a study conducted in our research center [38]. In pre-pubertal gilts, the peripheral blood concentrations of ZEN and its metabolites point to ongoing biotransformation processes that do not lead to hyperestrogenism, but compensate for a physiological deficiency of endogenous estrogens [39]. These observations have been confirmed by an analysis of the concentrations of the parent compound and its metabolites in gilts exposed to MABEL doses of ZEN [40]. Zearalenone metabolites were not identified in the first week of exposure, probably due to an inadequate supply of endogenous steroid hormones.

In contrast to the findings of other authors [37,40] and our previous research [21], β-ZEL was the predominant metabolite in the blood serum of gilts in successive weeks of exposure [38]. It could be speculated that the host organism tries to compensate for the physiological deficiency of endogenous estrogens (which are necessary for the essential life processes) [41], and its demand for compounds with high estrogenic activity (such as α-ZEL and ZEN) increases [40,42]. It is also possible that the seventh day of exposure to an undesirable substance such as ZEN marks the end of adaptive processes (adaptive immunity) [43]. Zearalenone could also be utilized as a substrate that regulates (in an inversely proportional manner) the expression of genes encoding HSDs—molecular switches modulating steroid hormone prereceptors [19,44,45]. Undesirable substances could also undergo enterohepatic recirculation before they are eliminated from the body [21,46], and/or exposure to ZEN could induce a specific response from the distal gut microbiota [11].

The above hypotheses, alone or in combination, could explain the peripheral blood concentrations of ZEN and its metabolites because this mycotoxin exerts multidirectional effects [21]. Zearalenone inhibits the synthesis and secretion of the follicle-stimulating hormone (FSH) [37] via negative feedback, thus decreasing steroid production [47,48].

During prolonged exposure to low ZEN doses, similar interdependences are observed between the average concentrations of ZEN and its metabolites in peripheral blood [37]. However, two differences were observed during prolonged (longer than seven days) exposure to ZEN. First, both ZEN metabolites were detected in peripheral blood. Next, the values of all evaluated parameters increased, probably due to the accumulation of ZEN and its metabolites (resulting from the saturation of active ERs and other factors that influence the levels of steroid hormones [47–49]), over time. In other studies investigating the effects of ZEN biotransformation in peripheral blood, animals were exposed to much higher doses of the mycotoxin [21,50,51]. These observations could suggest that in line with the hormesis paradigm [8,21], the exposure to very low doses of ZEN affects the synthesis and secretion of sex steroid hormones [18,39]. Therefore, the simultaneous processes of the biotransformation of very low ZEN doses are not identical, and the parent compound (ZEN) and its metabolites are utilized either completely or to a much larger extent (which was also the case during exposure to the MABEL dose) by the host organism [16]. The interactions between endogenous and exogenous (environmental) steroids could also be influenced by other endogenous factors, such as the accumulation of ZEN and its metabolites in intestinal tissues in the initial stages of biotransformation, the resulting expression of ERs and selected intestinal enzymes that participate in detoxification, which is accompanied by specific (but not clearly determined) accumulation of ZEN and its metabolites in intestinal tissues.

Undesirable substances such as ZEN are metabolized inside cells by two classes of enzymes. Phase I enzymes modify undesirable substances via several processes, including hydroxylation. These enzymes are known as cytochromes (CYP), they are abundant in the body and tissue-specific. Phase II enzymes, such as glutathione S-transferase (GST), conjugate metabolites through glucuronidation [52].

The P450 cytochrome (CYP) superfamily consists of several hundred isoenzymes that catalyze the oxidation of various substrates, including exogenous (xenobiotics) and endogenous (hormones, prostaglandins, and vitamins) compounds [53]. Many CYPs are inducible, which significantly increases their catalytic activity after exposure to specific chemical substances [54]. These compounds are ligands of specific receptors, such as the aryl hydrocarbon receptor (AhR) and ERs. Activated receptors are transferred to the nucleus, they undergo dimerization with nuclear partners, bind to specific sequences in subsequent promotors, and induce the transcription of target genes [55]. The above increases $mRNA$ levels and enhances the synthesis of CYP protein. This process ultimately boosts the enzymatic activity of specific CYPs [56].

In phase II, liver cells could become resistant to various substances due to the intensification of metabolic process and detoxification of undesirable compounds in feed [57]. The π isoform of glutathione S-transferase (GSTP1) is one of the molecules that elicit these types of mechanisms. In the body, GST occurs in the form of numerous isoenzymes, which have been divided into classes on the basis of their location in the cell, amino acid sequences, location of genes, and substrate specificity [58]. The role of GST is not limited to the detoxification of exogenous electrophilic toxins. The enzyme also protects the body against the harmful products of oxidative stress [59], and prevents damage to nucleic acids and lipids. Glutathione S-transferase participates in the metabolism of steroid hormones, biosynthesis of leukotriene C4 and prostaglandin E_2, and the maintenance of glutathione homeostasis [60].

The aim of the proposed study will be to determine in vivo the correlations between very low monotonic doses of ZEN (5, 10, and 15 μg ZEN/kg BW for 42 days), the carry-over of ZEN and its metabolites from the intestinal contents to the intestinal walls, the $mRNA$ expression of ERα and ERβ genes, and the $mRNA$ expression of genes modulating selected colon enzymes (CYP1A1 and GSTP1) in the intestinal mucosa of pre-pubertal gilts. The study will expand our understanding of the mechanisms underlying the expression of ERα and Erβ, which participate in both stages of mycotoxin (undesirable substance) biotransformation.

2. Materials and Methods

In our opinion, the research hypotheses could be effectively validated with the use of the methods deployed in precision medicine [14,33]. Precision medicine involves assessments of individual animals as well as entire populations, and the results of these observations play a very important role in clinical veterinary practice. Holistic methods have to be applied to deepen our understanding of pathological processes. These methods include technologies based on mass spectrometry or high-throughput molecular biology techniques.

2.1. Experimental Procedures

All procedures were carried out in compliance with Polish legal regulations for the determination of the terms and methods for performing experiments on animals and with the European Community Directive for the ethical use of experimental animals. The protocol was approved by the Local Ethics Committee for Animal Experimentation at the University of Warmia and Mazury in Olsztyn, Poland (opinion No. 42/2019 of 28 May 2019).

2.2. Experimental Animals and Feeding

An in vivo experiment will be performed at the Department of Veterinary Prevention and Feed Hygiene of the Faculty of Veterinary Medicine at the University of Warmia and Mazury in Olsztyn on 60 clinically healthy pre-pubertal gilts with initial BW of 14.5 ± 2 kg [10]. During the experiment, the animals will be housed in pens, they will be fed identical diets, and water will be available ad libitum. The gilts will be randomly divided into a control group (group C; n = 15) and three experimental groups (ZEN5, ZEN10, and

ZEN15; n = 15 each) [61,62]. Groups ZEN5, ZEN10, and ZEN15 will be administered ZEN (Sigma-Aldrich Z2125-26MG, St. Louis, MO, USA) *per os* at 5 μg/kg BW, 10 μg/kg BW, and 15 μg/kg BW, respectively. Each experimental group will stand in a separate pen and in the same building. The pens have an area of 25 m^2, which complies with the applicable cross compliance regulations (Regulation (EU) No 1306/2013 of the European Parliament and of the Council of 17 December 2013).

Analytical samples of ZEN will be dissolved in 96 μL of 96% ethanol (SWW 2442-90, Polskie Odczynniki SA, Poland) in weight-appropriate doses. Feed containing different amounts of ZEN in an alcohol solution will be placed in gel capsules. Before administration, the capsules will be stored at room temperature until the alcohol evaporates. Experimental group pigs will receive ZEN in gel capsules every day before morning feeding. The animals will be weighed at weekly intervals in order to adjust individual mycotoxin doses. Feed will be the carrier, and group C gilts will receive identical gel capsules without ZEN [10,11]. The feed will be supplied by the same producer. During the experiment, the gilts will be offered feed in friable form ad libitum twice daily (at 8:00 a.m. and 5:00 p.m.). The ingredient composition of complete diets will be specified by the manufacturer, as presented in Table 1.

Table 1. Declared composition of the complete diet.

Parameters	Composition Declared by the Manufacturer (%)
Soybean meal	16
Wheat	55
Barley	22
Wheat bran	4.0
Chalk	0.3
Zitrosan	0.2
Vitamin–mineral premix [1]	2.5

[1] Composition of the vitamin–mineral premix per kg: vitamin A—500.000 IU; iron—5000 mg; vitamin D3—100.000 IU; zinc—5000 mg; vitamin E (alpha-tocopherol)—2000 mg; manganese—3000 mg; vitamin K—150 mg; copper ($CuSO_4 \cdot 5H_2O$)—500 mg; vitamin B1—100 mg; cobalt—20 mg; vitamin B2—300 mg; iodine—40 mg; vitamin B6—150 mg; selenium—15 mg; vitamin B12—1500 μg; L-lysine—9.4 g; niacin—1200 mg; DL—methionine + cystine—3.7 g; pantothenic acid—600 mg; L-threonine—2.3 g; folic acid—50 mg; tryptophan—1.1 g; biotin—7500 μg; phytase + choline—10 g; ToyoCerin probiotic + calcium—250 g; antioxidant + mineral phosphorus and released phosphorus—60 g; magnesium—5 g; sodium and calcium—51 g.

The proximate chemical composition of the diets fed to gilts in groups C, ZEN5, ZEN10, and ZEN15 will be analyzed with the NIRS-DS2500 F monochromator-based NIR reflectance and transflectance analyzer with a scanning range of 850–2500 nm (FOSS, Hillerød, Denmark).

2.3. Toxicological Analyses

2.3.1. Determination of Mycotoxins in Feed

Feed will be analyzed for the presence of ZEN and DON (deoxynivalenol), and their concentrations will be determined by separation in immunoaffinity columns (Zearala-TestTM Zearalenone Testing System, G1012, VICAM, Watertown, MA, USA; DON-TestTM DON Testing System, VICAM, Watertown, MA, USA) and high-performance liquid chromatography (HPLC system, Agilent 1260)–mass spectrometry (MS, Agilent 6470) and chromatography columns (Atlantis T3 3 μm 3.0 150 mm Column No. 186003723, Waters, AN Etten-Leur, Ireland). Mycotoxins will be separated using a mobile phase of acetonitrile:water:methanol (46:46:8, $v/v/v$). The flow rate will be 0.4 mL/min. The limit of quantitation (LoQ) for ZEN will be 2 ng/g and 5 ng/g for DON. Zearalenone and its metabolites will be quantified at the Department of Veterinary Prevention and Feed Hygiene [63].

2.3.2. Biotransformation of ZEN

Tissue Samples

In each group, 5 animals will be euthanized on analytical dates 1 (D1—exposure day 7), 2 (D2—exposure day 21), and 3 (D3—exposure day 42) by the intravenous administration of pentobarbital sodium (Fatro, Ozzano Emilia BO, Italy) and bleeding. Immediately after cardiac arrest, tissue samples (approximately 1×1.5 cm) will be collected from entire intestinal cross-sections, from the following segments of the gastrointestinal tract: the duodenum—the first part (duodenal cap) and the horizontal or third part; the jejunum and ileum—middle parts; colon—middle parts of the ascending colon, transverse colon, and descending colon; the cecum—1 cm from the ileocecal valve. The samples will be rinsed with phosphate buffer and prepared for analyses [5,6].

Extraction and Purification

Zearalenone, α-ZEL, and β-ZEL will be extracted from tissues with the use of immunoaffinity columns (Zearala-TestTM Zearalenone Testing System, G1012, VICAM, Watertown, MA, USA) according to the manufacturer's recommendations. The obtained eluents will be placed in a water bath at 50 °C, and will be evaporated in a stream of nitrogen. The dry residue will be stored at –20 °C until chromatographic analysis. The procedure will be monitored with the use of internal standards, and the results will be validated by mass spectrometry.

Chromatographic Determination of the Concentrations of Zen and its Metabolites

The tissue concentrations of ZEN, α-ZEL, and β-ZEL will be determined with the Agilent 1260 liquid chromatograph (LC) and the Agilent 6470 mass spectrometer (MS). The prepared samples will be analyzed with the use of the Zorbax rapid resolution chromatographic column (2.1×50 mm; 1.8 micron Agilent Eclipse Plus C18) in gradient mode. The mobile phase will contain 0.1% (v/v) formic acid in water (solvent A) and 0.1% (v/v) formic acid in acetonitrile (solvent B). Gradient conditions will be as follows: initially, 20% B that increases to 100% B in 4.0 min and back to 20% B in 0.1 min.

Mycotoxin concentrations will be determined according to an external standard and will be expressed in ppb (ng/mL). The quantification process will involve matrix-matched calibration standards to eliminate matrix effects that can decrease sensitivity. Calibration standards will be dissolved in matrix samples based on the procedure described for the remaining samples. The material for preparing calibration standards will be free of mycotoxins. A signal-to-noise ratio of 3:1 will be used to estimate the limits of detection (LOD) for ZEN, α-ZEL, and β-ZEL. The LOQ will be estimated as the triple LOD value.

The specificity of the method will be determined by comparing the chromatograms of a blank sample with those corresponding to a spiked tissue sample.

Mass Spectrometric Conditions

The mass spectrometer was operate with ESI in the negative ion mode. The MS/MS parameters were opimized for each compoud. The linearity was tested by a calibration curve including six levels. Table 2 shows the optimized analysis conditions for the mycotoxins tested.

Table 2. Optimized conditions for mycotoxins tested.

Analyte	Precursor (m/z)	Production (m/z)	FragmentorVoltage (V)	Collision Energy (eV)	LOD (ng mL^{-1})	LOQ (ng mL^{-1})	Linearity (%R^2)
ZEN	317.1	273.3 187.1	160	25 33	0.03	0.1	0.999
α-ZEL	319.2	275.2 160.1	144	21 33	0.3	0.9	0.997
β-ZEL	319.2	275.2 160.1	144	21 33	0.3	1	0.993

A chromatogram of standard mixtures of all analytes is presented in Figure 1.

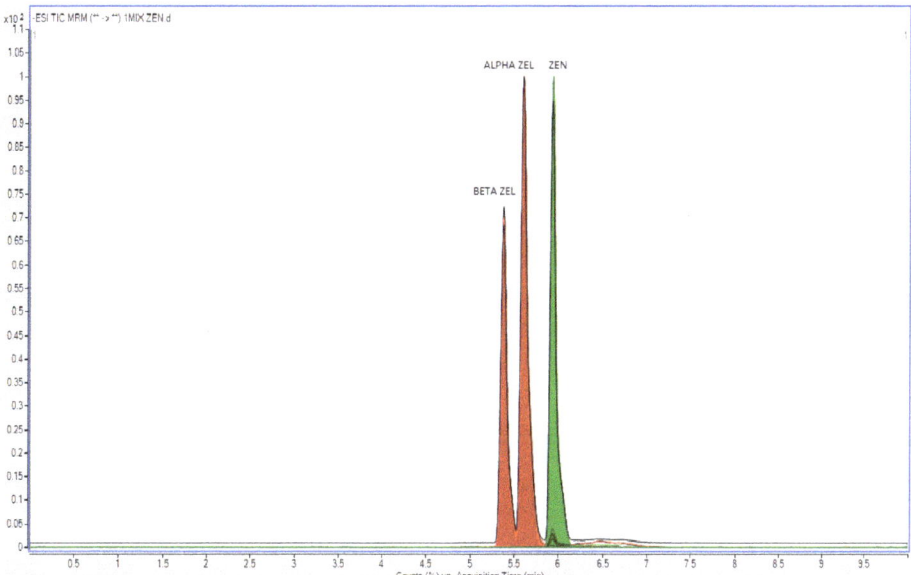

Figure 1. The chromatogram of standard solution.

Statistical Analysis

The results of the study will be processed at the Department of Discrete Mathematics and Theoretical Computer Science at the Faculty of Mathematics and Computer Science of the University of Warmia and Mazury in Olsztyn. The bioavailability of ZEN and its metabolites in the intestinal tissues of pre-pubertal gilts will be analyzed in three experimental groups and the control group, on different sampling dates. The results will be expressed as mean values ($\bar{x}$) and standard deviation (SD). The following tests will be carried out: (i) analyses of differences between the mean values in three experimental groups (receiving different doses of ZEN) and the control group on three analytical dates; (ii) analyses of differences between the mean values within groups (receiving the same ZEN dose) on each analytical date. In both tests, differences between mean values will be determined by one-way ANOVA. If the differences between groups are statistically significant, differences between pairs of means will be estimated by Tukey's multiple comparison test. If all values are below LOD (mean and variance are equal to zero) in any group, the values in the remaining groups will be processed by one-way ANOVA, and the differences between means in these groups will be compared with the population mean difference of zero in Student's t-test. Differences between groups will be estimated by Student's t-test. The results of each analysis will be considered to be highly significant at $p < 0.01$ (**) and significant at $0.01 < p < 0.05$ (*). Data will be analyzed in the Statistica v.13 program (TIBCO Software Inc., Silicon Valley, CA, USA, 2017).

2.4. Expression of ERα, ERβ, CYP1A1, and GSTP1 Genes

2.4.1. Collection and storage of samples for RNA Extraction

Immediately after cardiac arrest, tissue samples will be collected from the duodenum—the first part (duodenal cap) and the horizontal or third part; the jejunum and ileum—middle parts, and the colon—middle parts of the ascending colon, transverse colon, and descending colon. The samples will be stored in RNA*later* solution (Sigma-Aldrich; Germany), in accordance with the manufacturer's instructions. Tissue samples will be collected on the same dates.

2.4.2. Total RNA Extraction and CDNA Synthesis

Total RNA will be extracted from the tissues preserved in RNA*later* (approximately 20 mg per sample; $n = 3$ in each experimental group) using the Total RNA Mini isolation kit (A&A Biotechnology; Poland) according to the manufacturer's protocol. RNA samples will be incubated with RNase-free DNase I (Roche Diagnostics; Germany) to prevent contamination of genomic DNA. Total RNA quality and the purity of all samples will be estimated with the BioPhotometer (Eppendorf; Germany), and the results will be used to synthesize cDNA with the RevertAid™ First Strand cDNA Synthesis Kit (Fermentas; Canada). The cDNA synthesis reaction mixture for each sample will contain 1 µg of total RNA and 0.5 µg of oligo (dT)18 primers, and the reaction will be performed according to the manufacturer's protocol. The first synthesized cDNA strand will be stored at −20 °C for further analysis.

2.4.3. qPCR

Real-time PCR primers for ERα and ERβ mRNAs, and CYP1A1 and GSTP1 mRNAs will be designed using the Primer-BLAST tool based on the reference species (Table 3). β-actin will be used as the endogenous reference gene. The real-time PCR assay will be performed in the ABI 7500 real-time PCR system thermocycler (Applied Biosystems, Foster City, CA, USA) in singleplex mode. Further treatments will be applied as recommended by the manufacturer.

Table 3. Real-time PCR primers for the proposed study.

Primer		Sequence (5′→3′)	Amplicon Length (bp)	References
ERALFA	Forward	Agggaagctcctattgctcc	234	[64]
	Reverse	cggtggatgtggtccttctct		
ERBETA	Forward	Gcttcgtggagctcagcctg	262	[64]
	Reverse	aggatcatggccttgacacaga		
CYP1A1	Forward	cagagccgcagcagccaccttg	226	[48]
	Reverse	ggctcttgcccaaggtcagcac		
GSTP1	Forward	acctgcttcggattcaccag	178	[48]
	Reverse	ctccagccacaaagccctta		
β-Actin	Forward	catcaccatcggcaaaga	237	[65]
	Reverse	gcgtagaggtccttcctgatgt		

Quantitative cycle (Cq) values from qPCR will be converted to copy numbers using a standard curve plot (Cq versus log copy number) according to the methodology.

The rationale for using the standard curve is based on the assumption that unknown samples have equal amplification efficiency (usually above 90%), which is checked before unknown standards are extrapolated to the standard curve. To generate the standard curves, purified PCR products of each mRNA will be used to prepare a series of six 10-fold dilutions with known amounts of copy numbers, which will be used as templates in real-time PCR. The Cq values obtained for each dilution series will be plotted against the log copy number, and will be used to extrapolate unknown samples to copy numbers. mRNA copy numbers of the samples collected from all experimental groups in each exposure period will be divided by the averaged numbers from the control group, determined at the beginning of the experiment (control 0d), to obtain relative expression values, which will be presented as the expression ratio (R).

2.4.4. Statistical Analysis

The expression of ERα and ERβ in the digestive tract of gilts, and the expression of *CYP1A1* and *GSTP1* genes in the ascending colon and the descending colon will be presented as mean values ($\pm$) SD for each sample. The results will be analyzed using Statistica software (StatSoft Inc., USA). The mean values in the control and experimental groups will be compared by repeated-measures one-way ANOVA based on the ZEN dose administered to pre-pubertal gilts. If differences between groups are found, Tukey's post hoc test will be performed to determine which pairs of group means are significantly different. In ANOVA, group samples will be drawn from normally distributed populations characterized by the same variance. If the above assumptions are not met in all cases, the equality of group means will be tested using the Kruskal–Wallis test of ranks and the multiple comparisons test in ANOVA. Different group pairs will be identified by post hoc multiple comparisons of mean ranks for all groups.

3. Discussion

Mycotoxins have always been and will always be present in foodstuffs and feedstuffs—this is a banal truth. Higher mycotoxin doses can produce symptoms of mycotoxicosis (poisoning) in macroorganisms. However, little is known about the fate of mycotoxins and the responses of the host organism during exposure to low doses of mycotoxins in the range of NOAEL and MABEL doses [16]. Macroorganisms have developed various coping strategies that enable them to maintain homeostasis. These coping mechanisms can involve tolerance to very low mycotoxin doses [16]. Alternatively, mycotoxins can participate in vital life processes, as briefly noted in the Introduction. Mycotoxins are accumulated and absorbed not only in target tissues [66,67], which suggests that the intestinal mucosa containing ERs is the most exposed tissue and the first line of defense against undesirable substances [68]. Therefore, the relevant diagnostic tests and laboratory analyses will be performed in the proposed study.

Due to the general scarcity of published research into low-dose mycotoxicosis, additional in vivo data are needed to increase the safety of foodstuffs and feedstuffs, and minimize the risk of toxicity in the decision-making process [69]. The proposed study will attempt to determine whether low doses of ZEN can affect (i) the degree and site of β-ZEL accumulation in the porcine gastrointestinal tract at different exposure times; (ii) the expression of ERs in the porcine gastrointestinal tract, analyzed in vivo, in particular, the expression of Erα, which regulates intestinal function in the proximal segments of the gastrointestinal tract; (iii) the involvement of intestinal enzymes (expression effect) in the distal segment of the intestines in ZEN detoxification processes.

The results of the study will support the development of biomarkers of prolonged low-dose ZEN mycotoxicosis in pre-pubertal gilts within the framework of veterinary precision medicine.

Author Contributions: Conceptualization, M.G. and M.T.G.; methodology, P.B., E.O., Ł.Z. and K.L.-I.; software, Ł.Z.; validation, Ł.Z. and P.B.; formal analysis, A.B. and M.T.G.; investigation, P.B., Ł.Z., K.L.-I. and E.O.; data curation, M.G.; writing—original draft preparation, M.G., M.M., K.E.P. and M.T.G.; writing—review and editing, M.G., M.T.G., P.B. and A.B.; supervision, Ł.Z. and M.T.G.; project administration, Ł.Z.; funding acquisition, Ł.Z. and M.T.G. All authors have read and agreed to the published version of the manuscript.

Funding: The project was financially co-supported by the Minister of Science and Higher 613 Education under the program entitled "Regional Initiative of Excellence" for the years 2019–2022, 614 Project No. 010/RID/2018/19, amount of funding PLN 12,000,000.

Institutional Review Board Statement: Not applicable.

Informed Consent Statement: Not applicable.

Data Availability Statement: Not applicable.

Conflicts of Interest: The authors declare no conflict of interest.

References

1. Thielecke, F.; Nugent, A.P. Contaminants in Grain—A Major Risk for Whole Grain Safety? *Nutrients* **2018**, *10*, 1213. [CrossRef] [PubMed]
2. Fleetwood, J.; Rahman, S.; Holland, D.; Millson, D.; Thomson, L.; Poppy, G. As clean as they look? Food hygiene inspection scores, microbiological contamination, and foodborne illness. *Food Control* **2019**, *96*, 76–86. [CrossRef]
3. Alassane-Kpembi, I.; Pinton, P.; Oswald, I.P. Effects of Mycotoxins on the Intestine. *Toxins* **2019**, *11*, 159. [CrossRef]
4. Mahato, D.K.; Devi, S.; Pandhi, S.; Sharma, B.; Maurya, K.K.; Mishra, S.; Dhawan, K.; Selvakumar, R.; Kamle, M.; Mishra, A.K.; et al. Occurrence, Impact on Agriculture, Human Health, and Management Strategies of Zearalenone in Food and Feed: A Review. *Toxins* **2021**, *13*, 92. [CrossRef] [PubMed]
5. Piotrowska, M.; Sliżewska, K.; Nowak, A.; Zielonka, Ł.; Żakowska, Z.; Gajęcka, M.; Gajęcki, M. The effect of experimental fusarium mycotoxicosis on microbiota diversity in porcine ascending colon contents. *Toxins* **2014**, *6*, 2064–2081. [CrossRef]
6. Zachariasova, M.; Dzumana, Z.; Veprikova, Z.; Hajkovaa, K.; Jiru, M.; Vaclavikova, M.; Zachariasova, A.; Pospichalova, M.; Florian, M.; Hajslova, J. Occurrence of multiple mycotoxins in European feeding stuffs, assessment of dietary intake by farm animals. *Anim. Feed Sci. Technol.* **2014**, *193*, 124–140. [CrossRef]
7. Knutsen, H.-K.; Alexander, J.; Barregård, L.; Bignami, M.; Brüschweiler, B.; Ceccatelli, S.; Cottrill, B.; Dinovi, M.; Edler, L.; Grasl-Kraupp, B.; et al. Risks for animal health related to the presence of zearalenone and its modified forms in feed. *EFSA J.* **2017**, *15*, 4851. [CrossRef]
8. Calabrese, E.J. Hormesis: Path and Progression to Significance. *Int. J. Mol. Sci.* **2018**, *19*, 2871. [CrossRef] [PubMed]
9. Freir, L.; Sant'Ana, A.S. Modified mycotoxins: An updated review on their formation, detection, occurrence, and toxic effects. *Food Chem. Toxicol.* **2018**, *111*, 189–205. [CrossRef] [PubMed]
10. Rykaczewska, A.; Gajęcka, M.; Dąbrowski, M.; Wiśniewska, A.; Szcześniewska, J.; Gajęcki, M.T.; Zielonka, Ł. Growth performance, selected blood biochemical parameters and body weight of pre-pubertal gilts fed diets supplemented with different doses of zearalenone (ZEN). *Toxicon* **2018**, *152*, 84–94. [CrossRef] [PubMed]
11. Ciepliñska, K.; Gajęcka, M.; Dąbrowski, M.; Rykaczewska, A.; Zielonka, Ł.; Lisieska-Żołnierczyk, S.; Buliñska, M.; Gajęcki, M.T. Time-dependent changes in the intestinal microbiome of gilts exposed to low zearalenone doses. *Toxins* **2019**, *11*, 296. [CrossRef]
12. Ciepliñsk, K.; Gajęcka, M.; Nowak, A.; Dąbrowski, M.; Zielonka, Ł.; Gajęcki, M.T. The gentoxicity of caecal water in gilts exposed to low doses of zearalenone. *Toxins* **2018**, *10*, 350. [CrossRef]
13. Gajęcka, M.; Waśkiewicz, A.; Zielonka, Ł.; Goliñski, P.; Rykaczewska, A.; Lisieska-Żołnierczyk, S.; Gajęcki, M.T. Mycotoxin levels in the digestive tissues of immature gilts exposed to zearalenone and deoxynivalenol. *Toxicon* **2018**, *153*, 1–11. [CrossRef] [PubMed]
14. Tebani, A.; Afonso, C.; Marret, S.; Bekri, S. Omics-Based Strategies in Precision Medicine: Toward a Paradigm Shift in Inborn Errors of Metabolism Investigations. *Int. J. Mol. Sci.* **2016**, *17*, 1555. [CrossRef] [PubMed]
15. Celi, P.; Verlhac, V.; Pérez, C.E.; Schmeisser, J.; Kluenter, A.M. Biomarkers of gastrointestinal functionality in animal nutrition and health. *Anim. Feed Sci. Technol.* **2019**, *250*, 9–31. [CrossRef]
16. Schaller, T.H.; Snyder, D.J.; Spasojevic, I.; Gedeon, P.C.; Sanchez-Perez, L.; Sampson, J.H. First in human dose calculation of a single-chain bispecific antibody targeting glioma using the MABEL approach. *J. Immunother. Cancer* **2020**, *8*, e000213. [CrossRef]
17. Velmurugan, B.K.; Rathinasamy, B.; Lohanathan, B.P.; Thiyagarajan, V.; Weng, C.F. Neuroprotective Role of Phytochemicals. *Molecules* **2018**, *23*, 2485. [CrossRef]
18. Zhang, Q.; Caudle, W.M.; Pi, J.; Bhattacharya, S.; Andersen, M.E.; Kaminski, N.E.; Conolly, R.B. Embracing systems toxicology at single-cell resolution. *Curr. Opin. Toxicol.* **2019**, *16*, 49–57. [CrossRef]
19. Gajęcka, M.; Otrocka-Domagała, I. Immunocytochemical expression of 3β- and 17β-hydroxysteroid dehydrogenase in bitch ovaries exposed to low doses of zearalenone. *Pol. J. Vet. Sci.* **2013**, *16*, 55–62.
20. Gajęcka, M. The effect of low-dose experimental zearalenone intoxication on the immunoexpression of estrogen receptors in the ovaries of pre-pubertal bitches. *Pol. J. Vet. Sci.* **2012**, *15*, 685–691. [CrossRef]
21. Gajęcka, M.; Zielonka, Ł.; Gajęcki, M. Activity of zearalenone in the porcine intestinal tract. *Molecules* **2017**, *22*, 18. [CrossRef]
22. Dąbrowski, M.; Obremski, K.; Gajęcka, M.; Gajęcki, M.; Zielonka, Ł. Changes in the subpopulations of porcine peripheral blood lymphocytes induced by exposure to low doses of zearalenone (ZEN) and deoxynivalenol (DON). *Molecules* **2016**, *21*, 557. [CrossRef] [PubMed]
23. Silva-Campa, E.; Mata-Haro, V.; Mateu, E.; Hernández, J. Porcine reproductive and respiratory syndrome virus induces CD4+CD8+CD25+Foxp3+ regulatory T cells (Tregs). *Virology* **2012**, *430*, 73–80. [CrossRef] [PubMed]
24. Zielonka, Ł.; Jakimiuk, E.; Obremski, K.; Gajęcka, M.; Dąbrowski, M.; Gajęcki, M. An evaluation of the proliferative activity of immunocompetent cells in the jejunal and iliac lymph nodes of prepubertal female wild boars diagnosed with mixed mycotoxicosis. *Bull. Vet. Inst. Pulawy* **2015**, *59*, 197–203. [CrossRef]
25. Bryden, W.L. Mycotoxin contamination of the feed supply chain: Implications for animal productivity and feed security. *Anim. Feed Sci. Technol.* **2012**, *173*, 134–158. [CrossRef]
26. Grenier, B.; Applegate, T.J. Modulation of intestinal functions following mycotoxin ingestion: Meta-analysis of published experiments in animals. *Toxins* **2013**, *5*, 396–430. [CrossRef]
27. Gajęcka, M.; Zielonka, Ł.; Gajęcki, M. The effect of low monotonic doses of zearalenone on selected reproductive tissues in pre-pubertal female dogs—A review. *Molecules* **2015**, *20*, 20669–20687. [CrossRef]

28. Stopa, E.; Babińska, I.; Zielonka, Ł.; Gajęcki, M.; Gajęcka, M. Immunohistochemical evaluation of apoptosis and proliferation in the mucous membrane of selected uterine regions in pre-pubertal bitches exposed to low doses of zearalenone. *Pol. J. Vet. Sci.* **2016**, *19*, 175–186. [CrossRef]
29. Kramer, H.J.; van den Ham, W.A.; Slob, W.; Pieters, M.N. Conversion Factors Estimating Indicative Chronic No-Observed-Adverse-Effect Levels from Short-Term Toxicity Data. *Regul. Toxicol. Pharmacol.* **1996**, *23*, 249–255. [CrossRef]
30. Pastoor, T.P.; Bachman, A.N.; Bell, D.R.; Cohen, S.M.; Dellarco, M.; Dewhurst, I.C.; Doe, J.E.; Doerrer, N.G.; Embry, M.R.; Hines, R.N.; et al. A 21st century roadmap for human health risk assessment. *Crit. Rev. Toxicol.* **2014**, *44*, 1–5. [CrossRef]
31. Suh, H.Y.; Peck, C.C.; Yu, K.S.; Lee, H. Determination of the starting dose in the first-in-human clinical trials with monoclonal antibodies: A systematic review of papers published between 1990 and 2013. *Drug Des. Dev. Ther.* **2016**, *10*, 4005–4016. [CrossRef] [PubMed]
32. Vandenberg, L.N.; Colborn, T.; Hayes, T.B.; Heindel, J.J.; Jacobs, D.R.; Lee, D.-H.; Shioda, T.; Soto, A.M.; vom Saal, F.S.; Welshons, W.V.; et al. Hormones and endocrine-disrupting chemicals: Low-dose effects and nonmonotonic dose responses. *Endoc. Rev.* **2012**, *33*, 378–455. [CrossRef] [PubMed]
33. Dana, D.; Gadhiya, S.V.; Surin, L.G.S.; Li, D.; Naaz, F.; Ali, Q.; Paka, L.; Yamin, M.A.; Narayan, M.; Goldberg, I.D.; et al. Deep Learning in Drug Discovery and Medicine; Scratching the Surface. *Molecules* **2018**, *23*, 2384. [CrossRef]
34. Gupta, R.C. *Biomarkers in Toxicology*; Academic Press: Hopkinsville, Kentucky USA, 2019. [CrossRef]
35. Hickey, G.L.; Craig, P.S.; Luttik, R.; de Zwart, D. On the quantification of intertest variability in ecotoxicity data with application to species sensitivity distributions. *Environ. Toxicol. Chem.* **2012**, *31*, 1903–1910. [CrossRef]
36. Pinton, P.; Suman, M.; Buck, N.; Dellafiora, L.; De Meester, J.; Stadler, D.; Rito, E. Practical guidance to mitigation of mycotoxins during food processing. In *Report Commissioned by the Process-Related Compounds and Natural Toxins Task Force*; Report Series; ILSI Europe: Brussels, Belgium, 2019; ISBN 9789078637455. Available online: https://www.researchgate.net/publication/336533566 (accessed on 25 May 2019).
37. Zheng, W.; Feng, N.; Wang, Y.; Noll, L.; Xu, S.; Liu, X.; Lu, N.; Zou, H.; Gu, J.; Yuan, Y.; et al. Effects of zearalenone and its derivatives on the synthesis and secretion of mammalian sex steroid hormones: A review. *Food Chem. Toxicol.* **2019**, *126*, 262–276. [CrossRef] [PubMed]
38. Rykaczewska, A.; Gajęcka, M.; Onyszek, E.; Cieplińska, K.; Dąbrowski, M.; Lisieska-Żołnierczyk, S.; Bulińska, M.; Babuchowski, A.; Gajęcki, M.T.; Zielonka, Ł. Imbalance in the Blood Concentrations of Selected Steroids in Prepubertal Gilts Depending on the Time of Exposure to Low Doses of Zearalenone. *Toxins* **2019**, *11*, 561. [CrossRef]
39. Lawrenz, B.; Melado, L.; Fatemi, H. Premature progesterone rise in ART-cycles. *Reprod. Biol.* **2018**, *18*, 1–4. [CrossRef]
40. Bryła, M.; Waśkiewicz, A.; Ksieniewicz-Woźniak, E.; Szymczyk, K.; Jędrzejczak, R. Modified Fusarium Mycotoxins in Cereals and Their Products—Metabolism, Occurrence, and Toxicity: An Updated Review. *Molecules* **2018**, *23*, 963. [CrossRef]
41. Kowalska, K.; Habrowska-Górczyńska, D.E.; Piastowska-Ciesielska, A. Zearalenone as an endocrine disruptor in humans. *Environ. Toxicol. Pharmacol.* **2016**, *48*, 141–149. [CrossRef]
42. Yang, D.; Jiang, T.; Lin, P.; Chen, H.; Wang, L.; Wang, N.; Zhao, F.; Tang, K.; Zhou, D.; Wang, A.; et al. Apoptosis inducing factor gene depletion inhibits zearalenone-induced cell death in a goat Leydig cell line. *Reprod. Toxicol.* **2017**, *67*, 129–139. [CrossRef]
43. Benagiano, M.; Bianchi, P.; D'Elios, M.M.; Brosens, I.; Benagiano, G. Autoimmune diseases: Role of steroid hormones. *Best Pract. Res. Clin. Obstet. Gynaecol.* **2019**, *60*, 24–34. [CrossRef] [PubMed]
44. Gajęcka, M.; Rybarczyk, L.; Zwierzchowski, W.; Jakimiuk, E.; Zielonka, Ł.; Obremski, K.; Gajęcki, M. The effect of experimental, long-term exposure to low-dose zearalenone mycotoxicosis on the histological condition of ovaries in sexually immature gilts. *Theriogenology* **2011**, *75*, 1085–1094. [CrossRef] [PubMed]
45. Schoevers, E.J.; Santos, R.R.; Colenbrander, B.; Fink-Gremmels, J.; Roelen, B.A.J. Transgenerational toxicity of Zearalenone in pigs. *Reprod. Toxicol.* **2012**, *34*, 110–119. [CrossRef] [PubMed]
46. Hennig-Pauka, I.; Koch, F.J.; Schaumberger, S.; Woechtl, B.; Novak, J.; Sulyok, M.; Nagl, V. Current challenges in the diagnosis of zearalenone toxicosis as illustrated by a field case of hyperestrogenism in suckling piglets. *Porc. Health Manag.* **2018**, *4*, 1–9. [CrossRef]
47. He, J.; Wei, C.; Li, Y.; Liu, Y.; Wang, Y.; Pan, J.; Liu, J.; Wu, Y.; Cui, S. Zearalenone and alpha-zearalenol inhibit the synthesis and secretion of pig follicle stimulating hormone via the non-classical estrogen membrane receptor GPR30. *Mol. Cell. Endocrinol.* **2018**, *461*, 43–54. [CrossRef]
48. Zielonka, Ł.; Waśkiewicz, A.; Beszterda, M.; Kostecki, M.; Dąbrowski, M.; Obremski, K.; Goliński, P.; Gajęcki, M. Zearalenone in the Intestinal Tissues of Immature Gilts Exposed *per os* to Mycotoxins. *Toxins* **2015**, *7*, 3210–3223. [CrossRef]
49. Gajęcka, M.; Dabrowski, M.; Otrocka-Domagała, I.; Brzuzan, P.; Rykaczewska, A.; Cieplińska, K.; Barasińska, M.; Gajęcki, M.T.; Zielonka, Ł. Correlations between exposure to deoxynivalenol and zearalenone and the immunohistochemical expression of estrogen receptors in the intestinal epithelium and the mRNA expression of selected colonic enzymes in pre-pubertal gilts. *Toxicon* **2020**, *173*, 75–93. [CrossRef]
50. Demaegdt, H.; Daminet, B.; Evrard, A.; Scippo, M.L.; Muller, M.; Pussemier, L.; Callebaut, A.; Vandermeiren, K. Endocrine activity of mycotoxins and mycotoxin mixtures. *Food Chem. Toxicol.* **2016**, *96*, 107–116. [CrossRef]
51. Gajęcka, M.; Sławuta, P.; Nicpoń, J.; Kołacz, R.; Kiełbowicz, Z.; Zielonka, Ł.; Dąbrowski, M.; Szweda, W.; Gajęcki, M.; Nicpoń, J. Zearalenone and its metabolites in the tissues of female wild boars exposed *per os* to mycotoxins. *Toxicon* **2016**, *114*, 1–12. [CrossRef]

52. Sevior, D.K.; Pelkonen, O.; Ahokas, J.T. Hepatocytes: The powerhouse of biotransformation. *Int. J. Biochem. Cell Biol.* **2012**, *44*, 257–261. [CrossRef]
53. Agahi, F.; Juan, C.; Font, G.; Juan-García, A. In silico methods for metabolomic and toxicity prediction of zearalenone, α-zearalenone and β-zearalenone. *Food Chem. Toxicol.* **2020**, *146*, 111818. [CrossRef]
54. Piotrowska-Kempisty, H.; Klupczyńska, A.; Trzybulska, D.; Kulcenty, K.; Sulej-Suchomska, A.M.; Kucińska, M.; Mikstacka, R.; Wierzchowski, M.; Murias, M.; Baer-Dubowska, W.; et al. Role of CYP1A1 in the biological activity of methylated resveratrol analogue, 3,4,5,40-tetramethoxystilbene (DMU-212) in ovarian cancer A-2780 and non-cancerous HOSE cells. *Toxicol. Lett.* **2017**, *267*, 59–66. [CrossRef] [PubMed]
55. Freedland, J.; Cera, C.; Fasullo, M. CYP1A1 I462V polymorphism is associated with reduced genotoxicity in yeast despite positive association with increased cancer risk. *Mutat. Res. Genet. Toxicol. Environ. Mutagen.* **2017**, *815*, 35–43. [CrossRef] [PubMed]
56. Billat, P.A.; Roger, E.; Faure, S.; Lagarce, F. Models for drug absorption from the small intestine: Where are we and where are we going? *Drug Discov. Today* **2017**, *22*, 761–775. [CrossRef] [PubMed]
57. Basharat, Z.; Yasmin, A. Energy landscape of a GSTP1 polymorph linked with cytological function decay in response to chemical stressors. *Gene* **2017**, *609*, 19–27. [CrossRef] [PubMed]
58. Singh, H.O.; Lata, S.; Angadi, M.; Bapat, S.; Pawar, J.; Nema, V.; Ghate, M.V.; Sahay, S.; Gangakhedkar, R.R. Impact of GSTM1, GSTT1 and GSTP1 gene polymorphism and risk of ARV-associated hepatotoxicity in HIV-infected individuals and its modulation. *Pharm. J.* **2017**, *17*, 53–60. [CrossRef] [PubMed]
59. Lei, K.; Xia, Y.; Wang, X.C.; Ahn, E.H.; Jin, L.; Ye, K. C/EBPβ mediates NQO1 and GSTP1 antioxidative reductases expression in glioblastoma, promoting brain tumor proliferation. *Redox Biol.* **2020**, *34*, 101578. [CrossRef]
60. Kovacevic, Z.; Sahni, S.; Lok, H.; Davies, M.J.; Wink, D.A.; Richardson, D.R. Regulation and control of nitric oxide (NO) in macrophages: Protecting the "professional killer cell" from its own cytotoxic arsenal via MRP1 and GSTP1. *Biochim. Biophys. Acta* **2017**, *1861*, 995–999. [CrossRef]
61. Heberer, T.; Lahrssen-Wiederholt, M.; Schat, H.; Abraham, K.; Pyrembel, H.; Henning, K.J.; Schauzu, M.; Braeunig, J.; Goetz, M.; Niemann, L.; et al. Zero tolerances in food and animal feed—Are there any scientific alternatives? A European point of view on an international controversy. *Toxicol. Lett.* **2007**, *175*, 118–135. [CrossRef]
62. Smith, D.; Combes, R.; Depelchin, O.; Jacobsen, S.D.; Hack, R.; Luft, J.; Lammens, L.; von Landenberg, F.; Phillips, B.; Pfister, R.; et al. Optimising the design of preliminary toxicity studies for pharmaceutical safety testing in the dog. *Regul. Toxicol. Pharmacol.* **2005**, *41*, 95–101. [CrossRef]
63. Gajęcka, M.; Stopa, E.; Tarasiuk, M.; Zielonka, Ł.; Gajęcki, M. The expression of type-1 and type-2 nitric oxide synthase in selected tissues of the gastrointestinal tract during mixed mycotoxicosis. *Toxins* **2013**, *5*, 2281–2292. [CrossRef] [PubMed]
64. Pfaffl, M.W.; Lange, I.G.; Daxenberger, A.; Meyer, H.H.D. Tissue-specific expression pattern of estrogen receptors (ER): Quantification of ERa and ERb mRNA with real-time RT-PCR. *APMIS* **2001**, *109*, 345–355. [CrossRef] [PubMed]
65. Tohno, M.; Shimasato, T.; Moue, M.; Aso, H.; Watanabe, K.; Kawai, Y.; Yamaguchi, T.; Saito, T.; Kitazawa, H. Toll-like receptor 2 and 9 are expressed and functional in gut associated lymphoid tissues of presuckling newborn swine. *Vet. Res.* **2006**, *37*, 791–812. [CrossRef]
66. Śliżewska, K.; Nowak, A.; Gajęcka, M.; Piotrowska, M.; Żakowska, Z.; Zielonka, Ł.; Gajęcki, M. Cecal enzyme activity in gilts following experimentally induced Fusarium mycotoxicosis. *Pol. J. Vet. Sci.* **2015**, *18*, 191–197. [CrossRef] [PubMed]
67. Waśkiewicz, A.; Beszterda, M.; Kostecki, M.; Zielonka, Ł.; Goliński, P.; Gajęcki, M. Deoxynivalenol in the gastrointestinal tract of immature gilts under per os toxin application. *Toxins* **2014**, *6*, 973–987. [CrossRef] [PubMed]
68. Liew, W.P.P.; Mohd-Redzwan, S. Mycotoxin: Its impact on Gut health and microbiota. *Front. Cell. Infect. Microbiol.* **2018**, *8*, 60. [CrossRef]
69. Embry, M.R.; Bachman, A.N.; Bell, D.R.; Boobis, A.R.; Cohen, S.M.; Dellarco, M.; Dewhurst, I.C.; Doerrer, N.G.; Hines, R.N.; Moretto, A.; et al. Risk assessment in the 21st century: Roadmap and matrix. *Crit. Rev. Toxicol.* **2014**, *44*, 6–16. [CrossRef]

MDPI
St. Alban-Anlage 66
4052 Basel
Switzerland
www.mdpi.com

Toxins Editorial Office
E-mail: toxins@mdpi.com
www.mdpi.com/journal/toxins

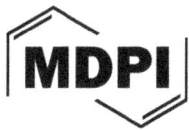

Disclaimer/Publisher's Note: The statements, opinions and data contained in all publications are solely those of the individual author(s) and contributor(s) and not of MDPI and/or the editor(s). MDPI and/or the editor(s) disclaim responsibility for any injury to people or property resulting from any ideas, methods, instructions or products referred to in the content.

www.ingramcontent.com/pod-product-compliance
Lightning Source LLC
LaVergne TN
LVHW070151120526
838202LV00013BA/910